Hormones and Pregnancy

Hormones and Pregnancy

Basic Science and Clinical Implications

Edited by

Felice Petraglia
University of Florence

Mariarosaria Di Tommaso
University of Florence

Federico Mecacci
University of Florence

CAMBRIDGE
UNIVERSITY PRESS

Shaftesbury Road, Cambridge CB2 8EA, United Kingdom

One Liberty Plaza, 20th Floor, New York, NY 10006, USA

477 Williamstown Road, Port Melbourne, VIC 3207, Australia

314–321, 3rd Floor, Plot 3, Splendor Forum, Jasola District Centre, New Delhi – 110025, India

103 Penang Road, #05–06/07, Visioncrest Commercial, Singapore 238467

Cambridge University Press is part of Cambridge University Press & Assessment, a department of the University of Cambridge.

We share the University's mission to contribute to society through the pursuit of education, learning and research at the highest international levels of excellence.

www.cambridge.org
Information on this title: www.cambridge.org/9781316516669

DOI: 10.1017/9781009030830

First published 2023

Printed in the United Kingdom by TJ Books Limited, Padstow Cornwall

A catalogue record for this publication is available from the British Library.

Library of Congress Cataloging-in-Publication Data
Names: Petraglia, F., editor. | Di Tommaso, Mariarosaria, editor. | Mecacci, Federico, editor.
Title: Hormones and pregnancy : basic science and clinical implications / edited by Felice Petraglia, Mariarosaria Di Tommaso, Federico Mecacci.
Description: Cambridge, United Kingdom ; New York, NY : Cambridge University Press, 2022. | Includes bibliographical references and index.
Identifiers: LCCN 2022011782 (print) | LCCN 2022011783 (ebook) | ISBN 9781316516669 (hardback) | ISBN 9781009030830 (epub)
Subjects: MESH: Pregnancy–physiology | Hormones–physiology | Hormones–metabolism | Pregnancy Complications | Endocrine System
  Diseases–complications
Classification: LCC RG525 (print) | LCC RG525 (ebook) | NLM WQ 205 | DDC 618.2–dc23/eng/20220404
LC record available at https://lccn.loc.gov/2022011782
LC ebook record available at https://lccn.loc.gov/2022011783

Cambridge University Press & Assessment has no responsibility for the persistence or accuracy of URLs for external or third-party internet websites referred to in this publication and does not guarantee that any content on such websites is, or will remain, accurate or appropriate.

Every effort has been made in preparing this book to provide accurate and up-to-date information that is in accord with accepted standards and practice at the time of publication. Although case histories are drawn from actual cases, every effort has been made to disguise the identities of the individuals involved. Nevertheless, the authors, editors, and publishers can make no warranties that the information contained herein is totally free from error, not least because clinical standards are constantly changing through research and regulation. The authors, editors, and publishers therefore disclaim all liability for direct or consequential damages resulting from the use of material contained in this book. Readers are strongly advised to pay careful attention to information provided by the manufacturer of any drugs or equipment that they plan to use.

Contents

Contributors

Yveline Ansaldi
Division of OB/GYN, University Hospital of
Geneva, Switzerland

Helen L. Barrett
Obstetric Medicine Department, The Royal
Hospital for Women, Randwick, Australia

Luigi Bartalena
Department of Medicine & Surgery, University of
Insubria, Italy

Nadia Berkane
Division of OB/GYN, University Hospital of
Geneva, Switzerland

John R. G. Challis
Departments of Physiology, Obstetrics, and
Gynecology, University of Toronto; Faculty of
Health Sciences, Simon Fraser University, British
Columbia

Philippe Chanson
Université Paris-Saclay, Inserm, Physiologie et
Physiopathologie Endocriniennes, Assistance
Publique-Hôpitaux de Paris, Hôpital Bicêtre,
Department of Endocrinology and Reproductive
Diseases, National Reference Center for Rare
Pituitary Diseases (HYPO), Le Kremlin-Bicêtre,
France

Vicki Lee Clifton
Mater Research Institute, Faculty of Medicine,
The University of Queensland, Australia

Mariarosaria Di Tommaso
Department of Health Sciences, Division of
Obstetrics and Gynecology, University of
Florence, Italy

Daniele Farsetti
Policlinico Casilino, University of Rome, Italy

Emily M. Frier
Clinical Research Fellow and Specialist Registrar
in Obstetrics and Gynecology, MRC Centre for
Reproductive Health, Queen's Medical Research
Institute, The University of Edinburgh, Scotland

Kiichiro Furuya
School of Biosciences, University of Nottingham;
Department of Obstetrics and Gynecology, Rinku
General Medical Centre, UK

Victor K. M. Han
Division of Neonatal-Perinatal Medicine,
Department of Pediatrics, Children's Health
Research Institute, Western University, Canada

Judith G. Hall
Departments of Medical Genetics and Pediatrics,
University of British Columbia, British
Columbia

Moshe Hod
Mor Women Health Care Center, Tel Aviv
University, Israel

Warrick Inder
Department of Diabetes and Endocrinology,
Princess Alexandra Hospital; Academy for
Medical Education, Faculty of Medicine, The
University of Queensland, Australia

Richard Ivell
School of Biosciences, Sutton Bonington Campus,
University of Nottingham, UK

Sailesh Kumar
Mayne Professor of Obstetrics & Gynecology,
Head of Mayne Academy of Obstetrics and
Gynaecology, Faculty of Medicine, The University
of Queensland; Mater Clinical School-University
of Queensland, Mater Health Services, Australia

Keiichi Kumasawa
Department of Obstetrics and Gynecology, Faculty of Medicine, The University of Tokyo, Japan

Adriana Lai
ASST dei Sette Laghi, Ospedale di Circolo, Italy

Jack Lockett
Department of Diabetes and Endocrinology, Princess Alexandra Hospital; Princess Alexandra-Southside Clinical Unit and Mater Research Institute, Faculty of Medicine, The University of Queensland, Australia

Anton Luger
Department of Medicine III, Medical University of Vienna, Italy

Stephen Lye
Executive Director Alliance for Human Development, Scotia Bank Scientist in Child and Adolescent Health, Lunenfeld-Tanenbaum Research Institute, Sinai Health System; Departments of Obstetrics and Gynecology, Physiology and Medicine, University of Toronto, Canada

Dominique Maiter
Department of Endocrinology and Nutrition, Cliniques Universitaires Saint Luc, Université Catholique de Louvain, Brussels, Belgium

Nicole E. Marshall
Department of Obstetrics and Gynecology, Oregon Health & Science University, Portland, Oregon, USA

David H. McIntyre
Head of Mater Clinical Unit, Faculty of Medicine, The University of Queensland, Australia

Federico Mecacci
Department of Health Sciences, University of Florence, Obstetrics and Gynecology, Careggi University Hospital, Italy

Sam Mesiano
William H. Weir MD Professor of Reproductive Biology, Department of Reproductive Biology, Cleveland, Ohio, USA

Leslie Myatt
Department of Obstetrics & Gynecology, Oregon Health & Science University, Portland, Oregon, USA

Yutaka Osuga
Department of Obstetrics and Gynecology, Faculty of Medicine, The University of Tokyo, Japan

Serena Ottanelli
Department of Health Sciences, University of Florence, Obstetrics and Gynecology, Careggi University Hospital, Italy

Irene Paternò
Department of Experimental, Clinical, and Biomedical Sciences, University of Florence, Careggi University Hospital, Italy

Felice Petraglia
Department of Experimental, Clinical, and Biomedical Sciences; Department of Obstetrics and Gynecology, University of Florence, Careggi University Hospital, Italy

Eliana Piantanida
Department of Medicine & Surgery, University of Insubria, Italy

Nicola Pluchino
Division of OB/GYN, University Hospital of Geneva, Switzerland

Jonathan Q. Purnell
Department of Medicine, Knight Cardiovascular Institute, Oregon Health & Science University, Portland, Oregon, USA

James M. Roberts
Magee-Womens Research Institute, Department of Obstetrics, Gynecology and Reproductive Science, Epidemiology, and Clinical and Translational Research, University of Pittsburgh, Pittsburgh, Pennsylvania, USA

Marie Helene Schernthaner-Reiter
Department of Medicine III, Medical University of Vienna, Italy

Viola Seravalli
Department of Health Sciences, Division of Obstetrics and Gynecology, University of Florence, Italy

Oksana Shynlova
Lunenfeld Tanenbaum Research Institute, Mount Sinai Hospital, Toronto, Canada; Departments of Obstetrics and Gynecology, and Physiology University of Toronto, Canada

Deborah M. Sloboda
Departments of Biochemistry and Biomedical Sciences, Obstetrics and Gynecology and Pediatrics, and Farncombe Family Digestive Health Research Institute, McMaster University, Canada

Roger Smith
Mothers and Babies Research Centre, Hunter Medical Research Centre, University of Newcastle, UK

Sarah J. Stock
Reader and Senior Clinical Lecturer in Maternal and Fetal Health & Honorary Consultant and Subspecialist in Maternal and Fetal Medicine, Welcome Trust Clinical Career Development Fellow Usher Institute, University of Edinburgh, Scotland

Noemi Strambi
Department of Health Sciences, Division of Obstetrics and Gynecology, University of Florence, Italy

Maria Laura Tanda
Department of Medicine & Surgery, University of Insubria, Italy

Kent L. R. Thornburg
Departments of Medicine, Knight Cardiovascular Institute; Obstetrics and Gynecology, Chemical Physiology and Biochemistry; Biomedical Engineering; Oregon Health & Science University, Portland, Oregon, USA

Herbert Valensise
Policlinico Casilino, University of Rome, Italy

Amy M. Valent
Department of Obstetrics and Gynecology, Oregon Health & Science University, Portland, Oregon, USA

Silvia Vannuccini
Department of Experimental, Clinical, and Biomedical Sciences, University of Florence, Careggi University Hospital, Italy

Greisa Vila
Department of Medicine III, Medical University of Vienna, Italy

Peter Wolf
Department of Medicine III, Medical University of Vienna, Italy

Chapter

1

The Neuroendocrinology of Pregnancy

Silvia Vannuccini, Irene Paternò, John R. G. Challis, and Felice Petraglia

1.1 Introduction

The neuroendocrine mechanisms involved in pregnancy are highly complex and include maternal, placental, and fetal systems, which are critical for implantation, maintenance of pregnancy, and timing of parturition (1), and for regulation of fetal-placental blood flow and fetal growth (2).

The brain and placenta are both central organs in the responses to stress (3), and maternal, fetal, and placental hypothalamus-pituitary-adrenal (HPA) axes play a significant role in controlling some of the adaptive mechanisms during pregnancy (4). The human placenta plays a primary role, as it may synthesize and release several neuroactive factors, including hypothalamus-like and pituitary-like hormones. The neurohormones produced by placental tissue act locally in modulating the release of the pituitary-like hormones, resembling the organization of the hypothalamus-pituitary-target gland axes. Furthermore, they are chemically identical and have the same biologic activities as their neuronal counterparts. Thus, the old concept considering the placenta as a passive organ, responsible only for exchange of gas and nutrients to the fetus, has been replaced by a new perspective where the placenta is a fully competent endocrine organ: Trophoblast, membranes, and maternal decidua produce a large variety of molecules including steroid hormones, hypothalamic-pituitary hormones, neuropeptides, growth factors, and cytokines (Table 1.1) (5). These hormones can exert their biologic effects acting as autocrine, paracrine, and endocrine factors (6, 7). However, the placenta also produces a number of hormones, such as human chorionic gonadotropin (hCG) and placental lactogen (hPL), that are not otherwise synthesized in the organism. Placental hormones enter the maternal and fetal circulation, where they are often present at concentrations far in excess of those found for similar hormones in the nonpregnant state, playing a pivotal role in the maternal-fetal

hormonal dialog. Thus, pregnancy represents a highly complex condition where three neuroendocrine systems (maternal, placental, fetal) are integrating their functions for an optimal pregnancy outcome (Figure 1.1).

1.2 Hypothalamus-Pituitary-Adrenal (HPA) Axis

The HPA axis plays a key role in the neuroendocrine response to stress via cortisol secretion, acting to restore homeostasis following stressful events for survival (8). Corticotropin-releasing hormone (CRH) represents the main regulator of the axis: Released from the hypothalamus, this neurohormone stimulates adrenocorticotropic hormone (ACTH) release from the anterior pituitary, and consequently glucocorticoid secretion from the adrenal cortex. Along with the maternal and fetal brain, the human placenta, decidua, chorion, and amnion produce CRH and urocortins (Ucns) peptides (9). In mammals, the CRH/Ucn family consists of at least four ligands: CRH, Ucn (10), Ucn2, and Ucn3, which are implicated as important neuroendocrine mediators in the physiology of early and late pregnancy and in the mechanisms of parturition (11).

1.2.1 Corticotropin-Releasing Hormone (CRH)

The secretion of maternal HPA axis hormones increases throughout pregnancy and is related to placental function, as circulating maternal CRH originates almost entirely from the placenta (6) (Figure 1.1). However, the responsiveness of the HPA axis to stressors is reduced during pregnancy, as shown by reduced ACTH and corticosteroids, in order to neutralize the impact of stress by minimizing stress-induced fetal exposure to maternal glucocorticoid (12). Unlike CRH, it is uncertain whether maternal plasma ACTH

1

Silvia Vannuccini et al.

Table 1.1. Neuroactive placental factors

Category	Factors
Hypothalamus-like hormones	• Corticotropin-releasing hormone (CRH) • Urocortins (Ucn1, Ucn2, Ucn3) • Gonadotropin-releasing hormone (GnRH) • Growth hormone-releasing hormone (GHRH) • Somatostatin (SST) • Thyrotropin-releasing hormone (TRH) • Oxytocin (OT)
Pituitary-like hormones	• Human chorionic gonadotropin (hCG) • Adrenocorticotropic hormone (ACTH) • Opioids (b-endorphin) • Placental growth hormone (PGH) • Human placental lactogen (hPL)
Neuropeptides	• Neuropeptide Y (NPY) • Chromogranin A (CgA) • Neurokinin B (NKB) • Monoamines
Neurosteroids	• Allopregnanolone
Neurotransmitters	• Dopamine • Epinephrine • Norepinephrine • Serotonin
Growth hormones	• Transforming growth factor-β (TGF-β) • Activin A • Follistatin • Follistatin-related gene (FLRG) • Inhibin A and B • Insulin-like growth factors (IGFs) • IGF-binding proteins (IGF-BPs) • Fibroblast growth factor (FGF) • Epidermal growth factor (EGF) • Vascular endothelial growth factor (VEGF)
Steroid hormones	• Progesterone • Estrogens
Vasoactive peptides	• Adrenomedullin (ADM) • Endothelins (ETs) • Calcitonin gene-related peptide (CGRP) • Parathyroid hormone-related peptide (PTH-rp)
Metabolic hormones	• Leptin • Ghrelin

originates from the maternal pituitary and/or from the placenta. Maternal ACTH and cortisol, but not CRH, undergo a typical circadian rhythmicity in the maternal circulation, suggesting that CRH is mostly of placental origin (13).

In the plasma of nonpregnant women, CRH concentrations are very low (around 15 pg/ml) or undetectable. The human placenta expresses large amounts of CRH (1000 times higher than in myometrium and choriodecidua) resulting in high CRH levels in maternal serum during pregnancy. Plasma CRH levels increase during the first trimester of pregnancy, then rise steadily until term (14). CRH levels are approximately 800 pg/ml during late third trimester and peak (2000–3000 pg/ml) during labor, becoming undetectable within 24 hours after delivery. In the fetal circulation, a linear correlation exists between maternal and fetal plasma CRH levels: CRH concentrations in umbilical venous plasma are higher than in the umbilical artery, supporting the notion that placenta is a major source of fetal plasma CRH (Figure 1.1).

Mechanisms regulating placental CRH release are not the same as those regulating hypothalamic release: prostaglandins (PGs), neurotransmitters (norepinephrine, acetylcholine), neuropeptides, and cytokines (IL-1) all stimulate CRH, whereas progesterone (P4), nitric oxide, and estrogens decrease placental CRH production. In the mother, cortisol inhibits hypothalamic CRH and ACTH release, with a negative feedback. In striking contrast, cortisol stimulates CRH release by the decidua, trophoblast, and fetal membranes, and it drives maternal and fetal HPA activation with a positive feedback loop (15). This positive feed-forward system is a unique feature of placental CRH, suggesting that it might not require such "safety switch-off" mechanisms, and the demand for the actions of CRH increases as pregnancy progresses toward term (4). In fact, at term and in labor, circulating levels of CRH, ACTH, and cortisol are increased (16), although they are not necessarily indicative of maternal HPA axis activation.

Placental CRH has complex effects including a role in the onset of labor (17, 18), resembling the timer of a biological clock counting from the early stages of gestation and signaling the timing of parturition (19). Interestingly, maternal CRH levels have been reported to be lower in women delivering post-term and higher in those who will deliver preterm compared to those in women

2

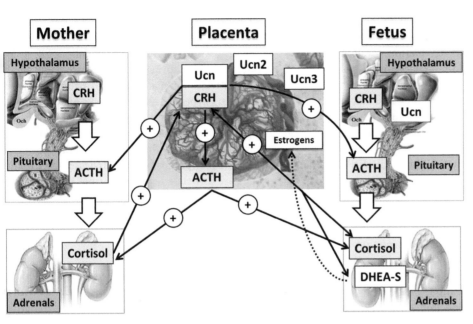

Figure 1.1 Maternal, placental, fetal neuroendocrine systems with three hypothalamus-pituitary-adrenal (HPA) axes integrating their functions. CRH, corticotropin-releasing hormone. ACTH, adrenocorticotropic hormone. Ucn, urocortin. DHEA-S, dehydroepiandrosterone sulfate.

delivering at term. These findings corroborate the important role of this neurohormone in regulating the placental "clock" of human pregnancy and in influencing its length (20).

Regarding endocrine functions, CRH regulates implantation, trophoblast cell growth and invasion, tissue remodeling through modulation of secretion of matrix metalloproteinases, and vascular tone through activation of the nitric oxide pathway, as well as inflammation through PGs release (2).

CRH also plays a pivotal role in regulating estrogen and progesterone production in the third trimester (21), corroborating the hypothesis that placental CRH levels are linked to the length of gestation in humans. The rapid rise of CRH in late pregnancy is associated with estriol (E3) surge and critically altered progesterone (P)/E3 and estriol/estradiol (E3/E2) ratios that create an estrogenic environment predisposing to the onset of labor (22). CRH also regulates myometrial contractility, exerting diverse roles at different stages of gestation. In fact, it mediates both relaxation and contraction of myometrium, depending on different patterns of expression and biologic effects of CRH receptors.

CRH and Ucn exert their actions by activating CRH receptors, named CRHR1 and CRHR2 (23). CRH has high affinity only for CRHR1, Ucn

shows approximately the same affinity for both receptors, whereas Ucn2 and Ucn3 bind with high affinity only to the CRHR2. Nonpregnant human myometrium expresses three CRHR subtypes: 1α, 1β, and 2β. As pregnancy progresses, the myometrium starts to express CRHR2α.

CRH-R1 and CRH-R2 stimulate divergent signaling pathways. CRH-R1 contributes to the maintenance of myometrial relaxation during pregnancy through activation of the adenylyl cyclase/cAMP pathway. In chorion trophoblast cells, CRH exerts a tonic stimulatory effect on 15-hydroxyprostaglandin dehydrogenase (PGDH) activity, an effect that may help to maintain a metabolic barrier that prevents bioactive PGs passing from the chorioamnion to the myometrium preventing myometrial activation during pregnancy (24). In contrast, at term, CRH induces phosphorylation of CRH-R2 variants, with subsequent stimulation of the phospholipase C/inositol triphosphate pathway and increase of myosin light chain phosphorylation, promoting myometrial contractility (25, 26). Furthermore, CRH induces stimulation of placental and membrane PGs output, and the inhibition of progesterone production (27).

CRH binding protein (CRH-BP) binds circulating CRH with high affinity, inhibiting its functions (28); in fact their interaction results in the dimerization of the protein and clearance of CRH from the circulation. Maternal serum CRHBP levels do not change significantly during most of gestation, but they fall during the final weeks of normal pregnancy and still further with the onset of labor (29). Significantly lower CRH and higher CRHBP levels are present in post-term pregnancies, suggesting that the lack of the reciprocal changes in CRH and CRHBP levels may delay the onset of labor.

Fetal stress responses are independent from those of the mother (30): The fetal hypothalamus releases CRH, together with placental CRH, inducing fetal pituitary ACTH secretion and the synthesis of cortisol by the fetal adrenal gland and maturation of the fetal lungs. In turn, the rising cortisol concentrations in the fetus stimulate placental CRH production through a positive feedback mechanism (Figure 1.1). ACTH in turn controls adrenocortical functional development, including angiogenesis and expression of steroidogenic enzymes.

The maturation of the fetal lungs as a result of increasing cortisol concentrations represents a fundamental aspect of fetal adaptive mechanisms to extra-uterine life activated in part by the stress of delivery. Moreover, fetal lung maturation is associated with increased production of surfactant protein A and phospholipids, both pro-inflammatory factors, that may stimulate myometrial contractility through increased production of PGs by fetal membranes and the myometrium itself. Thus, the fetus herself contributes to the onset of labor (15, 31).

Given its multiple effects on a number of placental functions, the role for CRH as a marker of pregnancy pathology has been proposed. CRH is abnormally secreted when obstetric complications occur, such as in pre-term birth (PTB), pre-eclampsia (PE), pregnancy-induced hypertension (PIH), and fetal growth restriction (FGR). In the case of miscarriage, CRH peptide has been found to be more expressed in the placenta in spontaneous abortion than in elective abortion of the same gestational age. In early pregnancy, high glucocorticoid secretion is associated with miscarriage compared with women with ongoing gestation, suggesting that maternal stress in the first trimester is associated with a higher risk for spontaneous abortion (32). Furthermore, CRH expression is significantly higher in preterm than in

term placentas (20) and maternal CRH levels at mid-gestation are higher in women who subsequently would have spontaneous PTB (33). Interestingly, chorioamnionitis associated with PTB activates the placental CRH pathway in vivo (34). In hypertensive disorders of pregnancy, maternal plasma and cord blood CRH levels are higher in women affected by PIH and PE compared to healthy women (35). Additional data confirm that pregnancies complicated by PE and FGR are associated with abnormal placental vascular resistance and abnormally high umbilical vein CRH levels.

1.2.2 Urocortins (Ucns)

Urocortin (Ucn) is synthesized and secreted by placental and fetal membranes, similar to CRH. However, urocortin is undetectable in maternal plasma during pregnancy, with no rise with increasing gestational age (36). Plasma levels are higher at labor, but they do not change significantly at the different stages of labor. Ucn has similar effects as CRH, augmenting matrix metalloproteinase, ACTH, and PGs secretion from cultured human placental cells, enhancing myometrial contractility. Ucn stimulates placental ACTH secretion, via a CRHR1-dependent mechanism, without any significant difference from CRH-induced ACTH release (37). Ucn has high affinity for CRHR1 and CRHR2 families and the CRH binding protein; particularly, Ucn exhibited greater affinity for CRHR2, acting as its natural ligand. Human myometrium expresses Ucn (38), which activates a number of intracellular signaling pathways that contribute to the activation of myometrial contractility.

Ucn2 and Ucn3 are localized in syncytiotrophoblast and extravillous trophoblast cells, while Ucn2 is also localized to blood vessel endothelial cells, leading to the suggestion of a role of Ucn2 in regulating the placental vascular endothelial behavior. In the fetal membranes, Ucn2 is distributed only in amnion, while Ucn3 is found in both amnion and chorionic cells (39). Ucn2 and Ucn3 modulate HPA axis activity at the hypothalamic level in a paracrine or autocrine fashion, but unlike CRH and Ucn, peripheral Ucn2 or Ucn3 administration does not increase either pituitary or placental ACTH secretion (39). Hypothalamic Ucn2 expression is increased by glucocorticoids and modulates basal HPA-axis circadian amplitude (40). Ucn2 plays a major role in the control of myometrial contractility during human pregnancy, involving the binding with CRHR2 (41).

Maternal plasma and cord blood Ucn levels have been found to be higher in women delivering pre-term compared to those delivering at term. Furthermore, Ucn levels in arterial cord blood are higher than in venous cord blood and in maternal plasma, suggesting a fetal rather than an exclusively placental source of the peptide at preterm parturition (42). Similarly, maternal plasma and cord blood Ucn levels are higher in women affected by hypertensive disorders of pregnancy associated with FGR compared with healthy women (43). Interestingly, early PE placental samples show stronger immunoreactivity for Ucn2 than for Ucn3, while Ucn3 immunostaining was stronger in late PE samples (44). Ucn has been found to contribute to the pathogenesis of FGR possibly through negative regulation of placental system A activity, which represents a placental amino acid transporter whose normal activity is fundamental for maintaining fetal growth (45).

1.3 Hypothalamus-Pituitary-Gonadal Axis: Gonadotropin-Releasing Hormone (GnRH)

The gonadotropin-releasing hormone (GnRH) is the main regulator of the hypothalamus-pituitary-gonadal axis. It acts on the anterior pituitary to induce the synthesis and secretion of luteinizing hormone (LH) and follicle-stimulating hormone (FSH), in turn exerting their actions on the ovaries.

From early pregnancy, the hypothalamus-pituitary-gonadal axis decreases its function, because of the rise of maternal serum inhibin levels during the first weeks of gestation and the secretion of maternal progesterone, limiting ovarian functioning in pregnancy.

However, GnRH is produced also by the human placental tissue and it is immunologically and chemically identical to hypothalamic GnRH (46). The total placental concentration of GnRH progressively increases during the first 24 weeks of gestation but declines later in pregnancy. Interestingly, placental and circulating GnRH levels increase during the first trimester, probably modulating human chorionic gonadotropin (hCG) production by trophoblast cells (47). Furthermore, it has been shown in animal models that GnRH causes a

significant decrease in the maximal contraction intensity of myometrium, inhibiting the release of placental prostaglandins. It has been observed that maternal circulating GnRH levels at 25–35 weeks of gestation were significantly higher in women who later had post-term pregnancies, and conversely, it was found to be significantly lower in those undergoing PTB.

1.4 Hypothalamus-Growth Hormone Axis: GH-Releasing Hormone (GHRH) and Somatostatin (SST)

Synthesis and secretion of pituitary growth hormone (GH) is regulated by two hypothalamic-releasing factors: GH-releasing hormone (GHRH) and somatostatin (SST), which has inhibitory properties (48). In women, circulating concentrations of GH-like immunoreactivity increase during pregnancy, although this is not associated with pituitary production. In fact, it rather reflects placental production of a bioactive GH variant (49).

During early pregnancy, pituitary GH is only measurable in maternal serum and it is secreted in a highly pulsatile pattern; conversely, in late pregnancy, 85 percent of circulating levels of bioactive GH derive from placenta, with relatively constant maternal serum concentrations. Placental GH, unlike pituitary GH, is unresponsive to hypothalamic GHRH, whereas glucose is the primary modulator of placental GH secretion. In fact, hypoglycemia induces placental GH synthesis with subsequent increase of maternal blood glucose level, protecting the fetus from nutrient deficiency (50). Placental GH stimulates insulin-like growth factor 1 (IGF-1) and its binding protein (IGFBP-3), reducing plasma clearance of IGF-1 and resulting in negative feedback suppression of maternal GH secretion.

SST levels in maternal circulation in pregnancy do not differ from nonpregnant state, suggesting a scarce placental contribution, while levels in fetoplacental circulation originate from the fetus.

1.5 Hypothalamus-Pituitary-Thyroid Axis

The hypothalamic thyrotropin-releasing hormone (TRH) regulates the release of thyroid-stimulating

5

hormone (TSH) by the anterior pituitary, representing the major effector on thyroid function. Human placenta shows immunoreactivity for TRH, although its bioactivity is still controversial. It seems that placental human chorionic gonadotropin (hCG) plays a major role is in regulating thyroid function in pregnancy. It is structurally similar to TSH and is able to bind TSH receptors with subsequent thyrotropic activity.

hCG belongs to the glycoprotein hormones family that also comprises LH, FSH and TSH. All members are heterodimers consisting of an α and a β subunit. The α subunit is common to all four glycoprotein hormones, while the β chains determine the biological activity and display extensive homology; that between hCG and LH about 80 percent. hCG is produced in large amounts by syncytiotrophoblasts. It is elaborated by all types of trophoblastic tissue, including that from hydatiform mole and choriocarcinoma.

The primitive trophoblast produces hCG very early in human pregnancy, since hCG is detectable 9 days after the midcycle LH peak. Maternal serum hCG peaks at 8–10 week and then declines to reach a plateau at 18–20 week of gestation (51). The elevation in circulating hCG seems to cause a transient fall in maternal serum TSH near the end of the first trimester in normal pregnancy. Thus, the lowering of TSH corresponds to a transient and partial blunting of the pituitary-thyroid axis associated with an increased hormonal output from the thyroid (52).

1.6 Oxytocin

Oxytocin (OT) is synthesized by neurons of the supraoptic and paraventricular nucleus in the hypothalamus and secreted by the posterior pituitary; its major target organs are the pregnant uterus and mammary glands, as it regulates myometrial contractility and milk ejection (53). Although placental expression and secretion of OT has been shown, their contribution to the mechanisms of parturition remains not fully elucidated. Placental OT secretion is increased by several paracrine factors such as CRH, activin A, and PGs operating within human intrauterine tissues.

Circulating OT levels gradually rise in pregnancy and become even higher during labor, when pulses of oxytocin become progressively bigger and more frequent. Basal levels of OT increased three- to four-fold during pregnancy and pulses increase in frequency, duration, and amplitude from late pregnancy through labor. A large oxytocin pulse occurs with the birth, and pulses continue afterwards, contributing to placenta expulsion and preventing postpartum bleeding (54). At the onset of labor, the uterine sensitivity to OT markedly increases in association with both an upregulation of OT receptor mRNA levels and a strong increase in the density of myometrial OT receptors, reaching a peak during early labor (53).

Given that the placental content of OT is approximately five times greater than in the posterior pituitary lobe, it is possible that the placenta might be the main source of OT during pregnancy. Estrogens are the major regulators of OT expression, inducing an increased expression of OT mRNA in decidua, chorion, and amnion in a concentration-dependent manner and with a bimodal response pattern. Indeed, nocturnal elevation of maternal plasma OT and estradiol concentrations correlate with circadian uterine activity (55).

Fetal membranes (amnion and chorion) and maternal decidua transmit hormonal signals to the myometrium and contribute to local changes in the estrogen-to-P4 ratio, suggesting that OT may act primarily as a local mediator and not as a circulating hormone during parturition (56).

During labor, OT is released into both the blood and brain, with high oxytocin levels in the cerebrospinal fluid, acting as a neuromodulator, with widespread central effects. OT enhances mood and wellbeing, promotes friendly social interactions, reduces anxiety and pain, lowering physiological and psychological stress. In addition, it reduces sympathetic nervous system activity ("fight or flight") and increases parasympathetic nervous system activity, playing a major role in influencing maternal behavior (54, 57).

1.7 Prolactin and Placental Lactogen (hPL)

Prolactin (PRL) is produced by lactotroph cells in the anterior pituitary gland under the inhibitory control of dopamine (DA). High circulating PRL levels are essential for maintaining pregnancy by providing luteotropic support to the corpus luteum, thereby stimulating progesterone secretion in early pregnancy (58).

The increasing PRL levels throughout gestation are linked to increasing estrogen levels, which also rise from early pregnancy. In humans, the placenta produces an increasing amount of placental lactogen (hPL) throughout pregnancy (59). hPL is structurally similar to PRL and binds to PRL receptors. Differently from PRL, hPL is not subjected to hypothalamic regulation by DA, hence providing a source of lactogenic hormones that is not subject to the normal negative feedback regulation (60).

The levels of hPL in maternal circulation are very low in early pregnancy and increase progressively, showing some correlation with placental weight. hPL accounts for 7–10 percent of proteins synthesized by the placenta at term, and the production rate of hPL increases as pregnancy progresses, approximately in proportion to placental mass with peak levels being reached during the last weeks of gestation. Thus, hPL represents one of the major metabolic and biosynthetic activities of the syncytiotrophoblast in humans (about 1g/day production near term) (61).

Maternal serum hPL levels reflect placental biosynthesis and are positively correlated with the size of the fetus (62), suggesting the possibility of using this hormonal marker for the screening of FGR. The rate of change of serial hPL measurements correlated well with intrauterine fetal growth velocity in the third trimester as estimated by ultrasound and to the deviation in birth weight (63). Elevated lactogen hormones contribute to regulating several functions: establishment of maternal behavior; food intake, suppression of stress responses during late pregnancy and lactation, to minimize the risk of adverse fetal programming from glucocorticoids; prevention of stress-induced hyperthermia; regulation of oxytocin neurons during parturition and lactation, hence contributing to myometrial contractility and milk ejection; and maternal recognition of the offspring, possibly by PRL-induced neurogenesis (64, 65).

1.8 Other Neuroendocrine Factors

1.8.1 Neuropeptide Y (NPY)

Neuropeptide Y (NPY) is a sympathetic neurotransmitter discovered in 1982 and has been shown to be involved in increased blood pressure, angiogenesis, and vasoconstriction. Sympathetic nerves and chromaffin cells of the adrenal glands have been hypothesized to be the major source of circulating NPY outside of pregnancy. In pregnant women, acidic extracts of human placental tissues collected at term contain high immunoreactive NPY (66).

NPY is present in cervical tissue from both early pregnant women and women at term, but no difference in intensity or distribution of NPY-containing nerves was demonstrated between early and term pregnant women or between women in labor and women before onset of labor. In pregnant women, maternal plasma NPY levels are higher than in nonpregnant women, without significant changes throughout gestation (67). Plasma NPY levels fall within a few hours after delivery, supporting the placental origin of the circulating NPY in pregnancy.

A role of NPY during labor at term and preterm is yet to be defined, but a functional association between the increase of NPY during labor and vaginal delivery is in accordance with the spontaneous labor-induced increase of other stress-related hormones such as catecholamines, cortisol and ACTH. It has been suggested that NPY is implicated in PE and PIH, as elevated maternal plasma NPY levels have also been reported in women affected by hypertensive disorders (68), whereas a reduced placental expression of NPY was observed, suggesting the involvement of the receptors in the abnormalities of placental angiogenesis (66).

1.8.2 Relaxin

Relaxin is a peptide hormone that is a member of the insulin family. In women, circulating relaxin is a product of the corpus luteum of pregnancy, but is also synthesized by other reproductive organs such as the uterus, decidua, and placenta, where relaxin acts locally. Circulating relaxin is secreted in a pattern similar to that of hCG.

Relaxin binds to its receptor RXFP1, which has been localized to a wide variety of reproductive and non-reproductive tissues. Relaxin has many uterotropic effects including stimulating uterine growth and vascularization, remodeling extracellular matrix components, and regulating vascular endothelial growth factor in preparation for implantation. Evidence also supports a role for relaxin in the systemic maternal vascular adaptations required for a healthy pregnancy.

Diminished relaxin levels in early pregnancy are linked with increased risks of miscarriage and the development of preeclampsia (69). Furthermore, it has been shown that women who are more likely to deliver preterm have increased circulating relaxin levels (70).

1.8.3 Parathyroid Hormone-Related Protein (PTHrP)

Parathyroid hormone-related protein (PTHrP) is an oncofetal protein that is expressed in many mammalian tissues. There is substantial evidence to support its role in pregnancy and labor as a placental calcium transport activator, potent vasorelaxant, and inhibitor of uterine contractions (71).

Human amnion is a major source of PTHrP and PTHrP mRNA abundance in amnion decreases during labor at term. Similarly, there is a dramatic decrease in amniotic fluid PTHrP concentrations associated with term labor, which is not evident in amniotic fluid obtained from preterm labor. These results suggest that at term, the dramatic decrease in PTHrP activity in tissue and amniotic fluid might be part of the physiological mechanism involved in the onset and/or progression of labor (72).

1.8.4 Opioids

Three families of opioid peptides are recognized: endorphin (END), enkephalin (ENK), and dynorphin (DYN). They derive from three prehormones: pro-opiomelanocortin (POMC) for β-END, proenkephalin (P-ENK) for ENK and prodynorphin (P-DYN) for DYN. Mu (μ), kappa (κ), and delta (δ) are the main opioid receptor types, but κ receptors are the more important type present in the placenta. Placental content of κ receptors increases with gestational age, and term placental content of κ receptors correlates with type of delivery.

CRH stimulates pro-opiomelanocortin hormone (POMC) release from human cultured placental cells, suggesting placental regulation of POMC secretion, somewhat similar to that occurring in pituitary cells. However, in contrast to the negative feedback activity of glucocorticoids, dexamethasone is not effective either in suppressing ACTH or b-END release from placental cells or in reducing the CRH-induced release of placental ACTH/b-END release. Indeed, there is abundant evidence to show that corticosteroids increase rather than decrease expression and synthesis of CRH from trophoblasts.

Many studies agree on a large increase of plasma b-END during labor and at parturition, although they do not indicate whether the peptide has pituitary or placental origin. Maternal plasma levels of ENK are not significantly different from those of nonpregnant women and do not change throughout pregnancy, supporting a local role of the peptide. On the contrary, maternal plasma DYN levels in the third trimester and at delivery are higher than in nonpregnant women and high levels are also detectable in amniotic fluid and in umbilical vein plasma (73).

1.8.5 Neurosteroids

The placenta is a source of several neurosteroids comprising progesterone itself, its derivatives 5a-pregnane-3a-ol-20- one (allopregnanolone) and 5a-dihydroprogesterone, and its precursor pregnenolone sulfate (74). Apart from progesterone, the role of placental neurosteroids in the physiology of pregnancy is largely unknown. These hormones may contribute to the neurochemical and behavioral changes of pregnancy and puerperium because they interfere with GABAergic circuits and have anxiolytic effects (75).

The levels of allopregnanolone in maternal serum increase progressively during gestation and, in contrast to progesterone, are augmented in hypertensive complications of pregnancy (76). In PE, there is an increased activity of tyrosine hydroxylase in placental tissue, and this is likely to contribute the higher levels of catecholamines in the maternal circulation (77). It is also a neuroactive hormone and may contribute to the psychological adaptation associated with pregnancy and puerperium. In fact, serum allopregnanolone levels were detectable postpartum and were significantly decreased in women with maternity "blues" (78).

A recent study showed that in healthy pregnant women, maternal serum allopregnanolone and progesterone levels significantly increased throughout gestation. No major changes were found at delivery, with the exception of a significant decrease of maternal and cord serum allopregnanolone levels during emergency cesarean section (76). This suggests the critical role of these steroids in maternal brain adaptation during pregnancy and perhaps in the development of the fetal brain. It has been suggested that allopregnanolone is brain protective during PTB or FGR, reducing the impact of hypoxia (79).

1.9 Conclusions

The neuroendocrine system in pregnancy involves highly complex maternal, fetal, and placental mechanisms, which are critical for the maintenance of pregnancy, the timing of parturition, fetal growth, and protection from adverse fetal programming. The brain and placenta are both central organs in the responses to stress, and the maternal, fetal, and placental hypothalamus–pituitary–adrenal (HPA) axes play a significant role in controlling some of the adaptive mechanisms during pregnancy. Indeed, the placenta, may be considered as a neuroendocrine organ rich in neurohormones, neuropeptides, and neurosteroids. Stress-related hormones, such as CRH, urocortins, oxytocin, and prolactin, are key placental neuroendocrine factors mediating both endocrine (metabolism, immune function, cardiovascular changes) and paracrine (uterine contractility, local hormone production) mechanisms involved in term and pre-term birth. Aberrations in neurohormones secretion, as an adaptive response of the feto-placental unit to adverse environmental conditions, may contribute to the development of gestational disorders, such as hypertensive disorders of pregnancy, intrauterine growth restriction, and gestational diabetes.

References

1. Vannuccini S, Bocchi C, Severi FM, et al. Endocrinology of human parturition. *Ann Endocrinol (Paris)*. 2016, 77 (2):105–113.

2. Voltolini C, and Petraglia F. Neuroendocrinology of pregnancy and parturition. In: *Handbook of Clinical Neurology*. 2014.

3. Behura SK, Dhakal P, Kelleher AM, et al. The brain-placental axis: Therapeutic and pharmacological relevancy to pregnancy. *Pharmacological Research*. 2019.

4. Petraglia F, Imperatore A, and Challis JRG. Neuroendocrine mechanisms in pregnancy and parturition. *Endocrine Reviews*. 2010, 31: 783–816.

5. Iliodromiti Z, Antonakopoulos N, Sifakis S, et al. Endocrine, paracrine, and autocrine placental mediators in labor. *Hormones*. 2012.

6. Petraglia F, Florio P, Nappi C, et al. Peptide signaling in human placenta and membranes: Autocrine, paracrine, and endocrine mechanisms. Vol., *Endocrine Reviews*. 1996, 17: 156–186.

7. Petraglia F, Florio P, and Torricelli M. Placental endocrine function. In: *Knobil and Neill's Physiology of Reproduction*. 2006.

8. Brunton PJ, and Russell JA. Endocrine induced changes in brain function during pregnancy. *Brain Research*. 2010.

9. Warren WB, and Silverman AJ. Cellular localization of corticotrophin releasing hormone in the human placenta, fetal membranes and decidua. *Placenta*. 1995.

10. Vaughan J, Donaldson C, Bittencourt J, et al. Urocortin, a mammalian neuropeptide related to fish urotensin I and to corticotropin-releasing factor. *Nature*. 1995.

11. Zoumakis E, Kalantaridou S, and Makrigiannakis A. CRH-like peptides in human reproduction. *Curr Med Chem*. 2009.

12. Welberg LAM, and Seckl JR. Prenatal stress, glucocorticoids and the programming of the brain. *Journal of Neuroendocrinology*. 2001.

13. Waddell BJ. The placenta as hypothalamus and pituitary: Possible impact on maternal and fetal adrenal function. *Reproduction, Fertility and Development*. 1993.

14. Florio P, Severi FM, Ciarmela P, et al. Placental stress factors and maternal-fetal adaptive response: The corticotropin-releasing factor family. *Endocrine*. 2002.

15. Challis JRG, Bloomfield FH, Booking AD, et al. Fetal signals and parturition. *Journal of Obstetrics and Gynaecology Research*. 2005.

16. Ochędalski T, Zylinńska K, Laudański T, et al. Corticotrophin-releasing hormone and ACTH levels in maternal and fetal blood during spontaneous and oxytocin-induced labour. *European Journal of Endocrinology*. 2001;

17. Vitoratos N, Papatheodorou DC, Kalantaridou SN, et al. "Reproductive" corticotropin-releasing hormone. In: *Annals of the New York Academy of Sciences*. 2006.

18. Challis JRG, Matthews SG, Gibb W, et al. Endocrine and paracrine regulation of birth at term and preterm. *Endocrine Reviews*. 2000.

19. McLean M, Bisits A, Davies J, et al. A placental clock controlling the length of

human pregnancy. *Nature Medicine*. 1995, 1(5):460–463.

20. Torricelli M, Ignacchiti E, Giovannelli A, et al. Maternal plasma corticotrophin-releasing factor and urocortin levels in post-term pregnancies. *European Journal of Endocrinology*. 2006.

21. Rainey WE, Rehman KS, and Carr BR. The human fetal adrenal: Making adrenal androgens for placental estrogens. *Seminars in Reproductive Medicine*. 2004.

22. Smith R, Smith JI, Shen X, et al. Patterns of plasma corticotropin-releasing hormone, progesterone, estradiol, and estriol change and the onset of human labor. *Journal of Clinical Endocrinology & Metabolism*. 2009, 94(6):2066–2074.

23. Grammatopoulos DK. Placental corticotrophin-releasing hormone and its receptors in human pregnancy and labour: Still a scientific enigma. In: *Journal of Neuroendocrinology*. 2008.

24. McKeown KJ, and Challis JRG. Regulation of 15-hydroxy prostaglandin dehydrogenase by corticotrophin-releasing hormone through a calcium-dependent pathway in human chorion trophoblast cells. *Journal of Clinical Endocrinology & Metabolism*. 2003.

25. Grammatopoulos DK, and Hillhouse EW. Role of corticotropin-releasing hormone in onset of labour. Vol. 354, *Lancet*. 1999, 1546–1549.

26. Simpkin JC, Kermani F, Palmer AM, et al. Effects of corticotrophin releasing hormone on contractile activity of myometrium from pregnant women. *BJOG: An International Journal of Obstetrics & Gynaecology*. 1999.

27. Jeschke U, Mylonas I, Richter DU, et al. Regulation of progesterone production in human term trophoblasts in vitro by CRH, ACTH and cortisol (prednisolone). *Archives of Gynecology and Obstetrics*. 2005.

28. Zhao XJ, Hoheisel C, Schauer J, et al. Corticotropin-releasing hormone-binding protein and its possible role in neuroendocrinological research. *Hormone and Metabolic Research*. 1997.

29. Florio P, Woods RJ, Genazzani AR, et al. Changes in amniotic fluid immunoreactive Corticotropin-Releasing Factor (CRF) and CRF-binding protein levels in pregnant women at term and during labor 1. *Journal of Clinical Endocrinology & Metabolism*. 1997.

30. Gitau R, Fisk NM, Teixeira JMA, et al. Fetal hypothalamic-pituitary-adrenal stress responses to invasive procedures are independent of maternal responses. *Journal of Clinical Endocrinology & Metabolism*. 2001.

31. Mesiano S, DeFranco E, Muglia, LJ. Parturition. In: *Knobil and Neill's Physiology of Reproduction: Two-Volume Set*. 2015.

32. Nepomnaschy PA, Welch KB, McConnell DS, et al. Cortisol levels and very early pregnancy loss in humans. *Proceedings of the National Academy of Sciences of the United States of America*. 2006.

33. Hobel CJ, Dunkel-Schetter C, Roesch SC, et al. Maternal plasma corticotropin-releasing hormone associated with stress at 20 weeks' gestation in pregnancies ending in preterm delivery. *American Journal of Obstetrics and Gynecology*. 1999.

34. Torricelli M, Novembri R, Bloise E, et al Changes in

placental CRH, urocortins, and CRH-receptor mRNA expression associated with preterm delivery and chorioamnionitis. *Journal of Clinical Endocrinology & Metabolism*. 2011.

35. Florio P, Imperatore A, Sanseverino F, et al. The measurement of maternal plasma corticotropin-releasing factor (CRF) and CRF-binding protein improves the early prediction of preeclampsia. *Journal of Clinical Endocrinology & Metabolism*. 2004.

36. Glynn BP, Welton A, Rodriguez-Linares B, et al. Urocortin in pregnancy. *American Journal of Obstetrics and Gynecology*. 1998.

37. Petraglia F, Florio P, Benedetto C, et al. Urocortin stimulates placental adrenocorticotropin and prostaglandin release and myometrial contractility in vitro. *Journal of Clinical Endocrinology & Metabolism*. 1999, 84(4):1420–1423.

38. Clifton VL, Qing G, Murphy VE, et al. Localization and characterization of urocortin during human pregnancy. *Placenta*. 2000, 21(8):782–788.

39. Imperatore A, Florio P, Torres PB, et al. Urocortin 2 and urocortin 3 are expressed by the human placenta, deciduas, and fetal membranes. *Am Journal of Obstetrics and Gynaecology*. 2006.

40. Hashimoto K, Nishiyama M, Tanaka Y, et al. Urocortins and corticotropin releasing factor type 2 receptors in the hypothalamus and the cardiovascular system. *Peptides*. 2004.

41. Karteris E, Hillhouse EW, and Grammatopoulos D. Urocortin II Is expressed in human pregnant myometrial cells and regulates myosin light chain phosphorylation: Potential role of the type-2 Corticotropin-

Releasing Hormone receptor in the control of myometrial contractility. *Endocrinology.* 2004;145(2):890–900.

42. Florio P, Torricelli M, Galleri L, et al. High fetal urocortin levels at term and preterm labor. *Journal of Clinical Endocrinology & Metabolism.* 2005.

43. Florio P, Torricelli M, De Falco G, et al. High maternal and fetal plasma urocortin levels in pregnancies complicated by hypertension. *Journal of Hypertension.* 2006.

44. Imperatore A, Rolfo A, Petraglia F, et al. Hypoxia and preeclampsia: Increased expression of urocortin 2 and urocortin 3. *Reproductive Sciences.* 2010.

45. Giovannelli A, Greenwood SL, Desforges M, et al. Corticotrophin-releasing factor and urocortin inhibit system a activity in term human placental villous explants. *Placenta.* 2011.

46. Sasaki K, and Norwitz ER. Gonadotropin-releasing hormone/gonadotropin-releasing hormone receptor signaling in the placenta. *Current Opinion in Endocrinology, Diabetes and Obesity.* 2011.

47. Lee HJ, Snegovskikh VV, Park JS, et al. Role of GnRH-GnRH receptor signaling at the maternal-fetal interface. *Fertility and Sterility.* 2010.

48. Sassolas G. Growth hormone-releasing hormone: Past and present. Hormone *Research.* 2000.

49. Frankenne F, Scippo ML, Van, BJ, et al. Identification of placental human growth hormone as the growth hormone-v gene expression product. *Journal of Clinical Endocrinology & Metabolism.* 1990.

50. Alsat E, Guibourdenche J, Couturier A, et al.

Physiological role of human placental growth hormone. *Molecular and Cellular Endocrinology.* 1998.

51. Davies S, Byrn F, and Cole LA. Human chorionic gonadotropin testing for early pregnancy viability and complications. *Clinics in Laboratory Medicine.* 2003.

52. Williams GR. Neurodevelopmental and neurophysiological actions of thyroid hormone. *Journal of Neuroendocrinology.* 2008.

53. Arrowsmith S, and Wray S. Oxytocin: Its mechanism of action and receptor signalling in the myometrium. *Journal of Neuroendocrinology.* 2014.

54. Uvnäs-Moberg K, Ekström-Bergström A, Berg M, et al. Maternal plasma levels of oxytocin during physiological childbirth - A systematic review with implications for uterine contractions and central actions of oxytocin. *BMC Pregnancy Childbirth.* 2019.

55. Bossmar T, Osman N, Zilahi E, et al. Expression of the oxytocin gene, but not the vasopressin gene, in the rat uterus during pregnancy: Influence of oestradiol and progesterone. *Journal of Endocrinology.* 2007.

56. FUCHS A-R, and FUCHS F. Endocrinology of human parturition: A review. *BJOG An International Journal of Gynecology & Obstetrics.* 1984.

57. Keverne EB. Central mechanisms underlying the neural and neuroendocrine determinants of maternal behaviour. *Psychoneuroendocrinology.* 1988.

58. Freeman ME, Kanyicska B, Lerant A, et al. Prolactin: Structure, function, and regulation of secretion. *Physiological Reviews.* 2000.

59. Ben-Jonathan N, LaPensee CR, and LaPensee EW. What can we learn from rodents about prolactin in humans? *Endocrine Reviews.* 2008.

60. Grattan DR, and Kokay IC. Prolactin: A pleiotropic neuroendocrine hormone. *Journal of Neuroendocrinology.* 2008.

61. Walker WH, Fitzpatrick SL, Saunders GF, et al. The human placental lactogen genes: Structure, function, evolution and transcriptional regulation. *Endocrine Reviews.* 1991.

62. Newbern D, and Freemark M. Placental hormones and the control of maternal metabolism and fetal growth. *Current Opinion in Endocrinology, Diabetes and Obesity.* 2011.

63. Sørensen S, Von Tabouillot D, Schiøler V, et al. Serial measurements of serum human placental lactogen (hPL) and serial ultrasound examinations in the evaluation of fetal growth. *Early Human Development.* 2000.

64. Shingo T, Gregg C, Enwere E, et al. Pregnancy-stimulated neurogenesis in the adult female forebrain mediated by prolactin. *Science (80-).* 2003.

65. Torner L, and Neumann ID. The brain prolactin system: Involvement in stress response adaptations in lactation. *Stress.* 2002.

66. Sahay A, Kale A, and Joshi S. Role of neurotrophins in pregnancy and offspring brain development. *Neuropeptides.* 2020.

67. Petraglia F, Coukos G, Battaglia C, et al. Plasma and amniotic fluid immunoreactive neuropeptide-Y level changes during pregnancy, labor, and at parturition. *Journal of Clinical Endocrinology & Metabolism.* 1989.

68. Khatun S, Kanayama N, Belayet HM, et al. Increased

concentrations of plasma neuropeptide Y in patients with eclampsia and preeclampsia. *American Journal of Obstetrics & Gynecology.* 2000.

69. Marshall SA, Senadheera SN, Parry LJ, et al. The role of relaxin in normal and abnormal uterine function during the menstrual cycle and early pregnancy. *Reproductive Sciences.* 2017.

70. Goldsmith LT, Weiss G, and Steinetz BG. Relaxin and its role in pregnancy. *Endocrinology and Metabolism Clinics of North America.* 1995.

71. Clemens TL, Cormier S, Eichinger A, et al. Parathyroid hormone-related protein and its receptors: Nuclear functions and roles in the renal and cardiovascular systems, the placental trophoblasts and the pancreatic islets. *British Journal of Pharmacology.* 2001.

72. Ferguson JE, Gorman JV, Bruns DE, et al. Abundant expression of parathyroid hormone-related protein in human amnion and its association with labor. *Proceedings of the National Academy of Sciences of the United States of America.* 1992.

73. Ahmed MS, Cemerikic B, and Agbas A. Properties and functions of human placental opioid system. *Life Sciences.* 1992.

74. Le Goascogne C, Eychenne B, Tonon MC, et al. Neurosteroid progesterone is up-regulated in the brain of jimpy and shiverer mice. *Glia.* 2000.

75. Dombroski RA, Casey ML, and MacDonald PC. 5α-dihydroprogesterone formation in human placenta from 5α-pregnan-3β/α-ol-20-ones and 5-pregnan-3β-yl-20-one sulfate. *Journal of Steroid Biochemistry and Molecular Biology.* 1997.

76. Luisi S, Petraglia F, Benedetto C, et al. Serum allopregnanolone levels in pregnant women: Changes during pregnancy, at delivery, and in hypertensive patients. *Journal of Clinical Endocrinology & Metabolism.* 2000.

77. Manyonda IT, Slater DM, Fenske C, et al. A role for noradrenaline in pre-eclampsia: Towards a unifying hypothesis for the pathophysiology. *BJOG: An International Journal of Obstetrics & Gynaecology.* 1998.

78. Nappi RE, Petraglia F, Luisi S, et al. Serum allopregnanolone in women with postpartum "blues." *Obstetrics & Gynecology.* 2001.

79. Pluchino N, Ansaldi Y, and Genazzani AR. Brain intracrinology of allopregnanolone during pregnancy and hormonal contraception. *Hormone Molecular Biology and Clinical Investigation.* 2019.

The Placenta as an Endocrine Organ/Placental Endocrinology

Roger Smith

2.1 The Placental Maturational Trajectory

The placenta is an unusual endocrine organ: It releases both steroid and peptide hormones. Unlike most endocrine glands the placenta does not release hormones in response to acute changes in the internal environment as the adrenal gland does for cortisol or adrenalin. The cells of the placenta do not store steroid or peptide hormones, but release the hormones as they are synthesized. In contrast to other endocrine glands which maintain homeostasis, the placenta is an agent of change. The placenta moves the mother's physiology from the nonpregnant equilibrium to a new trajectory, a new physiological setting in which the needs of the growing fetus distort her metabolism, her immune system, and even her behavior (1). The placenta does not respond to short term homeostasis demands; rather it is independent of the maternal environment and sends signals that are not controlled by the negative feedback processes found elsewhere in the endocrine system. Instead, the endocrinology of pregnancy is dependent on a placental maturational process that is epigenetically regulated.

The progressive maturation of the placenta leads to changes in the production of peptide hormones like human chorionic gonadotrophin (hCG), corticotrophin releasing hormone (CRH) and placental variant growth hormone. Equally maturation of the placenta leads to alterations in release of estrogens and progesterone. The fetus is also affected by placental maturation. The placenta metabolizes maternal cortisol, regulating its appearance in the fetal circulation. Placental peptide hormones also regulate fetal adrenal steroid synthesis. In addition, the placenta influences fetal thyroid hormone levels and calcium metabolism. Most maturational processes lead to sexual maturity which is followed by aging and an increased likelihood of death. In contrast, placental maturation is targeted towards birth of an infant capable of surviving in the ex-utero environment. Like other maturational processes such as puberty, placental maturation is not precisely timed, and women deliver at a range of gestations. Shorter gestations may lead to premature delivery of a fetus that is incapable of independent survival, while longer gestations may be associated with intrauterine death linked to deterioration of placental function as a consequence of the placenta reaching its full maturation and starting to deteriorate or age, before the delivery of the fetus (2). The absence of a negative feedback system regulating placental hormone production means that unfettered hormone release may overwhelm maternal metabolic processes and physiology leading to gestational diabetes, hyperemesis, cholestasis, thyrotoxicosis, vulnerability to viral infections, venous thromboembolism, and other pathologies. Placental signalling may also occur via recently discovered mechanisms such as the release of microparticles and exosomes containing peptide hormones and RNAs which may modulate maternal physiology and play a role in regulating the onset of labor (3).

It is possible that the maturational process of the placenta may give an insight into the maturational clocks of the associated fetus, such as timing of sexual maturity and even life expectancy. The products of conception give rise to both the placenta and the fetus. They are effectively twins following very different maturational pathways and marching to very different clocks – one lasts nine months, while the other may last ninety years. The placenta is a mammalian booster rocket that accelerates the development of mammalian offspring ensuring that they arrive in the world at a relatively advanced stage of development compared to most amniotes (a few lizards deliver live young). During pregnancy placental hormones also target the breast tissue, ensuring a source of nutrients for the infant following birth. Extended maternal care is a feature of mammalian parenting which contributes to offspring survival. Increasing evidence supports the view that maternal parenting is influenced by placental hormone effects on the maternal brain.

2.2 Placental Signaling of the Presence of the Pregnancy

The fusion of the sperm with the ovum creates the zygote. The zygote cell is totipotent as it is able to form all the tissues of the fetus and also of the placenta. A key method of regulating the expression of mammalian genes is DNA methylation. In this process, the DNA residue cytosine is methylated to form five methyl cytosine. Methyl cytosine marks genes to reduce their expression. Specific patterns of cytosine methylation create specific cell types by restricting which genes can be expressed. To generate the totipotent capabilities of the zygote the DNA derived from both the sperm and the ovum undergo a wave of demethylation that begins a process of development that is epigenetically regulated (4).

2.2.1 Expression of Syncytin and the Formation of the Trophectoderm

The wave of demethylation that occurs in the zygote releases retroviral elements from epigenetic silencing. In the human this leads to expression of the retroviral envelop proteins syncytin 1 and syncytin 2 (5). Retroviral proteins are remnants of viruses that incorporated into germline cells during infections in the distant evolutionary past and consequently are subsequently passed on from one generation to the next with reproduction. Retroviral proteins have been found in all mammals in which their presence has been sought (1). These retroviral proteins possess two critical domains, one that promotes immune suppression and one that promotes cell fusion. It seems likely that the immunosuppressive action of retroviral proteins is essential for mammalian pregnancy to suppress the maternal immune response that would otherwise occur to the allogenic fetus. These proteins are especially expressed in the trophectoderm that forms following the divisions of the zygote that leads to the formation of the morula.

2.2.2 Signaling the Presence of a Fertilized Ovum

The outer cells of the morula express syncytins which promote cell fusion and differentiation along a line leading to the trophectoderm which will form the placenta following implantation. Prior to implantation, the syncytin driven differentiation leads to expression of human chorionic gonadotrophin (6). The production of chorionic gonadotrophin is the key signal that allows the establishment of human pregnancy. The chorionic gonadotrophin has high homology with luteinizing hormone, and like luteinizing hormone stimulates the production of progesterone from the corpus luteum by acting on luteinizing hormone receptors. The combined action of chorionic gonadotrophin and progesterone suppress uterine contractility and allows implantation of the blastocyst (7).

2.3 Formation of the Cytotrophoblast and Syncytiotrophoblast Layers

With implantation the trophectoderm differentiates into the cytotrophoblast stem cell layer and the differentiated layer of syncytiotrophoblast. The fusion of cytotrophoblasts with the overlying layer of syncytiotrophoblast is mediated by the combined actions of syncytin 1 and syncytin 2. The generation of the syncytiotrophoblast layer is central to the endocrinology of pregnancy. The syncytiotrophoblast is in direct contact with the maternal blood and is able to release peptide and steroid hormones directly into the maternal circulation. There are multiple differences between the cytotrophoblast and the syncytiotrophoblast cells that reflect the change in function. Notably the mitochondria of the syncytiotrophoblast are numerous and small, likely linked to their key role in metabolizing cholesterol into progesterone (8). Transport of cholesterol to mitochondria is the rate limiting step in placental progesterone synthesis. This transfer of cholesterol is regulated by protein kinase A (9).

2.4 Regulation of Estrogen and Progesterone Synthesis

Within the mitochondria, cytochrome P450scc is located on the inner membrane and catalyzes the conversion of cholesterol into pregnenolone. 3b-hydroxysteroid-dehydrogenase-D4–5 isomerase type I in the inner membrane then transforms the pregnenolone into progesterone (10). The key role of protein kinase A in providing cholesterol to the mitochondria suggests that cyclic AMP pathways that are activated in the syncytiotrophoblast by multiple peptide hormones – including chorionic gonadotrophin – and by the syncytins create the environment for active placental progesterone synthesis and placental maintenance of pregnancy.

Estrogen production in human pregnancy is complex with four different estrogens – estradiol, estriol, estrone, and estetrol produced by the placenta using androgenic precursors from both the mother and fetus (11). The reticularis layer of the maternal adrenal produces the androgen dehydroepiandrostenedione (DHEA) and its sulphated form DHEAs. In the fetus a special fetal zone of the adrenal develops which also produces DHEAs. A specific feature of the fetal zone is its responsiveness to the peptide hormone corticotrophin releasing hormone (CRH) (12). CRH produced by the syncytiotrophoblast layer of the placenta is predominately released into the maternal circulation, but physiologically significant amounts are also released into the fetal circulation (13).

In the mother, placentally derived CRH stimulates the maternal pituitary, increasing ACTH production and melanocyte stimulating fragments of the pro-opiomelanocortin precursor peptide. The melanocyte stimulating actions of the pro-opiomelanocortin cause the darkening of skin sometimes seen in pregnancy including the linea nigra (14). Of more importance, the increased ACTH production leads to increased adrenal cortisol production and increased DHEA and DHEAs synthesis (15). The increased cortisol production is likely a key factor in reducing the sensitivity of maternal tissues to insulin and helping to divert glucose and fatty acids to the fetus. Thus high levels of placental CRH are associated with gestational diabetes (16). The maternal adrenally derived DHEA and DHEAs are substrates for placental estradiol production (Figure 2.1).

Within the fetus, placentally derived CRH likely acts on the fetal pituitary, and more importantly on the fetal zone of the adrenal. The effect of the CRH on the fetal pituitary appears modest as fetal ACTH and cortisol only rise late in pregnancy, and this appears more closely linked to maturation of the fetal hypothalamic regulation of the pituitary. In contrast, the fetal zone of the adrenal appears highly responsive to CRH, leading to increased DHEAs synthesis and release into the fetal circulation.

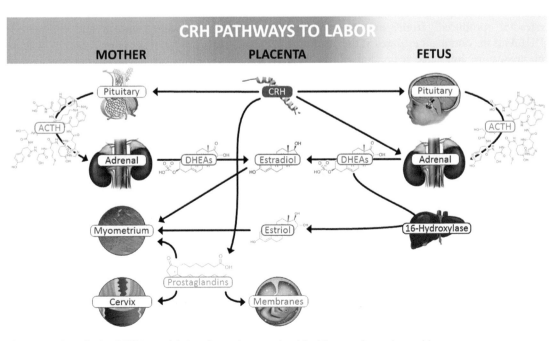

Figure 2.1 Pivotal role of CRH in modulating placental, maternal and fetal hormonal secretions at labor.

Fetal DHEAs are then subjected to 16 hydroxylation in the fetal liver.

The placenta is unable to synthesize estrogens *de novo*. Within the placenta, DHEAs of both maternal and fetal origin and 16 hydroxylated DHEAs of fetal origin can be desulphated by sulfatase. In the placenta, these androgens are then transformed by 3 beta hydroxysteroid dehydrogenase type 1 into androstenedione, and aromatase and 17 beta hydroxysteroid dehydrogenase convert the androstenedione into the estrogens of pregnancy. Androstenedione-derived DHEA is converted by aromatase into estrone, which is converted by 17 beta hydroxysteroid dehydrogenase into estradiol, while 16 hydroxylated DHEA is converted by the enzymes into estriol, and 16 hydroxy DHEA is converted by 15 hydroxylase in the fetal liver into estetrol.

2.5 The Presence of Four Different Estrogens: Why Is This Necessary?

Each of the four different estrogens found in maternal plasma during pregnancy (estradiol, estriol, estrone, and estetrol) are active at estrogen receptors. Each of the four estrogens of pregnancy are active at estrogen receptor alpha (ERα) receptors, which is the primary nuclear receptor expressed in the myometrium and other reproductive tissues. Estradiol is the most potent of the estrogens at the ERα. In terms of concentrations, estradiol produced from maternal adrenal DHEAs is the dominant estrogen at the beginning of pregnancy, but once formation of the fetal adrenal is complete all four estrogens increase in concentration across pregnancy through delivery (17). These data pose the question of the need for so many different estrogens. While all four estrogens are potent at the ERα receptor in vitro when tested alone, the results are different when studied together. Liganded nuclear estrogen receptors dimerize, translocate to the nucleus, and act as transcription factors recruiting co-activators to promoters with the estrogen response element sequences. However, Melamed et al. have shown that heterodimers formed when estradiol and estriol are both present block transactivation of estrogen responsive genes (18). So it seems the ratio of estrogens may be critical. Estriol is derived from fetal adrenal DHEAs precursors under stimulation from placental CRH, while estriol is predominantly derived from DHEAs of

maternal adrenal origin. As pregnancy advances estradiol is initially dominant, then estradiol and estriol are equimolar, and at the end of pregnancy, under the regulation of the exponentially increasing CRH, estriol becomes dominant. This pattern of altering estrogen ratios means that early in pregnancy there is an estrogenic environment which declines in mid-pregnancy only to return in late pregnancy. The CRH driven dominance of estriol in late pregnancy may be the signal for the onset of labor in humans. Intriguingly, estrogens can also act via a G protein coupled membrane receptor called GPR30. At the GPR30 receptor estradiol is an agonist while estriol is an antagonist (19), the physiological consequences of this antagonism is as yet unknown.

2.6 Regulation of Peptide Hormone Production

The syncytiotrophoblast layer of the placenta secretes a wide range of peptide hormones. These peptides mirror those produced by the pituitary and hypothalamus. In some cases the placental peptide is identical to the hypothalamic-pituitary hormone – as in the case of CRH – and in others is closely related and is a consequence of gene duplication, as in placental variant growth hormone. The transcription and translation of the placental hormones is stimulated primarily through the cAMP pathway, with activation of protein kinase A and phosphorylation of the transcription factor CREB. A number of the placental hormones interact with their cognate receptors on the surface of the syncytiotrophoblast. These receptors, such as the LHCG receptor and the CRH receptor R1, are G protein coupled receptors that activate adenylase cyclase, leading to increases in cAMP and further stimulation of the transcription and translation of the peptide hormone. This process generates a feedforward system, and in the case of CRH is linked to an exponential increase in CRH production throughout pregnancy (20). In the case of hCG, there is a rapid increase in release from the syncytiotrophoblast, but this is likely inhibited by rising levels of progesterone at the end of the first trimester (21). Other placental hormones whose transcription is increased by cAMP include GnRH, inhibins, calcitonin, human placental lactogen, and placental variant growth hormone.

2.7 Placental Release of Peptide Hormones

In most peptide secreting glands, the hormone is packaged into secretory vesicles and stored under the plasma membrane in preparation for secretion in response to stimuli. In contrast, in the placenta peptide hormones are channeled into the constitutive release pathway and are released as they are synthesized (22). Thus, in the placenta regulation of peptide secretion occurs at the transcriptional level.

2.8 Maternal Targets for Placental Signals

2.8.1 The Endometrium

The mother is the predominant target for the peptide and steroid hormones released from the placenta. A prime target is the endometrium. At the endometrium, placental hCG and progesterone (derived initially from the maternal ovary and later from the placenta) combine to promote decidualization of the uterine lining tissue (23). The decidualization facilitates implantation and the initial proliferation of endometrial glands to allow nutrient supply to the early trophoblast and embryo through the process of histiotrophic nutrition (24).

2.8.2 The Myometrium

Early in pregnancy the myometrium is targeted by trophectoderm derived human chorionic gonadotrophin and ovarian progesterone (stimulated by the hCG) to promote relaxation that promotes implantation (25). As pregnancy progresses placenta estrogen and progesterone programs the myometrium to grow through myometrial cell hyperplasia and hypertrophy that allows the uterus to accommodate the growing fetus. During the first and especially the second and third trimesters, peptide hormones such as CRH and hCG promote myometrial relaxation through their cognate receptors linked via g protein coupled receptors to adenylate cyclase. The activated adenylate cyclase promotes synthesis of cAMP that activates protein kinase A which phosphorylates CREB. Phosphorylated CREB maintains the transcriptome of the myometrium in a pro-pregnancy quiescent state (26). Late in pregnancy a rising ratio of estriol to estradiol activates estrogen receptors which are pro-contractile (27). CRH likely also targets fetal membranes (28) to promote prostaglandin synthesis which may drive myometrial inflammatory pathways that increase progesterone receptor A expression. Progesterone receptor A blocks the myometrial relaxation created by progesterone working through progesterone receptor B (29). The prostaglandins likely also create the inflammatory phenotype associated with NFkB mediated expression of 20 alpha dehydroxylase that metabolizes progesterone to inactive metabolites, helping to generate a pro-contractile phenotype (30). These late pregnancy endocrine changes promote the onset of human labor.

2.8.3 Maternal Metabolism

To facilitate fetal growth the placenta promotes mobilization of maternal metabolic resources and facilitates their transport across the placenta to the fetus. The placental peptide and steroid hormones target different aspects of maternal metabolism to promote mobilization of cholesterol, free fatty acids, glucose, and amino acids (31).

During the second and third trimesters of pregnancy, maternal plasma LDL cholesterol levels double. The rise in maternal cholesterol is predominately driven by increasing estrogen (32) and perhaps by progesterone; there is no evidence for an impact of CRH, placental variant GH, or placental lactogen on maternal cholesterol. This rise in maternal plasma cholesterol is key to providing the placenta with the substrate for de novo placental synthesis of progesterone and also for transport of cholesterol to the fetus for anabolic processes and the synthesis of fetal androgens that are substrates for placental estrogen synthesis.

To promote the supply of glucose to the fetus, placental hormones antagonize the action of maternal insulin. Key anti-insulin hormones of pregnancy include placental variant GH, placental lactogen, and CRH (16). CRH likely exerts its anti-insulin actions by stimulating maternal pituitary ACTH production which drives maternal adrenal cortisol synthesis. It is maternal cortisol that has potent anti-insulin effects, antagonizing the action of insulin at a post-receptor level. Placental variant GH also stimulates IGF1 levels during pregnancy, which also have post-receptor anti-insulin activity. The effects of placental variant GH and human placental lactogen additionally promote maternal lipolysis leading to increased maternal plasma free fatty acid concentrations which also have an anti-insulin effect.

Cortisol likely plays a major role in the catabolism of maternal tissues to mobilize amino acids for transport to the fetus, as similar rises in circulating amino acids and amino acid excretion are reported in Cushings disease (33).

2.8.4 Maternal Brain

Evidence in humans is limited, but in rodents clear evidence exists for placental hormone effects on maternal behavior (34). In the rat, prolactin and estradiol appear to play key roles (35). Unfortunately, there is little evidence available in the human regarding placental hormone effects on maternal behaviors, although effects on appetite during pregnancy, maternal anxiety, and behavior post-partum are likely. Post-natal

depression and psychosis are likely hormonally mediated (36).

2.8.5 Targeting the Breast

Estrogen and progesterone promote growth and maturation of the breast during pregnancy. Prolactin plays a key role in the development of lactational competency (37).

2.9 Summary

The placenta is a critical agent of the fetus that modifies the maternal environment to allow implantation, promote nutrient transfer from the mother to the fetus, orchestrate the onset of labor, promote breast development to allow breast feeding, and likely to modify maternal behavior to enhance the likelihood of infant survival. The consequences of the placental maturational program stay with the child long after the decomposition of the placenta.

References

1. Smith R, Paul JW, and Tolosa JM. Sharpey-Schafer Lecture 2019: From retroviruses to human birth. *Exp Physiol.* 2020, 105(4):555–561.

2. Sultana Z, Maiti K, Aitken J, et al. Oxidative stress, placental ageing-related pathologies and adverse pregnancy outcomes. *Am J Reprod Immunol.* 2017, 77(5).

3. Jin J, and Menon R. Placental exosomes: A proxy to understand pregnancy complications. *Am J Reprod Immunol.* 2018, 79(5):e12788.

4. Zeng Y, and Chen T. DNA methylation reprogramming during mammalian development. *Genes (Basel).* 2019, 10(4).

5. Tolosa JM, Schjenken JE, Clifton VL, et al. The endogenous retroviral envelope protein syncytin-1 inhibits LPS/PHA-stimulated cytokine responses in human blood and is sorted into placental exosomes. *Placenta.* 2012, 33 (11):933–941.

6. Cheng YH, and Handwerger S. A placenta-specific enhancer of the human syncytin gene. *Biol Reprod.* 2005, 73(3):500–509.

7. Makrigiannakis A, Vrekoussis T, Zoumakis E, et al. The role of HCG in implantation: A mini-review of molecular and clinical evidence. *Int J Mol Sci.* 2017, 18(6).

8. Fisher JJ, Bartho LA, Perkins AV, et al. Placental mitochondria and reactive oxygen species in the physiology and pathophysiology of pregnancy. *Clin Exp Pharmacol Physiol.* 2020, 47(1):176–184.

9. Gomez-Concha C, Flores-Herrera O, Olvera-Sanchez S, et al. Progesterone synthesis by human placental mitochondria is sensitive to PKA inhibition by H89. *Int. J. Biochem. Cell Biol.* 2011, 43(9):1402–1411.

10. Martinez F, Olvera-Sanchez S, Esparza-Perusquia M, et al. Multiple functions of syncytiotrophoblast

mitochondria. *Steroids.* 2015, 103:11–22.

11. Berkane N, Liere P, Oudinet JP, et al. From pregnancy to preeclampsia: A key role for estrogens. *Endocr Rev.* 2017, 38 (2):123–144.

12. Smith R, Mesiano S, Chan EC, et al. Corticotropin-releasing hormone directly and preferentially stimulates dehydroepiandrosterone sulfate secretion by human fetal adrenal cortical cells. *J Clin Endocrinol Metab.* 1998, 83 (8):2916–2920.

13. Nagashima K, Yagi H, Yunoki H, et al. Cord blood levels of corticotropin-releasing factor. *Biol Neonate.* 1987, 51(1):1–4.

14. Clark D, Thody AJ, Shuster S, et al. Immunoreactive alpha-MSH in human plasma in pregnancy. *Nature.* 1978, 273 (5658):163–164.

15. Sasaki A, Shinkawa O, and Yoshinaga K. Placental corticotropin-releasing hormone may be a stimulator of maternal pituitary adrenocorticotropic hormone

secretion in humans. *J Clin Invest.* 1989;84(6), 1997–2001.

16. Steine IM, LeWinn KZ, Lisha N, et al. Maternal exposure to childhood traumatic events, but not multi-domain psychosocial stressors, predict placental corticotrophin releasing hormone across pregnancy. *Soc Sci Med.* 2020, 266:113461.

17. Smith R, Smith JI, Shen X, et al. Patterns of plasma corticotropin-releasing hormone, progesterone, estradiol, and estriol change and the onset of human labor. *J Clin Endocrinol Metab.* 2009, 94(6):2066–2074.

18. Melamed M, Castano E, Notides AC, et al. Molecular and kinetic basis for the mixed agonist/antagonist activity of estriol. *Mol Endocrinol.* 1997, 11(12):1868–1878.

19. Lappano R, Rosano C, De Marco P, et al. Estriol acts as a GPR30 antagonist in estrogen receptor-negative breast cancer cells. *Mol Cell Endocrinol.* 2010, 320(1-2):162–170.

20. King BR, Smith R, and Nicholson RC. Novel glucocorticoid and cAMP interactions on the CRH gene promoter. *Mol Cell Endocrinol.* 2002, 194(1–2), 19–28.

21. Matsuo H, Maruo T, Hoshina M, et al. [Selective inhibition of synthesis and secretion of hCG by progesterone and its correlation with hCG (alpha, beta) mRNA levels]. *Nihon Naibunpi Gakkai Zasshi.* 1985, 61(9):882–892.

22. Morrish DW, Marusyk H, and Siy O. Demonstration of specific secretory granules for human chorionic gonadotropin in placenta. *J Histochem Cytochem.* 1987, 35 (1):93–101.

23. Gellersen B, Brosens IA, and Brosens JJ. Decidualization of the human endometrium: mechanisms, functions, and clinical perspectives. *Semin Reprod Med.* 2007, 25 (6):445–453.

24. Burton GJ, Jauniaux E, and Charnock-Jones DS. Human early placental development: potential roles of the endometrial glands. *Placenta.* 2007, 28 Suppl A:S64–9.

25. Doheny HC, Houlihan DD, Ravikumar N, et al. Human chorionic gonadotrophin relaxation of human pregnant myometrium and activation of the BKCa channel. *J Clin Endocrinol Metab.* 2003, 88 (9):4310–4315.

26. Karolczak-Bayatti M, Loughney AD, Robson SC, et al. Epigenetic modulation of the protein kinase A RIIalpha (PRKAR2A) gene by histone deacetylases 1 and 2 in human smooth muscle cells. *J Cell Mol Med.* 2011, 15(1):94–108.

27. Anamthathmakula P, Kyathanahalli C, Ingles J, et al. Estrogen receptor alpha isoform ERdelta7 in myometrium modulates uterine quiescence during pregnancy. *EBioMedicine.* 2019, 39:520–530.

28. Jones SA, and Challis JR. Effects of corticotropin-releasing hormone and adrenocorticotropin on prostaglandin output by human placenta and fetal membranes. *Gynecol Obstet Invest.* 1990, 29(3):165–168.

29. Mesiano S, Chan EC, Fitter JT, et al. Progesterone withdrawal and estrogen activation in human parturition are coordinated by progesterone receptor A expression in the myometrium. *J Clin Endocrinol Metab.* 2002, 87(6):2924–2930.

30. Nadeem L, Balendran R, Dorogin A, et al. Pro-inflammatory signals induce 20alpha-HSD expression in myometrial cells: A key mechanism for local progesterone withdrawal. *J Cell Mol Med.* 2021.

31. Brizzi P, Tonolo G, Esposito F, et al. Lipoprotein metabolism during normal pregnancy. *Am J Obstet Gynecol.* 1999, 181 (2):430–434.

32. Angelin B, Olivecrona H, Reihner E, et al. Hepatic cholesterol metabolism in estrogen-treated men. *Gastroenterology.* 1992, 103 (5):1657–1663.

33. Faggiano A, Pivonello R, Melis D, et al. Evaluation of circulating levels and renal clearance of natural amino acids in patients with Cushing's disease. *J Endocrinol Invest.* 2002, 25 (2):142–151.

34. Bridges RS, Robertson MC, Shiu RP, et al. Endocrine communication between conceptus and mother: placental lactogen stimulation of maternal behavior. *Neuroendocrinology.* 1996, 64 (1):57–64.

35. Bridges RS. Neuroendocrine regulation of maternal behavior. *Front Neuroendocrinol.* 2015, 36:178–196.

36. Schiller CE, Meltzer-Brody S, and Rubinow DR. The role of reproductive hormones in postpartum depression. *CNS Spectr.* 2015, 20(1):48–59.

37. Macias H, and Hinck L. Mammary gland development. *Wiley Interdiscip Rev Dev Biol.* 2012, 1(4):533–557.

Chapter

3

The Role of Oxytocin in Pregnancy

Kiichiro Furuya and Richard Ivell

3.1 Introduction

3.1.1 Oxytocin Biosynthesis

Oxytocin is a small peptide hormone comprising nine amino acids constrained by a cystine sulphydryl bridge between amino acids 1 and 7 (Figure 3.1). The last amino acid is amidated, which in part protects the molecule from unspecific rapid degradation in the blood. Oxytocin is the product of a small gene on human chromosome 20p12.2, which encodes a larger precursor polyprotein also including an oxytocin carrier protein called neurophysin I. Although oxytocin is largely associated with strictly mammalian physiologies, such as viviparity and birth of live young – as well as lactation – evolutionarily it is a very ancient hormone with relatives controlling gamete extrusion even in worms. Like the structurally related hormone vasopressin, the peptide responsible for most of its systemic endocrine actions is made by only a few thousand specialized cells within the hypothalamus of the brain. These magnocellular neurones are localized to two symmetrical regions (called the paraventricular [PVN] and supraoptic [SON] nuclei) close to the third ventricle of the brain. Both the oxytocinergic as well as the vasopressinergic neurones have long axons which leave the base of the brain, passing through the pituitary stalk, to terminate in the well vascularized posterior lobe of the pituitary gland [1].

When the oxytocin gene is expressed, the resulting mRNA is attached to the rough endoplasmic reticulum (ER) and the translated precursor protein transferred to the ER lumen and hence to the Golgi apparatus and the regulated secretory pathway, where it is processed to cleave out the active peptide hormone which, together with its carrier protein neurophysin I, is packaged into dense-core secretory granules. Importantly, most of these secretory granules are then transported

Figure 3.1 Scheme to show the synthesis and transport of oxytocin (OT) within the magnocellular neurones of the hypothalamus. The oxytocin gene is transcribed to mRNA within the cell bodies on the PVN and SON and translated to generate the precursor protein, which comprises a signal peptide, oxytocin and its carrier neurophysin I (Np I). Processing of the precursor occurs within the secretory granules during their transport down the axons to the nerve endings in the posterior pituitary, from which oxytocin is released into the bloodstream upon electrical stimulation.

down the nerve axons via the pituitary stalk to the posterior pituitary, where they are stored until specifically released by a nerve impulse from the cell bodies in the hypothalamus. Not all oxytocin is released from the posterior pituitary; some is also released from the cell bodies and dendrites within the hypothalamus itself. However, this hormone secretion is largely achieved by the release of intracellular Ca^{2+} stores within the magnocellular neurones, and not by nerve impulses, indicating that a differential regulation of oxytocin secretion is possible. In this way, central effects of oxytocin – for example on behavior or satiety – may be differently regulated from the release of endocrine oxytocin into the bloodstream in association with labor and breast-feeding [2].

3.1.2 Pulsatile Secretion of Oxytocin

The delivery of a hormone in a pulsatile fashion is a very effective way of encoding biological information, particularly for hormones acting at a long distance from their source. It is the physiological equivalent of digitally encoding music or images and allows for much more faithful informational flow, with less disruptive "noise." It has the added advantage that much less hormone is required (see later), which for oxytocin, being produced by only a few thousand cells in the brain, is an important factor. Peptide-containing granules are transported to the nerve terminals in the posterior pituitary where they are stored and only released upon receipt of a nerve impulse from the cell bodies. Thus, the regulated train of nerve impulses can precisely control the dosage of hormone entering the bloodstream. Together with the relatively short half-life of oxytocin in the blood (2–20 minutes, depending on physiology; the expression of the enzyme oxytocinase during pregnancy effectively shortens oxytocin half-life) this ensures a faithful digitally encoded signal. Although other pulsatile hormone systems depend for informational accuracy upon the rate of receptor desensitization, this may be less important for the oxytocin system, where being able to optimize (minimize) the amount of hormone released when this is in limited supply may be more significant.

3.1.3 Decoding at the Oxytocin Receptor

The receptor for oxytocin is a class I 7-transmembrane domain G-protein-coupled receptor (GPCR) with only a short N-terminal extracellular domain [1]. It is encoded by a relatively small gene, with only three exons, on human chromosome 3p25. The small peptide with its relatively rigid three-dimensional structure interacts with both the receptor N-terminus as well as the extracellular loops of the transmembrane domains to elicit signal transduction on the cytoplasmic side. This involves recruitment of an inhibitory G protein and activation of PI3-kinase

with ensuing release of Ca^{2+} from intracellular stores, and possibly also promotion of Ca^{2+} entry into the cells through so-called L-channels [2]. Importantly, the oxytocin receptor appears to desensitize only slowly in myometrial cells naturally expressing the receptor, suggesting that β-arrestin associated receptor internalization may not play a big role in oxytocin receptor function. More relevant perhaps is that the expression and function of the oxytocin receptor appears to be amplified by a range of different mechanisms at times and in tissues when it is most needed. Receptor gene expression increases dramatically at term of pregnancy (see below), but also it appears to evoke further expression of Ca^{2+}-releasing uterotonic prostaglandins in the same tissues. Moreover, it is reported to increase tight junction formation between cells, thereby concerting uterotonic action, as well as promoting positive feedback loops, such as the Ferguson reflex (see below) which leads to more oxytocin release from the posterior pituitary.

A further important regulatory aspect involves uterine quiescence. It is experimentally established that increasing cAMP in myometrial cells can prevent spontaneous or oxytocin-induced contraction. In some species (rodents, pigs) this may be achieved by the peptide hormone relaxin, though this appears not to be the case for the human. Progesterone may also promote signalling pathways which discourage contraction. However, modulating membrane stiffness can achieve a similar effect. The oxytocin receptor is preferentially localized in cell membranes to highly mobile lipid rafts. By increasing the amount of cholesterol in the membranes (as may occur in obese women), or even of relatively inactive steroids such as 17OH-progesterone, the ability of the oxytocin receptor to respond to the hormone is greatly diminished, thereby also inducing quiescence.

3.2 Oxytocin and Reproductive Physiology

Oxytocin is involved in several pregnancy-related and perinatal events including parturition and breastfeeding, but also the maintenance of pregnancy. However, other roles of oxytocin in reproductive physiology – including implantation, gamete function and mating, reproductive behavior, and early embryogenesis – have also been demonstrated.

3.2.1 Conception and the Initiation of Pregnancy

Although traditionally oxytocin has been recognized as a "labor-related hormone," involved both in uterine contractions at term as well as in lactation, recent research has revealed that oxytocin also has important roles in the initiation of pregnancy, including reproductive behavior and copulation, as well as in fertility. In the human, circulating oxytocin levels increase during intercourse in both males and females. This increasing oxytocin appears to contribute to penile erection and ejaculation, as well as to orgasm [3,4]. However, it is important to note that there may be species-specific differences. For example, reproductive behavior in rodents appears to be less affected by a lack of oxytocin. *In vivo* studies using oxytocin-knockout (OT-KO) mice indicate that their reproductive behavior is still appropriate, and that they are able to become pregnant normally [5].

From other *in vivo* research, rodents appear not always to need oxytocin for copulation, even though peripheral oxytocin or oxytocin in cerebrospinal fluid (CSF) still appears to facilitate reproductive behaviour. In the female, several studies have looked at the relationship between circulating oxytocin profiles and female reproductive behavior, sexual arousal, and fertility. Measuring the oxytocin profile across the human menstrual cycle showed cyclic changes with lowest oxytocin levels in the luteal phase [6]. Unlike in rodents, in the human oxytocin appears to have an essential role during male penile erection and ejaculation as well as in female orgasm in association with copulation and appropriate reproductive behavior [7]. Sexual arousal-induced serum oxytocin levels show marked peaks at the moment of orgasm. However, the physiological relationship between sexual arousal and increasing serum oxytocin level is unclear as to whether the hormone is in any way causative or merely a response to sexual arousal or natural physiological events [8]. Oxytocin receptor expression in multiple male and female reproductive organs strongly suggests that oxytocin may indeed have an important role in both intercourse and orgasm, such as ejaculation and uterine peristalsis – the essential components of reproductive physiology for receiving and transporting sperm from male ejaculation.

In a monkey model, both oxytocin and the oxytocin receptor are also expressed exclusively within preovulatory follicles and form part of a paracrine system promoting follicle maturation and luteinisation consequent to the LH surge [9]. Following successful fertilization, oxytocin additionally contributes to the development of the early embryo. Furuya and colleagues revealed oxytocin receptor expression on the cumulus cells surrounding human oocytes, suggesting a role for oxytocin also in early embryogenesis [10], with expression from the oocyte through to the blastocyst stage. Oxytocin levels increase by the 4-cell stage, and rapidly fall from the 8-cell to the blastocyst stage.

3.2.2 Maintenance of Pregnancy

Maintaining "uterine quiescence" after fertilization and implantation is particularly important for the successful progress of pregnancy to term gestation and normal labor. If the uterus acquires inappropriate contractility and oxytocin-responsiveness, both the fetus and the mother face the risk of fetal prematurity and/or, in the event of delayed labor and post-term gestation, serious utero-placental conditions including intrauterine fetal death. Thus, the regulation of oxytocin-responsiveness, such as appropriate oxytocin receptor expression in the myometrium, is essential for feto-maternal safety and a healthy outcome.

Although oxytocin has been recognized as a main factor in the onset of labor, the serum concentration of oxytocin during natural parturition does not increase further in women following the second stage of labor [11]. In contrast, Wathes and colleagues revealed that oxytocin receptor expression sharply increases just before the onset of labor [12]. Similarly, Kimura and colleagues showed a marked increase in the mRNA encoding the oxytocin receptor in term myometrium compared to pre-term [13]. Fuchs and colleagues also investigated the comparison of oxytocin receptor expression at the protein level between early and term pregnancy and showed that expression in term myometrium increases at least twelve-fold compared with that in early pregnancy. These findings indicate that it is the upregulation of oxytocin receptor expression which is regulating the timing of labor [14,15] and that this is occurring largely at the transcriptional level [13].

An additional factor may be the secretion of fetal oxytocin. The difference in serum oxytocin levels between the fetal pituitary gland and the umbilical artery suggests that oxytocin may also be produced and released from the fetus, possibly reaching the placenta.

The maintenance of myometrial quiescence throughout pregnancy until the initiation of labor may involve several factors influencing myometrial signalling or cell membrane properties. For example, it is known that progesterone is able to attenuate the myometrial intracellular response. Clinically, progesterone agents are administered intramuscularly or vaginally to prevent a threatened preterm delivery and suppress uterine contraction. In rodents, luteolysis and progesterone withdrawal in the late gestational period appear to be involved in the increasing sensitivity towards uterine contraction and labor. However, in the human, progesterone withdrawal does not occur and the source of most progesterone, the placenta, is ejected only after delivery. The human myometrium expresses two protein subtypes of the progesterone receptor (PR), PRA and PRB. Though they are both the products of the same gene, the former acts as a transcriptional inhibitor, whereas the latter stimulates the transcription of progesterone-responsive genes. Several studies have shown that in the myometrium PRA is more highly expressed just after the onset of labor [16]. This induction of the PRA protein would have the same effect as progesterone withdrawal. In a human myometrium sample obtained from caesarean section without labor, the expression of the PRA/PRB mRNA ratio was clearly correlated to the expression of oxytocin receptor mRNA [17]. These findings suggest that there is a kind of "functional" progesterone withdrawal in the human myometrium which helps to regulate the oxytocin receptor and other proteins involved in uterine activation.

3.2.3 Parturition

One of the best-known roles of oxytocin is to contribute to uterine contraction during parturition. In particular, the expression of the oxytocin receptor in the myometrium can increase by up to 100-fold at term and reaches a peak at the beginning of labor. This increase in oxytocin receptor expression appears to parallel the increased sensitivity of the myometrium in respect of oxytocin. However,

several studies have indicated that oxytocin alone may not always be essential for the initiation of labor and parturition. Nishimori and colleagues [5] used OT-KO mice to study the effects of oxytocin on labor and pregnancy and were able to show that inactivation of the oxytocin gene did not lead to any deficit in fertility, pregnancy, initiation of labor, or parturition. The results confirmed that, irrespective of the presence or not of oxytocin, luteolysis and the release of prostaglandin F2-alpha (PGF2α) at the end of pregnancy was a key factor in the initiation of labor, at least in rodents [5]. Moreover, the action of oxytocin on the uterus depends on the location of the oxytocin receptors in the myometrium, with their spatial expression changing across gestation. Only the oxytocin receptors, which are expressed mainly in the corpus and fundus of the uterus, appear to be important in the expulsion of the fetus.

As mentioned earlier, oxytocin is secreted from the posterior pituitary in a notably pulsatile fashion; this makes single measurements of the hormone problematic. Hence, simple assessment of circulating oxytocin may not always seem compatible with the progression of labor and could explain the variations seen simply as a result of sampling methodology (18). Figure 3.2 illustrates continuous blood sampling for OT measurement over two days at pre-term and term in the cow and highlights the extreme pulsatility in this period. Furthermore, one needs to consider the positive feedback circumstances which drive the expulsion of the fetus: Not only are oxytocin pulses increasing in frequency, and receptors are progressively more up-regulated, but there is concomitant expression of uterotonic PGF2α, as well as the Ferguson reflex, whereby distension of uterine smooth muscle cells feeds back neurally to the hypothalamus to increase the oxytocin output.

3.2.4 Postpartum

Oxytocin contributes not only to labor and parturition, but also subsequently to the expulsion of the placenta and the attenuation of postpartum hemorrhage in the third stage of labor by persistent uterine contraction. Breast-feeding at this time assists uterine involution by encouraging further oxytocin release. The pattern of release in this phase remains pulsatile in the early postpartum period, but the oxytocin secretion profile

Figure 3.2 Pattern of pulsatile oxytocin measured at 15 minute intervals within the ovarian vein of a cow before and during labor. Annotation indicates the behavior of the cow as well as the different stages of delivery of the calf and placenta (reproduced from [20] with permission).

gradually changes into a so-called long-lasting type with continued breastfeeding [20]. The mechanisms involved in the changing pattern of uterine contraction from pulsatile during labor to continuous during uterine involution remain unclear. From a clinical perspective it is known that the uterus reduces in size by about 1–2 cm per day upon manual examination, finally recovering its normal size after about one month. Comparing the intervals of uterine involution between primiparous and multiparous women over 60 days showed that while the period of uterine involution was not significantly different between the two groups, the minimum size of the uterus achieved by multiparous women was greater than for primipara.

3.2.5 Breastfeeding

Studies using OT-KO mice have shown that oxytocin is essential for breastfeeding and lactation, but not for fetal expulsion [5]. In these mice,

parturition appeared normal, but the OT-KO mice failed to breastfeed and also neglected infant care, resulting in offspring death. Oxytocin is a key component of the milk-ejection reflex. Infant suckling at the nipple activates afferent neurons which in turn stimulate oxytocin release from the posterior pituitary into the peripheral blood. This oxytocin interacts with oxytocin receptors on the smooth muscle cells of the mammary alveolar wall leading to milk letdown [21].

Profiles of serum oxytocin concentration during breastfeeding have been investigated by meta-analysis. The oxytocin secretion is pulsatile and increases with the period of breastfeeding [22–24]. After about 10 minutes, the peaks of oxytocin merge together, resulting in a prolonged oxytocin plateau. Oxytocin levels return to baseline approximately 20 minutes after cessation of breastfeeding. Furthermore, the skin contact between mother and child additionally increased oxytocin levels. In summary, the number of oxytocin pulses are associated with milk yield, breastfeeding duration, and maternal stress in the postpartum period [25,26]. Moreover, it should be recalled that the oxytocin released on breastfeeding also promotes postpartum uterine contraction and reconstruction [22].

There is currently no evidence to suggest that oxytocin administration is helpful for disorders of breastfeeding, such as breast engorgement, though it has been speculated that oxytocin infusion during labor may be associated with some postpartum problems with breastfeeding and maternal response [27].

3.2.6 Infant Care, Parenting (Bonding), and Motherhood

It is well known that it is important to encourage breastfeeding and mother-infant interaction as soon as possible in the postpartum period. While an understanding of parenting and motherhood is part of this equation, it appears that persistent expression of oxytocin from the hypothalamus and posterior pituitary gland is also a key aspect in the establishment of mother-infant bonding. Recent obstetrical research has revealed that oxytocin has an essential role in regard to maternal behavior including infant care, parenting, and bonding [5,26,28]. By impacting on increasing prolactin (PRL), decreasing stress-related hormones, facilitating social interaction, and attenuating anxiety, the central release of oxytocin during breast-feeding facilitates the psychological adaptation of the mother against postpartum psychophysical stress [29]. Other animal studies also indicate that oxytocin promotes the initiation of motherhood and maternal behavior. OT-KO mice have shown that the genetic lack of oxytocin disrupts maternal behavior and virgin female mice given exogenous oxytocin start showing maternal behavior, such as nest-building and infant care. In contrast, postpartum mice given an oxytocin receptor antagonist show decreased maternal behavior and neglect their offspring. Similarly, in vivo studies in macaques show that administration of oxytocin or an oxytocin receptor antagonist can influence maternal behavior [30]. Several animal studies have shown that abnormal peripheral oxytocin levels may be associated with a deficiency in maternal behavior [31]. Together, such studies confirm that oxytocin is a key factor for ensuring an adequate maternal response in the perinatal period. However, further research is needed to elaborate the precise mechanisms involved in how oxytocin is able to promote the establishment of motherhood.

3.3 Clinical Application of Oxytocin

3.3.1 Oxytocin Administration for the Induction of Labor

Oxytocin preparations have been routinely used for many decades for the induction and augmentation of labor as an essential medication in obstetrical practice. The sensitivity of the myometrium towards oxytocin varies depending on parity, gestational period, degree of uterine cervical ripening (Bishop scoring), and spontaneous contractility before oxytocin administration. The effect of giving oxytocin usually emerges within 3 to 5 minutes, finally reaching constant contractility 40 minutes after administration. Oxytocin administration should be discontinued immediately when uterine tachysystole (more than 5 contractions per 10 minutes on cardiotocography) is found. As the half-life of oxytocin at this time is approximately 3 to 5 minutes, excessive uterine contractility due to oxytocin will disappear quickly and tachysystole should be improved. The mode of oxytocin administration includes low-dose or high-dose infusion [32], as well as "rest and break" administration [33]. With regard

to efficacy and safety, internationally the low-dose continuous infusion regimen is generally approved. Whilst pulsatile oxytocin administration has been developed and implemented [34], it is rarely used because of the special equipment required and there appears to be little clinical benefit with respect to labor induction. For the formulation of the oxytocin solution, 5 units (1IU = ~1.68 µg pure peptide) of oxytocin should be added in 500 mL of saline or 5 percent glucose solution (final concentration 10 mU/mL). Traditionally, oxytocin intravenous infusion should begin at 1–2 mU/min, increasing by a further 1–2 mU/min by 30 minutes. The maximum oxytocin dose has been established by national clinical guidelines. Effective uterine contraction that is essential for appropriate labor progression is defined as 150–350 Montevideo Units (MU: accumulation of intrauterine pressure amplitude directly measured by intrauterine pressure catheter over a 10-minute period by cardiotocography). Prior to rupture of membranes (ROM) the obstetrician should recognize appropriate contraction extra-abdominally only by the frequency of contraction, but after ROM, MU can be used to monitor contractions. MU is particularly warranted to assess uterine contraction together with iatrogenic ROM for obese pregnant women. In order to avoid the risk of fetal hypoxia, oxytocin infusion should be discontinued immediately when contractions exceed 5 over a 10 minute period and/or they are accompanied by abnormal fetal heart rate. The medical indications for labor induction using oxytocin are: (1) post-term pregnancy, (2) pre-labor rupture of membrane, (3) stillbirth, (4) hypertensive disorders of pregnancy (HDP), (5) gestational diabetes (GDM), (6) fetal growth restriction (FGR), (7) oligo/polyhydramnios, (8) infection in utero (i.e. endometritis in pregnancy), (9) *abruptio placentae*, and (10) twins [35].

Predictive factors for a successful induction of labor include cervical ripening (Bishop score) and noncervical factors such as: multiparity, low BMI, tall maternal height, low estimated fetal weight (EFW), and no comorbidities associated with placental dysfunction (including preeclampsia). Amniotomy, the iatrogenic rupture of the amniotic membrane, is also effective in inducing/augmenting uterine contraction by increasing myometrial oxytocin sensitivity, thereby shortening total labor time [36]. The "ARRIVAL study," one of the largest to analyze the elective induction of labor among low-risk primiparous women, looked at the appropriate gestational period for initiation of induction. This study indicated that induction of labor at 39 weeks of gestation was safer and resulted in a lower rate of caesarean section [37].

3.3.2 Oxytocin Administration to Facilitate Breastfeeding

Postpartum breastfeeding is not always successful, and some women may need clinical help to facilitate proper breast function. Delayed breastfeeding can lead to mastitis due to the obstruction of milk ejection. Initially, manual and mechanical breast pumping can help to prevent mastitis. However, these procedures may be painful, hence pharmacological approaches are being looked at. The clinical use of intranasal oxytocin spray administration as a galactogogue has been assessed [38], also in the context of possible autism and psychological disorders, as well as for adopting mothers desiring to breastfeed [39]. However, the results showed that such an intranasal oxytocin spray had no significant effect to obviate mastitis [40] or facilitate breastfeeding in postpartum women over the first five postpartum days [38,41]. In contrast, clinical research has indicated that intrapartum oxytocin administration to induce labor may have a negative effect on subsequent breastfeeding. Intravenous oxytocin infusion dose-dependently reduces the endogenous oxytocin levels on day two postpartum, though without affecting the incidence of mastitis, as also when combined with epidural analgesia. Intrapartum oxytocin infusion may also increase serum prolactin [18].

3.3.3 Oxytocin Administration for Prevention of Postpartum Hemorrhage (PPH)

As described above, oxytocin contributes not only to labor but also to assisting placental ejection and preventing PPH. More than 500 mL/min of rapid and massive bleeding can result from exposed spiral arteries opening to the surface of the placental detachment site just after placental expulsion and can lead to hemorrhagic shock. Physiologically, this is normally prevented by

further contraction of the uterine myometrium immediately after parturition. Clinically, the "acceptable" amount of labor-related hemorrhage is defined as less than 500 mL for vaginal delivery and as less than 1000 mL for caesarean section [42]. As insufficient contraction of the myometrium following parturition can result in a fatal hemorrhagic shock, obstetricians may routinely administer intravenous oxytocin immediately postpartum also to facilitate placental delivery. In 2012, the WHO recommended four uterotonic options to alleviate postpartum hemorrhage: oxytocin, misoprostol, ergometrine/methylergometrine, and the fixed-dose combination of oxytocin and ergometrine. Especially, the use of oxytocin (10 IU, IM/IV) is recommended as first choice for the prevention of PPH on all births. Intravenous (IV) administration acts immediately and increases with peak concentration after 30 minutes. Intramuscular (IM) administration acts more slowly but produces a longer lasting clinical effect up to one hour. Prophylactic oxytocin administration in the third stage of labor was shown to reduce PPH >500 mL and the need for additional uterotonic agents [43,44]. A 2018 meta-analysis showed that, although there was no significant difference in the amount of bleeding or the incidence of PPH between IV and IM administration, the IV route significantly reduced the requirement for further uterotonic drugs [45].

3.3.4 Oxytocin Application for Autism, Maternal Depression, and Mental Disorders

Oxytocin receptor expression has been identified in numerous organs of the body besides the uterine myometrium. In particular, oxytocin is not only a hormone of the reproductive system but also has active roles in the brain, where it can influence physiological functions, as well as reproductive and social behavior. Oxytocin has a role in attenuating stress responses, including the HPA axis, inflammatory responses, and anxiety-related behavior [46–49], whereas reduced peripheral oxytocin concentration may contribute to depression, nervous mood, and PTSD (post-traumatic stress disorder) [50].

Several prospective clinical trials have suggested that an intranasal oxytocin spray can improve social skills and relieve mood in patients suffering mental disorders [49], though such studies are not without controversy [51]. Moreover, a mutation in the oxytocin receptor gene has been linked to familial autism spectrum disorder (ASD) and oxytocin administration may improve several symptoms in ASD patients, together implying that oxytocin receptor agonists could theoretically act as novel psychological therapeutics.

Pregnancy and childbirth are also associated with clinical psychological problems; with particularly primiparous mothers reacting to the significant changes in their environment due to the stress of infant care and the hormonal changes in the postpartum period. New parents are faced with economic problems, the difficulty of organizing their work and infant care, socio-economic isolation due to lack of support from family and aged parents, and expectation stereotypes in regard to motherhood.

These all exacerbate the physical, social, and psychological stress on new mothers, often resulting in depression, or "maternity blues", which affect some 20 percent of postpartum women. Oxytocin may act to neutralize stress hormones, such as anti-inflammatory factors, and to attenuate anxiety, fear, and depressive mood as a brain factor influencing oxytocin receptors in the amygdala, hippocampus, and cerebral cortex. The sharply rising oxytocin levels during parturition may therefore play a protective role as part of a maternal adaptive response against stress in the perinatal period and peripheral oxytocin concentration has been linked to maternal depression [31,52,53]. However, this does not mean that exogenously applied oxytocin can alleviate such symptoms [51].

3.4 Oxytocin Receptor Antagonists for Obstetric Use

3.4.1 Oxytocin Receptor Antagonists

Three synthetic oxytocin receptor antagonists are commonly used in the clinic or in research: atosiban, barusiban, and retosiban (Figure 3.3). Atosiban antagonizes both oxytocin receptors and also V1A vasopressin receptors, and is effective on endometrial and myometrial cells with a relatively short half-life of 0.21 (initial) to 1.7 (final) hours. Thereby it also inhibits oxytocin-induced PGF2α release and consequent uterine

contraction, thus also increasing the chance of embryo implantation. Barusiban is an oxytocin receptor-specific antagonist with a half-life of 2.2–2.8 hours, and hence a longer-lasting action, inhibiting myometrial contraction in a similar way to atosiban. In vivo studies in mice show that barusiban dose-dependently supports implantation by inhibiting spontaneous uterine contraction. Retosiban (half-life 1.45 hours) is a novel, high-affinity oxytocin receptor antagonist, developed to prevent preterm birth by inhibiting inappropriate uterine contraction.

3.4.2 Effects of Oxytocin Receptor Antagonists in ART: Prevention of Spontaneous Abortion

Because the oxytocin receptor antagonist atosiban appears to have no toxicity or other impact on sperm or the early embryo, it has recently been applied also to prevent spontaneous miscarriage following in vitro fertilization and embryo transfer (IVF-ET). In one study the antagonist was administered to women who had become pregnant following oocyte donation. The number of spontaneous uterine contractions as well as their amplitude were significantly reduced in the atosiban-treated groups [54]. Similarly, atosiban treatment significantly improved pregnancy and implantation rates after IVF-ET [55].

3.4.3 Effects of Oxytocin Receptor Antagonists on Tocolysis: Prevention of Preterm Labor

Preterm labor is a major cause of prenatal death as well clinically significant neonate morbidity. Both mortality and morbidity of offspring are inversely related to the length of gestation. For potential preterm birth between 23 and 26 weeks, every day that pregnancy can be extended increases the survival rate of the fetus by 3 percent. Since prenatal glucocorticoid administration for 48 hours is important to mature fetal lung function, tocolysis to prevent preterm birth is essential. While previously beta (β)-agonists have been the tocolytic agent of choice to reduce uterine contraction, their use in the USA and EU has been decreasing due to serious side-effects, such as palpitation, pulmonary edema, and leukopenia.

Atosiban
Ki 6.4nM
equipotent at V1a, V1b, V2 receptors

Barusiban (FE-200440)
Ki 0.64 nM
300-fold selectivity vs V1a receptors

Retosiban (GSK-221149A)
Ki 0.65nM
1400-fold selectivity vs Via receptors

Oxytocin
Ki 6.8nM
10-fold selectivity vs V1a receptors

Figure 3.3 The structures of the three oxytocin receptor antagonists: atosiban, barusiban, and retosiban, together with the structure of the natural ligand, oxytocin, also indicating their experimentally determined association constants (Ki) at the human oxytocin receptor.

Atosiban is approved for clinical use in the EU to prevent preterm birth due to its limited side effects [56]. The APOSTEL III-trial compared atosiban and a Ca²⁺-blocker, nifedipine. Similar preventative effects were found in both groups, but adverse effects were significantly increased only in the nifedipine group [57].

For the other oxytocin receptor antagonists, it was demonstrated that barusiban has a dose-dependent tocolytic effect in the macaque but not in women [58]. In a phase II trial of the high-affinity oxytocin receptor antagonist retosiban in women with spontaneous preterm labor, it was shown that the antagonist achieved a greater than one week increase in time to delivery compared with placebo, a significant reduction in the number of preterm deliveries, a nonsignificant increase in uterine quiescence, and a favorable safety profile [59]. These findings prompt a wide application for the prevention of preterm birth.

3.5 Alternative Applications of Oxytocin and Oxytocin Receptor Antagonists: Clinical Potential and Possibilities

3.5.1 Effect of Oxytocin Administration on Male Infertility

For the clinician, oxytocin is generally associated with uterine contraction and breastfeeding, and its applications have traditionally focused on the female and maternal physiology. However, oxytocin also contributes to male reproductive function, including penile erection and ejaculation [60–62]. In the male, oxytocin is also involved in spermiation and sperm transport through effects on the myoid cells of the seminiferous tubules and the ductus deferens, respectively [63], and while circulating oxytocin still derives from the posterior pituitary, it is also produced locally within the testes [64].

A number of studies have looked at a role for oxytocin in the context of male infertility with animal studies suggesting an improvement in spermiation following oxytocin administration. Taken together, the findings suggest that oxytocin may have promising applications in regard to the improvement of sperm transport, penile erection, proliferation of prostate cells, and as a potential marker of prostate cancer [65].

3.5.2 Oxytocin and Pain Relief

Besides its role in the periphery, oxytocin is also secreted within the brain, in particular within the hypothalamus, with oxytocin neurons projecting to numerous brain centers influencing mood, anxiety, and sensation, including the response to pain [1]. Moreover, oxytocin is able to attenuate inflammatory responses including modulation of the HPA-axis and the systemic stress response, as well as anxiety-related behaviors [46,47,49,66]. As a result the oxytocin/oxytocin receptor system has attracted attention as a promising therapeutic

target in the context of analgesia [67,68]. Oxytocin administration stimulated oxytocinergic projections from the paraventricular nucleus of the hypothalamus [62] and it is suggested that subcutaneous injection of oxytocin is able to reduce long-lasting acute pain [68,69]. Mostly intranasal administration of oxytocin has been used since it is believed that this may increase levels of oxytocin within the central nervous system. However, it appears unlikely that the peptide can cross the blood-brain barrier via the nasal mucosa [51], so that it is more likely that such effects are mediated via a peripheral impact of oxytocin. Moreover, the results of human studies are inconsistent [68]. Thus oxytocin may be able to influence pain perception in two ways: by regulation of emotional anxiety in the cortex and amygdala, and by possibly having an analgesic effect at the level of the spinal cord and peripheral nerves [68,69], but more research is needed.

3.5.3 Control of Food Intake

Oxytocin also appears to be involved in the regulation of food intake [62]. Animal and human studies suggest that oxytocin administration has an anorexigenic effect, leading to a reduction in food intake. Also, hypothalamic oxytocin mRNA expression appears to decrease with fasting, and some research indicates that food components may have an important role in regard to the activation of oxytocinergic neurons. There appears to be a close relationship between oxytocin and the gastrointestinal hormone cholecystokinin (CCK) in regard to appetite and fat digestion. CCK facilitates pancreatic and bile secretion, leading to appetite reduction. Oxytocin is considered to be downstream of such anorexigenic factors (including CCK, leptin, and estrogen), with CCK administration *in vivo* leading to activation of oxytocinergic neurons in the hypothalamus via the vagus nerve. Although oxytocin administration has been shown to result in decreased food intake, meta-analysis suggests that this may not be significant. Oxytocin does appear to suppress carbohydrate intake, but not that of fat [70].

3.6 Conclusion

In its traditional area of clinical application, there is no doubt that the oxytocin/oxytocin receptor system is intimately involved in uterine contraction and the promotion of labor. However, oxytocin may not always be essential to trigger the initiation of labor. Furthermore, inducing uterine contraction by oxytocin contributes to the prevention of postpartum hemorrhage with uterine involution. Recent clinical trials have also shown that oxytocin receptor antagonists are able to suppress uterine contraction in the context of IVF-ET, as well as to preempt threatened preterm labor, thereby contributing to improved pregnancy rates in ART and the prevention of preterm birth.

Recent studies have suggested a new role for oxytocin as a neuropeptide. The projection of oxytocinergic neurons within the brain and the central nervous distribution of oxytocin receptors suggest that oxytocin may be able to modulate emotion, anxiety, mood, and possibly pain, besides having roles in maternal behavior and food intake, although how such brain systems can be pharmaceutically addressed remains unclear. For the future, oxytocin receptor agonists and antagonists should be considered important choices in modulating uterine function, the initiation of labor, delivery, and possibly mood and maternal behavior.

References

1. Ivell R, Ludwig M, Tribe RM, et al. Oxytocin. *In* M. K. Skinner (Ed.), *Encyclopedia of Reproduction*. vol. 2, 2018; 597–606. Academic Press: Elsevier.

2. Arrowsmith S, and Wray S. Oxytocin: Its mechanism of action and receptor signalling in the myometrium. *J Neuroendocrinol*. 2014, 26: 356–369.

3. Borrow AP, and Cameron NM. The role of oxytocin in mating and pregnancy. *Horm Behav*. 2012, 61 :266–276.

4. Giraldi A, Marson L, Nappi R, et al. Physiology of female sexual function: Animal models. *J Sexual Med*. 2004, 1: 237–253.

5. Nishimori K, Young LJ, Guo Q et al. Oxytocin is required for nursing but is not essential for parturition or reproductive behavior. *Proc Natl Acad Sci USA*. 1996, 93: 11699–11704.

6. Salonia A, Nappi RE, Pontillo M, et al. Menstrual cycle-related changes in plasma oxytocin are relevant to normal sexual function in healthy women. *Horm Behav*. 2005, 47: 164–169.

7. Veening JG, de Jong TR, Waldinger MD, et al. The role of oxytocin in male and female reproductive behavior. *Eur J Pharmacol*. 2015, 753: 209–228.

8. Carmichael MS, Warburton VL, Dixen J, et al. Relationships among cardiovascular, muscular, and oxytocin responses during human sexual activity. *Arch Sexual Behav*. 1994, 23: 59–79.

9. Einspanier A, Ivell R, and Hodges JK. Oxytocin: A follicular luteinisation factor in the marmoset monkey. *Adv Exp Med Biol*. 1995, 395: 517–522.

10. Furuya K, Mizumoto Y, Makimura N, et al. A novel biological aspect of ovarian oxytocin: Gene expression of oxytocin and oxytocin receptor in cumulus/luteal cells and the effect of oxytocin on embryogenesis in fertilized oocytes. *Adv Exp Med Biol*. 1995, 395: 523–528.

11. Fuchs AR, Romero R, Keefe D, et al. Oxytocin secretion and human parturition: pulse frequency and duration increase during spontaneous labor in women. *Am J Obstet Gynecol*. 1991, 165: 1515–1523.

12. Wathes DC, Borwick SC, Timmons PM, et al. Oxytocin receptor expression in human term and preterm gestational tissues prior to and following the onset of labour. *J Endocrinol*. 1999, 161: 143–151.

13. Kimura T, Takemura M, Nomura S, et al. Expression of oxytocin receptor in human pregnant myometrium.

Endocrinology. 1996, 137: 780–785.

14. Soloff MS, Alexandrova M, and Fernstrom MJ. Oxytocin receptors: Triggers for parturition and lactation? *Science*. 1979, 204: 1313–1315.

15. Fuchs AR, Fuchs F, Husslein P, et al. Oxytocin receptors in the human uterus during pregnancy and parturition. *Am J Obstet Gynecol*. 1984, 150: 734–741.

16. Pieber D, Allport VC, Hills F, et al. Interactions between progesterone receptor isoforms in myometrial cells in human labour. *Mol Hum Reprod* 2001, 7: 875–879.

17. Mesiano S, Chan EC, Fitter JT, et al. Progesterone withdrawal and estrogen activation in human parturition are coordinated by progesterone receptor A expression in the myometrium. *J Clin Endocrinol Metab*. 2002, 87: 2924–2930.

18. McNeilly AS, Robinson IC, Houston MJ, et al. Release of oxytocin and prolactin in response to suckling. *Br Med J*. 1983, 286: 257–259.

19. Uvnäs-Moberg K, Widström AM, Werner S, et al. Oxytocin and prolactin levels in breast-feeding women. Correlation with milk yield and duration of breast-feeding. *Acta Obstet Gynecol Scand*. 1990, 69: 301–306.

20. Fuchs AR, Ivell R, Ganz N, et al. Secretion of oxytocin in pregnant and parturient cows: Corpus luteum may contribute to plasma oxytocin at term. *Biol. Reprod.* 2001, 65: 1135–1141.

21. Christensson K, Nilsson BA, Stock S, et al. Effect of nipple stimulation on uterine activity and on plasma levels of oxytocin in full term, healthy, pregnant women. *Acta Obstet Gynecol Scand.* 1989, 68: 205–210.

22. Jonas W, Johansson LM, Nissen E, et al. Effects of intrapartum oxytocin administration and epidural analgesia on the concentration of plasma oxytocin and prolactin, in response to suckling during the second day postpartum. *Breastfeeding Med.* 2009, 4: 71–82.

23. Nissen E, Uvnäs-Moberg K, Svensson K, et al. Different patterns of oxytocin, prolactin but not cortisol release during breastfeeding in women delivered by caesarean section or by the vaginal route. *Early Hum Devel.* 1996, 45: 103–118.

24. Yokoyama Y, Ueda T, Irahara M, et al. Releases of oxytocin and prolactin during breast massage and suckling in puerperal women. *Eur J Obstet Gynecol Reprod Biol.* 1994, 53: 17–20.

25. Uvnas Moberg K, Ekstrom-Bergstrom A, Buckley S, et al. Maternal plasma levels of oxytocin during breastfeeding – A systematic review. *PLoS ONE* 2020, 15: e0235806.

26. Bell AF, Erickson EN, and Carter CS: Beyond labor: The role of natural and synthetic oxytocin in the transition to motherhood. *J Midwifery Womens Health.* 2014, 59: 35–42.

27. Odent MR. Synthetic oxytocin and breastfeeding: Reasons for testing an hypothesis. *Med Hypotheses.* 2013, 81: 889–891.

28. Williams GL, Gazal OS, Leshin LS, et al. Physiological regulation of maternal behavior in heifers: roles of genital stimulation, intracerebral oxytocin release, and ovarian steroids. *Biol Reprod.* 2001, 65: 295–300.

29. Carter CS, Altemus M, and Chrousos GP. Neuroendocrine and emotional changes in the post-partum period. *Prog Brain Res.* 2001, 133: 241–249.

30. Boccia ML, Goursaud AP, Bachevalier J, et al. Peripherally administered non-peptide oxytocin antagonist, L368,899, accumulates in limbic brain areas: a new pharmacological tool for the study of social motivation in non-human primates. *Horm Behav.* 2007, 52: 344–351.

31. Gordon I, Zagoory-Sharon O, Leckman JF, et al. Oxytocin and the development of parenting in humans. *Biol Psychiatry.* 2010, 68: 377–382.

32. Budden A, Chen LJ, and Henry A. High-dose versus low-dose oxytocin infusion regimens for induction of labour at term. *Cochrane Database Syst Rev.* 2014, Cd009701.

33. Saccone G, Ciardulli A, Baxter JK, et al. Discontinuing oxytocin infusion in the active phase of labor: A systematic review and meta-analysis. *Obstet Gynec.* 2017, 130: 1090–1096.

34. Tribe RM, Crawshaw SE, Seed P, et al. Pulsatile versus continuous administration of oxytocin for induction and augmentation of labor: Two randomized controlled trials. *Am J Obstet Gynecol.* 2012, 206 (230):e231–238.

35. ACOG Practice Bulletin No. 107: Induction of labor. *Obstet Gynecol.* 2009, 114: 386–397.

36. Smyth RM, Markham C, and Dowswell T. Amniotomy for shortening spontaneous labour. *Cochrane Database Syst Rev.* 2013, Cd006167.

37. Grobman WA, Rice MM, Reddy UM, et al. Labor induction versus expectant management in low-risk nulliparous women. *N Engl J Med.* 2018, 379: 513–523.

38. Winterfeld U, Meyer Y, Panchaud A, et al. Management of deficient lactation in Switzerland and Canada: A survey of midwives' current practices. *Breastfeeding Med.* 2012, 7: 317–318.

39. Cazorla-Ortiz G, Obregón-Guitérrez N, Rozas-Garcia MR, et al. Methods and success factors of induced lactation: A scoping review. *J Hum Lact.* 2020, 36: 739–749.

40. Mangesi L, and Zakarija-Grkovic I. Treatments for breast engorgement during lactation. *Cochrane Database Syst Rev.* 2016, Cd006946.

41. Fewtrell MS, Loh KL, Blake A, et al. Randomised, double blind trial of oxytocin nasal spray in mothers expressing breast milk for preterm infants. *Arch Dis Child Fetal Neonatal Ed.* 2006, 91: F169–174.

42. Practice Bulletin No. 183: Postpartum Hemorrhage. *Obstet Gynecol.* 2017, 130: e168–e186.

43. Salati JA, Leathersich SJ, Williams MJ, et al. Prophylactic oxytocin for the third stage of labour to prevent postpartum haemorrhage. *Cochrane Database Syst Rev.* 2019, Cd001808.

44. Westhoff G, Cotter AM, and Tolosa JE. Prophylactic oxytocin for the third stage of labour to prevent postpartum haemorrhage. *Cochrane Database Syst Rev.* 2013, Cd001808.

45. Durocher J, Dzuba IG, Carroli G, et al. Does route matter?

Impact of route of oxytocin administration on postpartum bleeding: A double-blind, randomized controlled trial. *PLoS ONE.* 2019, 14: e0222981.

46. Windle RJ, Shanks N, Lightman SL, et al. Central oxytocin administration reduces stress-induced corticosterone release and anxiety behavior in rats. *Endocrinology.* 1997, 138: 2829–2834.

47. Petersson M, Wiberg U, Lundeberg T, et al. Oxytocin decreases carrageenan induced inflammation in rats. *Peptides.* 2001, 22: 1479–1484.

48. Neumann ID. Brain oxytocin: A key regulator of emotional and social behaviours in both females and males. *J Neuroendocrinol.* 2008, 20: 858–865.

49. Churchland PS, and Winkielman P. Modulating social behavior with oxytocin: how does it work? What does it mean? *Horm Behav.* 2012, 61: 392–399.

50. Cyranowski JM, Hofkens TL, Frank E, et al. Evidence of dysregulated peripheral oxytocin release among depressed women. *Psychosom Med.* 2008, 70: 967–975.

51. Leng G, and Ludwig M. Intranasal oxytocin: Myths and delusions. *Biol Psychiatry.* 2016, 79: 243–250.

52. Saxbe D, Khaled M, Horton KT, et al. Maternal prenatal plasma oxytocin is positively associated with prenatal psychological symptoms, but method of immunoassay extraction may affect results. *Biol Psychol* 2019. 147: 107718.

53. Bosch OJ, Meddle SL, Beiderbeck DI, et al. Brain oxytocin correlates with maternal aggression: Link to anxiety. *J Neurosci.* 2005, 25: 6807–6815.

54. Craciunas L, Kollmann M, Tsampras N, et al. Oxytocin antagonists for assisted reproduction. *Cochrane Database Syst Rev.* 2016, Cd012375.

55. Moraloglu O, Tonguc E, Var T, et al. Treatment with oxytocin antagonists before embryo transfer may increase implantation rates after IVF. *Reprod Biomed Online.* 2010, 21: 338–343.

56. Kam KY, and Lamont RF. Developments in the pharmacotherapeutic management of spontaneous preterm labor. *Expert Opin Pharmacother.* 2008, 9: 1153–1168.

57. van Vliet EOG, Nijman TAJ, Schuit E, et al. Nifedipine versus atosiban for threatened preterm birth (APOSTEL III): A multicentre, randomised controlled trial. *Lancet.* 2016, 387: 2117–2124.

58. Thornton S, Goodwin TM, Greisen G, et al. The effect of barusiban, a selective oxytocin antagonist, in threatened preterm labor at late gestational age: A randomized, double-blind, placebo-controlled trial. *Am J Obstet Gynecol.* 2009, 200 (627): e621–610.

59. Thornton S, Miller H, Valenzuela G, et al. Treatment of spontaneous preterm labour with retosiban: A phase 2 proof-of-concept study. *Br J Clin Pharmacol.* 2015, 80: 740–749.

60. Ogawa S, Kudo S, Kitsunai Y, et al. Increase in oxytocin secretion at ejaculation in male. *Clin Endocrinol.* 1980, 13: 95–97.

61. Carmichael MS, Humbert R, Dixen J, et al. Plasma oxytocin increases in the human sexual response. *J Clin Endocrinol Metab.* 1987, 64: 27–31.

62. Melis MR, Argiolas A, andGessa GL. Oxytocin-induced penile erection and yawning: site of action in the brain. *Brain Res.* 1986, 398: 259–265.

63. Filippi S, Vannelli GB, Granchi S, et al. Identification, localization and functional activity of oxytocin receptors in epididymis. *Mol Cell Endocrinol.* 2002, 193: 89–100.

64. Ivell R, Balvers M, Rust W, et al. Oxytocin and male reproductive function. *Adv Exp Med Biol.* 1997, 424: 253–264.

65. Thackare H, Nicholson HD, and Whittington K. Oxytocin - Its role in male reproduction and new potential therapeutic uses. *Hum Reprod Update.* 2006, 12: 437–448.

66. Neumann ID, Wigger A, Torner L, et al. Brain oxytocin inhibits basal and stress-induced activity of the hypothalamo-pituitary-adrenal axis in male and female rats: Partial action within the paraventricular nucleus. *J Neuroendocrinol.* 2000, 12: 235–243.

67. Goodin BR, Anderson AJB, Freeman EL, et al. Intranasal oxytocin administration is associated with enhanced endogenous pain inhibition and reduced negative mood states. *Clin J Pain.* 2015, 31: 757–767.

68. Boll S, Almeida de Minas AC, Raftogianni A, et al. Oxytocin and pain perception: From animal models to human research. *Neuroscience.* 2018, 387: 149–161.

69. Tracy LM, Georgiou-Karistianis N, Gibson SJ, et al. Oxytocin and the modulation of pain experience: Implications for chronic pain management. *Neurosci Biobehav Rev.* 2015, 55: 53–67.

70. Onaka T, and Takayanagi Y. Role of oxytocin in the control of stress and food intake. *J Neuroendocrinol.* 2019, e12700.

Chapter

4

The Role of Human Chorionic Gonadotropin in Pregnancy

Keiichi Kumasawa and Yutaka Osuga

4.1 Human Chorionic Gonadotropin (hCG)

4.1.1 Placental Hormones

hCG is a gonadotropin that is mainly produced in human trophoblasts and placentas. The production of hormones by human trophoblasts is greater in both quantity and diversity than that of any single endocrine tissue in all mammalian species.

4.1.2 Gonadotropin

Gonadotropins are a group of glycoprotein hormones secreted by gonadotropic cells of the anterior pituitary of vertebrates (1). This hormone family includes the mammalian follicle-stimulating hormone (FSH), luteinizing hormone (LH), and hCG (2). These hormones are central to the endocrine system that regulates normal growth, sexual development, and reproductive function via positive or negative feedback (3). Both LH and FSH are secreted by the anterior pituitary gland, whereas hCG is secreted by the placenta of pregnant humans (4). Gonadotropins exert influence on the gonads, controlling gamete and sex hormone production.

4.1.3 hCG

4.1.3.1 Biosynthesis

Chorionic gonadotropin is a glycoprotein with biological activity similar to that of LH. Both LH and FSH act via the same LH-hCG receptor.

hCG has a molecular weight of 36,000 to 40,000 Da and has the highest carbohydrate ratio, approximately 30 percent, of all human hormones. The carbohydrate component, especially the terminal sialic acid, prevents the hormone from being catabolized. Thus, the 36-h plasma half-life of intact hCG is much longer than the 2-h plasma half-life of LH. The hCG molecule comprises two dissimilar subunits named α- and β-subunits and includes thyroid stimulating hormone (TSH), LH, and FSH.

The two types of subunits are noncovalently linked and are held together by electrostatic and hydrophobic forces. Isolated subunits cannot bind the LH-hCG receptor and thus lack biological activity.

hCG is produced almost exclusively in the placenta; however, it is also synthesized at low levels in the fetal kidneys. A tiny amount of hCG is produced in normal tissues of nonpregnant women and sometimes men, primarily in the anterior pituitary gland (5).

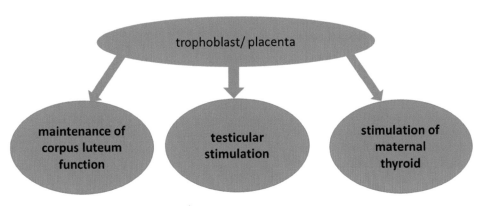

Figure 4.1 hCG keep pregnancy successful in various ways

33

The hCG hormone is, as stated above, structurally related to three other glycoprotein hormones: LH, FSH, and TSH. All four glycoproteins share a common α-subunit. However, each of the β-subunits, although sharing certain similarities, is characterized by a distinctively different amino acid sequence, leading to different biological mechanisms.

Synthesis of the α- and β-subunits of hCG is regulated separately. A single gene located on chromosome 6 encodes α-subunit. Seven genes on chromosome 19 encode for the β-hCG-β-LH family of subunits. Among the seven genes, six encode for β-hCG and one for β-LH (6). Both subunits are synthesized as large precursors, which are then cleaved by endopeptidases to mature forms. Intact hCG is then assembled and rapidly released by secretory granule exocytosis (7).

There are two types of hCG molecules with different immunoreactivity. Both have the same amino acid sequence; however, there is a difference in their carbohydrate content. hCG with a smaller amount of carbohydrate content is produced in the syncytiotrophoblast, whereas hCG with a larger amount of carbohydrate is produced in the cytotrophoblast, promoting invasion of the fertilized ovum into the endometrium during the early stage of pregnancy (8). hCG with a larger amount of carbohydrate is also secreted in choriocarcinoma and is related to the degree of malignancy.

There are multiple forms of hCG in the maternal plasma and urine that vary enormously in bioactivity and immunoreactivity. Some result from enzymatic degradation and others from modifications during molecular synthesis and processing.

Before five weeks of gestation, hCG is expressed both in syncytiotrophoblasts and cytotrophoblasts (9). Later during the first trimester, when maternal serum levels peak, at approximately nine to ten weeks of gestation, hCG is produced almost solely in the syncytiotrophoblast (10). At this time, mRNA concentrations of both α- and β-subunits in the syncytiotrophoblast are greater than those at term (11). Because the hCG trend in normal pregnancy is known, we can adopt hCG as a screening procedure to identify abnormal fetuses.

Circulating free levels of the β-subunit are too low to be detectable throughout pregnancy. In part, this is because of the difference in synthesis of α- and β-subunits. Free α-subunits that do not combine with β-subunits are found in placental tissue and maternal plasma. Levels of the α-subunit increase gradually until they plateau at approximately 36 weeks' gestation. Therefore, they account for only 30–50 percent of the hormones (12). This is because α-hCG secretion corresponds to placental mass, whereas complete hCG molecule secretion is maximal at eight to ten weeks' gestation, corresponding to peak serum hCG levels.

4.1.3.2 Serum and Urine Concentrations

The hCG molecule is detectable in the plasma of pregnant women seven to nine days after the LH surge followed by ovulation. Thus, hCG enters the maternal circulation at the time of blastocyst implantation. After that, plasma levels increase rapidly, doubling every two days until they peak at approximately nine to eleven weeks' gestation. To date, many studies of serum hCG trends have been undertaken, and they have revealed the same trend despite the diversity of multiple forms (Table 4.1). Intact hCG circulates as multiple highly-related isoforms with variable cross-reactivity between different commercial assays. Thus, the calculated serum hCG levels can vary considerably among the numerous available assays, even in the same plasma. This variability emphasizes the need to use the same assay type when measuring serial plasma hCG levels. Peak maternal plasma levels reach approximately 50,000–100,000 mIU/mL between 60 and 80 days after the last menstrual day. At 10–12 weeks of gestation, plasma levels begin to decline

Table 4.1. Trend and range of serum hCG level (two significant digits)

Gestational week	Range (mIU/mL)
3	0–50
4	20–500
5	500–5000
6	3000–20000
8	14,000–170,000
12	16,000–160,000
24	2500–82,000
36	2400–50,000

rapidly until about 14 weeks of gestation and remain low during the remainder of the pregnancy.

The hCG appearance trend in fetal blood is similar to that in the mother. However, fetal plasma levels are only approximately 3 percent of those in the mother. In contrast, the amniotic fluid hCG level during early pregnancy is similar to that in the maternal plasma. As the pregnancy progresses, the hCG concentration in the amniotic fluid decreases faster than that in the mother, and around near term the levels are only approximately 20 percent of those in the maternal plasma.

Maternal urine contains the same variety of hCG degradation products as maternal plasma. The principal urinary form is the terminal product of hCG degradation, the β-core fragment. Concentrations of this fragment follow the same trend as in the maternal plasma, peaking at approximately 10 weeks' gestation. Importantly, the β-subunit antibody commercially used to detect pregnancy reacts with both intact hCG, the major form in the plasma, and hCG fragments, the major form in the urine.

4.1.3.3 Regulation of hCG

The placental gonadotropin-releasing hormone (GnRH) has strong effects on the regulation of hCG formation. Both GnRH and its receptor are expressed by cytotrophoblasts and syncytiotrophoblasts (13). GnRH administration elevates plasma hCG levels, and trophoblast cells, in vitro, respond to GnRH treatment and increase hCG secretion. Pituitary GnRH production is also regulated by inhibin and activin. Placental cell experiments have revealed that activin stimulates and inhibin inhibits GnRH and hCG production (14).

Renal clearance of hCG accounts for only 30 percent of its total metabolic clearance. The remainder is cleared by liver metabolism (15). Clearances of α- and β-subunits are approximately 10- and 30-fold greater than that of intact hCG, respectively. Despite 30 percent contribution, in pregnancies complicated by chronic renal disease, hCG clearance can be markedly decreased.

4.2 Biological Functions

hCG is mainly produced in the cytotrophoblast and placenta. Therefore, hCG is thought to be essential for pregnancy. Since the 1970s, many researchers and clinicians have examined its functions; however, many unknown factors remain to be elucidated. For example, both α- and β-subunits are required for binding to the LH-hCG receptor in the corpus luteum and fetal testis. LH-hCG receptors are present in various tissues; however, their roles have not been elucidated. Here, we focus on three main functions Almost all the functions are involved in the maintenance of a successful pregnancy.

4.2.1 Maintenance of Corpus Luteum Function

The best-known biological function of hCG is to maintain the corpus luteum function, such as continuous progesterone production. However, an additional explanation is provided for the physiological function of hCG in pregnancy. Peak plasma hCG levels are attained well after the end of progesterone secretion from hCG-stimulated corpus luteum. Specifically, luteal progesterone synthesis begins to decline at approximately six weeks of gestation despite continued and increasing hCG production.

4.2.2 Testicular Stimulation

Another major role of hCG is the stimulation of fetal testicular testosterone secretion, which reaches the highest level when hCG levels reach a peak. Thus, at a critical time in male sexual differentiation, hCG enters the fetal plasma from the syncytiotrophoblast. In the fetus, it acts as an LH surrogate to stimulate Leydig cells and for cell replication and testosterone synthesis to promote male sexual differentiation(16).

Fetal Leydig cells produce high levels of testosterone. There is circumstantial evidence that placental production of hCG peaks at approximately 10 weeks' gestation and maintains a higher level until approximately 14 weeks' gestation, controlling early fetal gonadal steroidogenesis (17). The testicular capacity of hCG binding reaches a peak at 15–20 weeks' gestation (18). Studies of steroidogenic enzymes and steroidogenic enzyme gene expression have shown that the cholesterol side-chain cleavage enzyme (P-450scc), adrenodoxin, and P-450c17 genes are highly expressed in the fetal testes, mainly at approximately 15 weeks' gestation. After 16 weeks' gestation, P-450c17 mRNA decreases more rapidly than

35

P-450scc mRNA. This gestational week-related pattern of P-450scc and P-450c17 mRNA expression is similar to that of fetal testicular and serum testosterone concentrations (19) and is associated with hCG production. These findings suggest that the expression of steroidogenic genes is directly regulated by circulating hCG. The P-450Arom (aromatase gene) is poorly expressed in the fetal testis. The lack of significant local estradiol production might explain the nondesensitization of the fetal Leydig cells in the presence of high hCG levels (20). Before approximately 16 weeks' gestation, there is no vascularization of the fetal anterior pituitary from the hypothalamus. Thus, pituitary LH secretion is minimal, and hCG acts as LH before this time. After that, as hCG levels fall, pituitary LH maintains modest testicular stimulation.

4.2.3 Stimulation of the Maternal Thyroid

Another major role of hCG is stimulation of the maternal thyroid, especially during the absence of fetal synthesis of the thyroid hormone.

4.2.3.1 hCG and TSH

The maternal thyroid gland is also stimulated by hCG. In some women with gestational trophoblastic disease, biochemical and clinical evidence of hyperthyroidism sometimes develops, but declines after therapy.

This used to be attributed to the formation of chorionic thyrotropins by neoplastic trophoblasts. However, it has been discovered that certain forms of hCG bind to TSH receptors on thyrocytes (21). Exogenous hCG treatment in adult men increases thyroid activity. The thyroid-stimulatory activity in the plasma of pregnant women during the first trimester differs appreciably between individuals. Modifications of hCG oligosaccharides are involved in the ability of hCG to stimulate thyroid function. For example, acidic isoforms stimulate thyroid activity, and some more basic isoforms stimulate iodine uptake (22). The LH-hCG receptor is expressed by thyrocytes; therefore, hCG stimulates thyroid activity via LH-hCG and TSH receptors (23).

Transient biochemical features of hyperthyroidism are observed in 2–15 percent of women during early pregnancy (24). Many women with hyperemesis gravidarum have abnormally high serum thyroxine levels and low TSH levels, resulting from TSH-receptor stimulation from high (normal for pregnancy) hCG concentration. This transient condition is also termed gestational transient thyrotoxicosis. Even if associated with hyperemesis, antithyroid drugs are not effective. The degree of hCG elevation does not correlate with thyroxine and TSH values, which become more normal during mid-pregnancy (25).

4.2.3.2 Thyroid Hormones and Fetal Brain Development

During the nineteenth century, data showed that normal thyroid function was associated with brain development. Since then, numerous studies involving rats, sheep, and humans have reinforced this concept, usually by the effects of fetal or maternal thyroid deficiencies (26). Thyroid hormones have their most significant effects on the terminal stages of brain differentiation, including synaptogenesis, dendrite and axon growth, myelination, and neuronal migration.

For educational achievement, there have been controversial studies undertaken. For example, Nelson et al. reported that maternal low-level thyroxin at the end of the first trimester was associated with reduced performance in an arithmetic test, but not in a language test, in five-year-old offspring (27). However, in another study, maternal thyroid dysfunction during early pregnancy did not have a clinically important association with impaired child performance at school or for educational achievement (28). Owing to the influence of environmental factors, including education, it is difficult to draw conclusions regarding the link between thyroid hormone levels and infant development.

4.2.3.3 Mechanism of Thyroid Effect on the Fetal Brain

Thyroid hormones act by binding to nuclear receptors and modulating the transcription of responsive genes. Thyroid hormone receptors are widely distributed in the fetal brain, which also occurs prior to the time the fetus can synthesize thyroid hormones. It is difficult to identify how the molecular targets for thyroid hormones act in the developing brain; however, some progress has been made. For example, the promoter of the myelin basic protein gene directly responds to thyroid hormones and contains the expected hormone response element. This matches the observation that induced hypothyroidism in rats leads to the diminished synthesis of mRNAs for several myelin-associated proteins(29).

4.2.3.4 Other Functions of hCG

Three other functions of hCG are discussed here. One is the promotion of relaxin secretion by the corpus luteum. LH-hCG receptors are found in the myometrium and uterine vascular tissue. It has been hypothesized that hCG might promote uterine vascular vasodilation and myometrial smooth muscle relaxation (30). Another function is regulating the expansion of dNK cell numbers by chronic gonadotropin during the early stage of placentation, leading to pregnancy (31). The third function is to suppress lymphocyte cell division and proliferation, in vitro, and maintain a successful pregnancy (32). These three functions are associated with pregnancy, which is reasonable based on the period and location of hCG expression.

4.3 Clinical Application

4.3.1 Pregnancy Tests

Rapid and accurate pregnancy determination is essential to identify an ectopic pregnancy that sometimes leads to massive intraperitoneal bleeding. Current pregnancy tests adopt enzyme-linked immunosorbent assays for the β-subunit of hCG.

After pregnancy test results, an initial transvaginal sonography (TVS) is typically performed to identify the gestation location. If a yolk sac, embryo, or fetus is identified within the uterus or the adnexa, a diagnosis can be made. However, in many cases, one TVS is not enough for diagnosis, and tubal pregnancy could still be a possibility. In such cases, neither normal nor ectopic pregnancies are identified. The term pregnancy of unknown location is used until additional clinical information allows the determination of the pregnancy location.

4.3.1.1 Measurement of hCG

hCG is a glycoprotein with a high carbohydrate content. The general structure of hCG is a heterodimer composed of two dissimilar subunits, α and β, which are noncovalently linked. The α-subunit is identical to those of LH, FSH, and TSH; however, the β-subunit is structurally distinct. Thus,

antibodies have been developed with high specificity for the hCG β-subunit. Such specificity allows for its detection, and numerous commercial immunoassays are available for measuring serum and urine hCG levels. Although each immunoassay detects a slightly different mixture of hCG variants, its free subunits, or metabolites, are all appropriate for pregnancy testing (33). Depending on the assay used, the sensitivity of the laboratory detection limit of hCG in serum is 1.0 mIU/mL or lower (34).

False-positive hCG test results are, at present, rare (35). Some women have circulating serum factors that might bind to the test antibody directed to hCG in an assay. The most common factors are heterophilic antibodies that bind to the animal-derived test antibodies used in an immunoassay. Thus, women who have worked closely with animals are more likely to obtain these antibodies. Elevated hCG levels might also reflect molar pregnancy and its associated cancers. Other rare causes of positive assays without pregnancy are (1) exogenous hCG injection used for weight loss, (2) renal failure with impaired hCG clearance, (3) physiological pituitary hCG, and (4) hCG-producing tumors originating from various organs such as the gastrointestinal site, ovary, bladder, or lungs (36).

4.3.1.2 Home Pregnancy Tests

Commercially available pregnancy test kits have been available since the early 1970s, and millions are sold annually in the United States. Currently, over 60 different test kits are for sale in the United States (37). However, to date, many of these are not as accurate as advertised (38). For example, Cole et al. showed that a detection limit of 12.5 mIU/mL would be required to diagnose 95 percent of all pregnancies at the time of missed menses; however, they reported that only one brand met this degree of sensitivity (39). Two other commercial kits revealed false-positive or invalid results. With an hCG concentration of 100 mIU/mL, positive results were displayed in only 44 percent of all brands. Thus, only approximately 15 percent of pregnancies could be diagnosed at the time of missed menses. Some manufacturers of newer home urine assays describe greater than 90 percent accuracy of test kits performed on the expected day of menses.

Some cases were detected as early as four days before the expected menstrual date. However, careful analysis suggests that these assays are often not as sensitive as advertised. To avoid the misjudgment of pregnancy, in case of negative signs using a commercial kit, it is important to repeat the test several days later.

In addition, when the test kits show a positive sign of pregnancy, those women are required to go to a hospital or clinic to be examined. To rule out an ectopic pregnancy or chorionic disease, a TVS is required, sometimes more than once.

4.3.2 Abnormally High or Low Levels

There are several clinical circumstances where even higher maternal plasma hCG levels are found. Some examples are multifetal pregnancy, erythroblastosis fetalis associated with fetal hemolytic anemia, and gestational trophoblastic disease. Relatively higher hCG levels may be found in women carrying a fetus with Down syndrome (40). This observation is used in biochemical screening tests. The reason for the elevation is not clear; however, reduced placental maturity has been speculated. Various malignant tumors also produce hCG, sometimes in large amounts, especially in cases of trophoblastic neoplasms(41).

Relatively low hCG plasma levels are found in women with early pregnancy loss, including ectopic pregnancy.

4.3.2.1 Ectopic Pregnancy

An ectopic tubal pregnancy that undergoes repeated minor ruptures instead of a single episode of rapid massive bleeding frequently develops into a pelvic hematocele. The hematocele, which contains old blood, clots, and gestational tissue, is surrounded by adhesions and is misleadingly called a "chronic" ectopic pregnancy. The term "chronic" describes only the appearance of the pelvic mass and does not imply the duration. The incidence has been reported in 28 percent of all ectopic pregnancies (42). The more common acute ectopic pregnancy has a high serum β-hCG level and rapid growth, leading to a timely diagnosis, and a higher risk of tubal rupture. With a chronic ectopic pregnancy, the abnormal trophoblast dies during the early stage, and thus, negative or low static serum β-hCG levels are observed (43). Chronic ectopic pregnancies typically rupture late, if at all; however, they commonly form a complex pelvic mass, which is often the reason for diagnostic surgery. A total of 50 percent of patients with chronic ectopic pregnancy have shown a negative serum β-hCG level, which has a sonographic appearance that is distinctly different from acute ectopic pregnancy (42).

4.3.2.2 Chorionic Disease

Gestational trophoblastic disease contains a group of uncommon but interrelated conditions derived from placental trophoblasts. Gestational trophoblastic disease is the appropriate collective name for a hydatidiform mole, whereas the term gestational trophoblastic neoplasia is reserved for cases with persistent plasma hCG levels even after evacuation or removal of the hydatidiform mole, metastatic disease, or choriocarcinoma. Although the pathology and clinical behavior of the complete and partial moles are different, the initial management of both conditions is surgical evacuation by suction, determination of the baseline, and follow-up with plasma hCG level (44).

In the diagnosis of pregnancy, clinicians must consider an abnormal pregnancy when there are abnormal plasma hCG levels.

4.4 Multimodality Diagnosis

4.4.1 β-hCG

hCG is produced in very small amounts in normal tissues of men and nonpregnant women, primarily in the anterior pituitary gland. Therefore, the detection of hCG in blood or urine almost always indicates pregnancy. β-hCG is a critical subunit that distinguishes β-hCG and LH and FSH. Thus, β-hCG plays an important clinical role.

4.4.2 β-hCG Levels above the Discriminatory Threshold

Several investigators have described discriminatory β-hCG levels above which failure to visualize a uterine pregnancy indicates that the pregnancy is either not alive or is ectopic (45). Some institutions set their discriminatory threshold at $\geq$1500 mIU/mL, whereas others adopt $\geq$2000 mIU/mL. Moreover, other groups have suggested an even higher threshold, adding that with live intrauterine pregnancies, a gestational sac was seen 99 percent of the time with a discriminatory level of $\geq$3510 mIU/mL (43).

If the initial β-hCG level exceeds the discriminatory level and no evidence of an intrauterine pregnancy is detected by TVS, then an ectopic pregnancy is almost certain. The diagnosis is narrowed down to a failing intrauterine pregnancy, a recent complete abortion, or an ectopic pregnancy. Early multifetal gestation also remains a possibility. Without clear evidence of an ectopic pregnancy, serial β-hCG level assessment is undertaken, and the level is checked 48 hours later. This procedure prevents unnecessary methotrexate admission and avoids harm to an early, normal multifetal pregnancy. In cases of a greater possibility of ectopic gestation, dilation and evacuation is another option to distinguish ectopic from failing intrauterine pregnancy. Importantly, each decision should be made carefully and appropriately.

4.4.3 β-hCG Levels below the Discriminatory Zone

If the initial β-hCG level is below the set discriminatory value, pregnancy location is not technically discernible with TVS. With these pregnancies of unknown locations, serial β-hCG assays are performed to identify patterns that indicate either growing or failing intrauterine pregnancy (IUP). When β-hCG levels increase or decrease outside the normal range, there is a concern of ectopic pregnancy. With early normal progressing IUPs, Barnhart and colleagues reported a minimum increase in hCG of 24 percent in 24 hours and a 53 percent increase in 48 hours (46). Seeber and

colleagues revealed an even more conservative ratio, with a minimal 35 percent increase in 48 hours in normal IUPs(47). Even with multifetal gestation, the same increase of plasma β-hCG level is expected (48). Despite the guidelines, Silva and colleagues pointed out that a third of women with an ectopic pregnancy had a 53 percent increase in plasma β-hCG levels at 48 hours (49). Moreover, they reported that ectopic pregnancies show various trends in plasma β-hCG levels, and that approximately half of the ectopic pregnancies show decreasing plasma β-hCG levels, whereas the other half have increasing levels. Despite a declining plasma β-hCG level, a resolving ectopic pregnancy may rupture.

With a failing IUP, plasma β-hCG levels can also be anticipated. Following spontaneous abortion, rates decline by 21–35 percent at 48 hours and 68 to 84 percent at 7 days, which are clinically useful data for observing this process (46).

In pregnancies without these expected increases or decreases in β-hCG levels, discrimination between a nonliving IUP and an ectopic pregnancy might be supported by repeated evaluation of plasma β-hCG levels (50). Delayed β-hCG levels indicate a risk of rupture. In such cases, dilation and evacuation is a useful option and provides a quicker diagnosis balanced against normal pregnancy interruption. Before dilation and evacuation, a second TVS examination might be undertaken, which could help informative findings, leading to better treatment.

References

1. Pierce, JG, and Parsons, TF. Glycoprotein hormones: Structure and function. *Annu Rev Biochem*. 1981, 50: 465–495.

2. Stockell Hartree, A, and Renwick, AG. Molecular structures of glycoprotein hormones and functions of their carbohydrate components. *Biochem J*. 1992, 287(Pt 3): 665–679.

3. Godine, JE, Chin, WW, and Habener, JF. Alpha Subunit of rat pituitary glycoprotein hormones. Primary structure of the precursor determined from the nucleotide

sequence of cloned cDNAs. *J Biol Chem*. 1982, 257, 8368–8371,

4. Golos, TG, Durning, M, and Fisher, JM. Molecular cloning of the rhesus glycoprotein hormone alpha-subunit gene. *DNA Cell Biol*. 1991, 10, 367–380.

5. McGregor, WG, Kuhn, RW, and Jaffe, RB. Biologically active chorionic gonadotropin: Synthesis by the human fetus. *Science*. 1983, 220, 306–308.

6. Miller-Lindholm, AK, LaBenz, CJ, Ramey, J, et al. Human chorionic gonadotropin-beta gene expression in first trimester placenta.

Endocrinology. 1997, 138, 5459–5465.

7. Morrish, DW, Manickavel, V, Jewell, LD, et al. Immunolocalization of alpha and beta chains of human chorionic gonadotropin, placental lactogen and pregnancy-specific beta-glycoprotein in term placenta by a touch preparation method. *Histochemistry*. 1987, 88, 57–60.

8. Hoshina, M, Ashitake, Y, and Tojo, S. Immunohistochemical interaction on antisera to HCG and its subunits with chorionic tissue of early gestation. *Endocrinol Jpn*. 1979, 26, 175–184.

9. Maruo, T, Ladines-Llave, CA, Matsuo, H, et al. A novel change in cytologic localization of human chorionic gonadotropin and human placental lactogen in first-trimester placenta in the course of gestation. *Am J Obstet Gynecol.* 1992, 167, 217–222.

10. Beck, T, Schweikhart, G, and Stolz, E. Immunohistochemical location of HPL, SP1 and beta-HCG in normal placentas of varying gestational age. *Arch Gynecol.* 1986, 239, 63–74.

11. Hoshina, M, Boothby, M, and Boime, I. Cytological localization of chorionic gonadotropin alpha and placental lactogen mRNAs during development of the human placenta. *J Cell Biol.* 1982, 93, 190–198

12. Cole, LA. Immunoassay of human chorionic gonadotropin, its free subunits, and metabolites. *Clin Chem.* 1997, 43, 2233–2243.

13. Wolfahrt, S, Kleine, B, and Rossmanith, WG. Detection of gonadotrophin releasing hormone and its receptor mRNA in human placental trophoblasts using in-situ reverse transcription-polymerase chain reaction. *Mol Hum Reprod.* 1998, 4, 999–1006.

14. Petraglia, F, Vaughan, J, and Vale, W. Inhibin and activin modulate the release of gonadotropin-releasing hormone, human chorionic gonadotropin, and progesterone from cultured human placental cells. *Proc Natl Acad Sci USA.* 1989, 86, 5114–5117.

15. Wehmann, RE, and Nisula, BC. Renal clearance rates of the subunits of human chorionic gonadotropin in man. *J Clin Endocrinol Metab.* 1980, 50, 674–679.

16. Zirkin, BR, and Papadopoulos, V. Leydig cells: Formation, function, and regulation. *Biol Reprod.* 2018, 99, 101–111.

17. Clements, JA, Reyes, FI, Winter, JS, et al. Studies on human sexual development. III. Fetal pituitary and serum, and amniotic fluid concentrations of LH, CG, and FSH. *J Clin Endocrinol Metab.* 1976, 42, 9–19.

18. Molsberry, RL, Carr, BR, Mendelson, CR, et al. Human chorionic gonadotropin binding to human fetal testes as a function of gestational age. *J Clin Endocrinol Metab.* 1982, 55, 791–794.

19. Tapanainen, J, Kellokumpu-Lehtinen, P, Pelliniemi, L, et al. Age-related changes in endogenous steroids of human fetal testis during early and midpregnancy. *J Clin Endocrinol Metab.* 1981, 52, 98–102.

20. Leinonen, PJ, and Jaffe, RB. Leydig cell desensitization by human chorionic gonadotropin does not occur in the human fetal testis. *J Clin Endocrinol Metab.* 1985, 61, 234–238.

21. Hershman, JM. Human chorionic gonadotropin and the thyroid: Hyperemesis gravidarum and trophoblastic tumors. *Thyroid.* 1999, 9, 653–657.

22. Kraiem, Z, Sadeh, O, Blithe, DL, et al. Human chorionic gonadotropin stimulates thyroid hormone secretion, iodide uptake, organification, and adenosine 3',5'-monophosphate formation in cultured human thyrocytes. *J Clin Endocrinol Metab.* 1994, 79, 595–599.

23. Tomer, Y, Huber, GK, and Davies, TF. Human chorionic gonadotropin (hCG) interacts directly with recombinant human TSH receptors. *J Clin Endocrinol Metab.* 1992, 74, 1477–1479.

24. Fitzpatrick, DL, and Russell, MA. Diagnosis and management of thyroid disease in pregnancy. *Obstet Gynecol Clin North Am.* 2010, 37, 173–193.

25. Nathan, N, and Sullivan, SD. Thyroid disorders during pregnancy. *Endocrinol Metab Clin North Am.* 2014, 43, 573–597.

26. Oppenheimer, JH, and Schwartz, HL. Molecular basis of thyroid hormone-dependent brain development. *Endocr Rev,* 1997, 18, 462–475.

27. Noten, AM, Loomans, EM, Vrijkotte, TG, et al. Maternal hypothyroxinaemia in early pregnancy and school performance in 5-year-old offspring. *Eur J Endocrinol.* 2015, 173, 563–571.

28. Nelson, SM, Haig, C, McConnachie, A, et al. Maternal thyroid function and child educational attainment: Prospective cohort study. *BMJ.* 2018, 360, k452.

29. Remaud, S, Gothie, JD, Morvan-Dubois, G, et al. Thyroid hormone signaling and adult neurogenesis in mammals. *Front Endocrinol (Lausanne).* 2014, 5, 62.

30. Kurtzman, JT, Wilson, H, and Rao, CV. A proposed role for hCG in clinical obstetrics. *Semin Reprod Med.* 2001, 19, 63–68.

31. Kane, N, Kelly, R, Saunders, PT, et al. Proliferation of uterine natural killer cells is induced by human chorionic gonadotropin and mediated via the mannose receptor. *Endocrinology.* 2009, 150, 2882–2888.

32. Han, T. Inhibitory effect of human chorionic gonadotrophin on lymphocyte blastogenic response to mitogen, antigen and allogeneic cells. *Clin Exp Immunol.* 1974, 18, 529–535.

33. Braunstein, GD. The long gestation of the modern home pregnancy test. *Clin Chem.* 2014, 60, 18–21.

34. Wilcox, AJ, Baird, DD, Dunson, D, et al. Natural limits

of pregnancy testing in relation to the expected menstrual period. *JAMA.* 2001, 286, 1759–1761.

35. Braunstein, GD. False-positive serum human chorionic gonadotropin results: Causes, characteristics, and recognition. *Am J Obstet Gynecol.* 2002, 187, 217–224.

36. Montagnana, M, Trenti, T, Aloe, R, et al. Human chorionic gonadotropin in pregnancy diagnostics. *Clin Chim Acta.* 2011, 412, 1515–1520.

37. Grenache, DG. Variable accuracy of home pregnancy tests: Truth in advertising? *Clin Chem Lab Med.* 2015, 53, 339–341.

38. Johnson, S, Cushion, M, Bond, S, et al. Comparison of analytical sensitivity and women's interpretation of home pregnancy tests. *Clin Chem Lab Med.* 2015, 53, 391–402.

39. Cole, LA. The utility of six over-the-counter (home) pregnancy tests. *Clin Chem Lab Med.* 2011, 49, 1317–1322.

40. Banerjee, S, Smallwood, A, Chambers, AE, et al. A link between high serum levels of human chorionic gonadotrophin and chorionic expression of its mature functional receptor (LHCGR) in Down's syndrome pregnancies. *Reprod Biol Endocrinol.* 2005, 3, 25.

41. Stenman, UH, Alfthan, H, and Hotakainen, K. Human chorionic gonadotropin in cancer. *Clin Biochem.* 2004, 37, 549–561.

42. Bedi, DG, Moeller, D, Fagan, CJ, et al. Chronic ectopic pregnancy. A comparison with acute ectopic pregnancy. *Eur J Radiol.* 1987, 7, 46–48.

43. Brennan, DF, Kwatra, S, Kelly, M, et al. Chronic ectopic pregnancy – Two cases of acute rupture despite negative beta hCG. *J Emerg Med.* 2000, 19, 249–254.

44. Smith, HO, Kohorn, E, and Cole, LA. Choriocarcinoma and gestational trophoblastic disease. *Obstet Gynecol Clin North Am.* 2005, 32, 661–684.

45. Barnhart, K, Mennuti, MT, Benjamin, I, et al. Prompt diagnosis of ectopic pregnancy in an emergency department setting. *Obstet Gynecol.* 1994, 84, 1010–1015.

46. Barnhart, K, Sammel, MD, Chung, K, et al. Decline of serum human chorionic gonadotropin and spontaneous complete abortion: Defining the normal curve. *Obstet Gynecol.* 2004, 104, 975–981.

47. Seeber, BE, Sammel, MD, Guo, W, et al. Application of redefined human chorionic gonadotropin curves for the diagnosis of women at risk for ectopic pregnancy. *Fertil Steril.* 2006, 86, 454–459.

48. Chung, K, Sammel, MD, Coutifaris, C, et al. Defining the rise of serum HCG in viable pregnancies achieved through use of IVF. *Hum Reprod.* 2006, 21, 823–828.

49. Silva, C, Sammel, MD, Zhou, L, et al. Human chorionic gonadotropin profile for women with ectopic pregnancy. *Obstet Gynecol.* 2006, 107, 605–610.

50. Zee, J, Sammel, MD, Chung, K, et al. Ectopic pregnancy prediction in women with a pregnancy of unknown location: Data beyond 48 h are necessary. *Hum Reprod.* 2014, 29, 441–447.

Chapter

5

The Role of Estrogens in Pregnancy

Nadia Berkane, Yveline Ansaldi, and Nicola Pluchino

5.1 Introduction

The importance of estrogens during pregnancy, and particularly estradiol (E2), stems from their role in the development and maturation of trophoblast cells and maternal adaptation to pregnancy. Pregnancy is characterized by a significant increase in maternal estrogen levels. E2 increases from 376pmol/L during the luteal phase of the menstrual cycle to greater than 11,000 pmol/L at the end of pregnancy (1).

E2 plays a crucial role in the establishment and maintaining of pregnancy, as demonstrated by the fact that a reduction or blockage of estrogen results in reduced blastocyst implantation and higher rates of miscarriage.

The present chapter reviews current knowledge on the role of estrogens in normal pregnancy as well as in most frequent pathological conditions.

5.2 Site of Estrogens Synthesis during Pregnancy

In early human pregnancy, estrogens are mainly synthesized by the corpus luteum, with a hormonal ovary-to-placenta shift occurring at approximately nine weeks of gestation (2), which results in placental production of E2 and blunting of the gonadotrope axis. Placental macrophages (Hofbauer cells) may synthetize estrogens, but syncytiotrophoblasts (ST) are the main source of estrogens (3). Estrogen production during pregnancy as a result of testosterone aromatization is insignificant due to a much higher affinity of aromatase for $D4$-androstenedione (4). E2 can also be produced in maternal adipose tissue and may contribute, albeit in a minor way, to maternal estrogen concentrations (3).

Human placenta does not express 17a-hydroxylase-17,20 lyase and is thus unable to convert pregnenolone and progesterone into the estrogen precursors, dehydroepiandrosterone (DHEA) and $D4$-androstenedione respectively (3,5). To synthesize estrogens, placenta requires external DHEA, which is provided by maternal and fetal adrenal glands as DHEAS. DHEAS is a product of sulfonation of DHEA by sulfotransferase 2A1, expressed in maternal and fetal adrenal glands and liver (6).

Placental production of E2 from DHEAS requires four key cell-specific enzymes:

(1) Sulfatases expressed by STs which convert DHEAS into DHEA
(2) Type I 3b-hydroxysteroid dehydrogenase (HSD)/$D5D4$isomerase (HSD3B1), expressed by STs and invasive CTs, converts DHEA into $D4$-androstenedione.
(3) Aromatase converts $D4$-androstenedione into E1.
(4) 17-b-HSD type 1 (HSD17B1) converts E1 into E2.

Plasma concentrations of $D4$-androstenedione increase gradually throughout pregnancy and at delivery (3). $D4$-androstenedione is subsequently irreversibly converted into estrone by aromatase. Aromatase, encoded by the CYP19 gene, is expressed in numerous tissues (gonads, brain, fetal liver, vascular smooth muscle cells, endothelial cells, macrophages, adipocytes, and connective tissues) (7) and is widely expressed in the placenta by STs (8). An autocrine loop enhances placental aromatase expression by E2 via ER (9). Estrone (E1) can be sulfonated, resulting in E1S, which is reversibly convertible to E1 and has a longer half-life. E1 is converted into E2 by 17-b-HSD type 1 (HSD17B1). Besides placental estrogen production, there is local synthesis of E2 within the uterine arteries as uterine artery smooth muscle cells express aromatase and invasive CTs express 17-b-HSD type 1 (10). E1 and E2 can be further catabolized as described hereafter.

E3 is mainly derived from 16a-hydroxylated DHEAS, a fetal liver product, and can also be produced by the 16a-hydroxylation of E2 in the fetal liver (11). E3 is therefore a marker of fetal liver function which is synthesized in large amounts in pregnancy (12). Conversion of E2 into E3 is mainly considered irreversible, although conversion via an intermediate 16-keto E2 has been described (3,13).

E4 is the product of 15a/16a-hydroxylation of E2 by 15a-hydroxylase, an enzyme which is specific to the fetal liver and which is not expressed after birth (14). The concentration of E4 is therefore much higher in the fetal than maternal circulation, and E4 is no longer produced after birth (14). The late-pregnancy maternal E4 concentrations are approximately in the 3 nanomolar levels ($\sim$1 ng/mL). E4 produces biological changes in the rodent uterus, such as weight increase, progesterone receptor stimulation, enzyme induction, and histological and ultrastructural changes. It also binds to the human endometrial estrogen receptor. The biochemical, histological, and ultrastructural responses of the immature rat uterus to E4 reveal a tendency toward cell differentiation, in contrast to the typical mitotic responses that are observed after E2 treatment (15). However, the specific role of this estrogen remains unknown, but it probably acts as a selective estrogen receptor modulator (15).

Catecholestrogens are produced by the irreversible hydroxylation of C-2 or C-4 of E1 and E2, mediated by cytochrome P450 (CYP450) isoforms mostly expressed in the placenta and liver. In the placenta, CYP1A1 and CYP3A4 are involved (3). The resulting active hydroxylated estrogens metabolites (2-OH- E2, 4-OH-E2, 2-OH-E1, and 4-OH-E1) display genomic and nongenomic effects (3,16).

Catecholestrogens are converted by catechol-O-methyltransferase (COMT) into methoxyestrogens, one of which is 2-methoxyestradiol (2-ME2). The soluble form of COMT is expressed by maternal arterial endothelial and decidual cells and increases throughout pregnancy (3).

Estrogens may also undergo reversible sulfation, glucuronidation or quinone synthase processes resulting in inactive metabolites which can be excreted into the bile and/or urine (3,17).

Sulfation is mediated by cytosolic sulfotransferases (SULTs), producing water-soluble deactivated sulfated estrogens with a high albumin-binding affinity, rendering them unable to bind to estrogen receptors (ERs) and thus biologically inactive (18). SULT1E1 (also called EST), is one of the main SULTs involved in the sulfation of estrogens and has a strong affinity for E1 and E2 at the nanomolar concentrations found in pregnancy (19). SULT1E1is synthesized by STs, as well as in other maternal and fetal tissues (3). SULT1E1 knockout mice display excess estrogen leading to placental thrombosis and excess fetal death (20). Placental thrombosis may be prevented by anti-estrogen or anticoagulant treatment (20).

As the placenta lacks 17α-hydroxylase, the precursors for estrogen synthesis are mainly derived from the maternal and fetal adrenal glands. The fetus provides DHEA sulfate, which is essential to the production of estrogen, and the placenta stimulates the synthesis of its own precursor DHEA sulfate by lowering fetal cortisol through the upregulation of placental HSD11B2 which converts maternal cortisol in cortisone (fetal cortisol is mainly maternal cortisol) (21). Tight control mechanisms exist to protect adrenal glands against very low or excess estrogen levels (3). Placentas from pre-eclamptic women which exhibit lower HSD11B2 expression and activity induce a vicious circle (22).

5.3 From Pre-implantation to Myometrial Invasion

The synchronous interaction between a competent embryo and a receptive endometrium is a complex molecular process indispensable for successful implantation. The endometrium acquires receptivity to embryo implantation in response to progesterone (P) action on an appropriately primed endometrium.

Estrogenic stimulation results in endometrial proliferation and the induction of P receptors (3). In response to P, the endometrium undergoes profound conformational and biochemical changes, from proliferative to secretory, with a concomitant induction of endometrial receptivity and opening of the window of implantation. Successful implantation requires estrogen functioning. Blocking estrogen signaling using ICI 182780, an estrogen receptor antagonist, prevents blastocyst implantation if administered during days 1, 2, and 3 after fecundation in female rats (23).

Six days after fertilization, the blastocyst reaches the uterine cavity. The blastocyst is composed of an inner cell mass – the future embryo – and an outer ring cell layer, called the

43

trophectoderm, which combines with the maternal endometrium to contribute to the formation of the future placenta. The trophectoderm attaches onto the uterine endometrium before the blastocyst penetrates the endometrium (3). The trophoblast derived from the trophectoderm is composed of a cytotrophoblast inner layer of mononuclear cells (CTs) which multiply and fuse to form an outer multinucleated layer, the syncytiotrophoblast (ST), after adhesion to the endometrium. Estradiol promotes trophoblast cell proliferation but also stimulates villous CT differentiation into ST (24,25).

ST invades the endometrium leading to penetration of the blastocyst into the decidua. Trophoblastic development consists in the formation of villi. The distal parts of anchoring villi are composed of CTs, which proliferate to form CT shells which are in direct contact with maternal uterine cells and vessels (3). ST is involved in gas exchanges, fetal nourishment, and protection, as well as playing an essential endocrine function secreting HCG, estrogens, P, and several other hormones. Interestingly, the synthesis of estradiol is characterized by a positive feedback loop as estradiol upregulates its own production (24,25).

The remodeling process of the uterine arteries is marked by spreading and migration of invasive CTs (Extra-villous trophoblast cells), into the decidua and the first third of the myometrium (3). This step is essential to the growth of the fetoplacental unit and to normal placental function.

5.4 Uterine Artery Remodeling

Uterine artery remodeling results in a complete loss of vascular tone and reduced responsiveness to vasoactive substances, as well as widening of the vascular lumen promoting high blood flow (26). Estradiol and its metabolites are involved and promote the upregulation of cell proliferation, differentiation, and migration of invasive CTs (3). The remodeling starts by penetration of CTs into maternal vessels. The interaction between CTs and the artery wall leads to a disruption and loss of the smooth muscle cells and replacement by EVTs and fibrinoid deposits.

During the first wave of trophoblast invasion, spiral artery lumina are filled by a transient accumulation of EVT plugs, creating localized hypoxia

with overexpression of hypoxia inducible factor-1a (HIF-1a), which stimulates VEGF synthesis (27), thus promoting vasculogenesis, angiogenesis, and placental development (28). A normtoxic local state, which is crucial for further placental and fetal development, is established after the progressive disappearance of the plugs. Insufficient trophoblast development and abnormal angiogenesis, due to low E2 levels, further promote a reduction in estrogen production, resulting in a vicious cycle of hormonal imbalance and disrupted implantation (3).

5.5 Angiogenesis and Placenta Development

Estrogens play multiple and essential roles during pregnancy. They promote placental development through proliferation, differentiation, and migration of trophoblast cells, and stimulate migration and proliferation of endothelial cells and uterine angiogenesis (28). This contributes to the expansion of the maternofetal surface.

Estradiol has strong angiogenic properties when it binds to estrogen receptor alpha (ERα). Vascular endothelial growth factor (VEGF) is an important angiogenic factor and a key mediator for angiogenesis during pregnancy. There is a growing body of evidence concerning the links between VEGF and estradiol 29. Estradiol promotes VEGF, and the expression of its membrane receptors VEGFR-1 and VEGFR-2 and shares similar signaling (i.e., phosphatidylinositol-3 kinase/protein kinase B) and activation of c-Fos and c-Jun (3,29).

Estradiol-mediated angiogenesis is finely controlled by the interactions between estradiol and ERα/β (29). Thus, estradiol binding to ERβ prevents angiogenesis and the placenta is known to express ERβ. Differentiated placental cells such as multinucleated syncytiotrophoblast and other cells express Erβ (3). In addition, a decrease in ERα expression by senescent or hypoxic placenta or during preeclampsia, has also been described (25). The irreversible hydroxylation of carbon 2 of estradiol leads to 2-OH E2 formation, which should be considered as an antiproliferative molecule given its low affinity to ERs 2-OH E2 is quickly metabolized by the COMT enzyme into 2-ME2, a potent anti-proliferative anti-angiogenic factor, which decreases VEGF expression and inhibits vascular tubule formation (3,30). These conversions are mediated by several enzymes specifically distributed in the placenta, the uterus and other maternal organs.

5.6 Estrogens, Uterine Blood Flow, and Systemic Vasodilation

The significant increase of uterine blood flow during pregnancy from 94.5 ml/min to 342 ml/min is essential for the rapid development of the fetoplacental unit. Uterine blood flow accounts for around 3.5 percent of the cardiac output in early pregnancy and increases to 4 times more at the end of gestation (31). This is possible due to the combination of decreased uterine artery resistance, increased plasma volume, and increased maternal cardiac output (32). The 2-ME2 metabolite is an important contributor to the increase of uterine blood flow, through its promotion of migration and invasion of extra villous cytotrophoblasts which induce uterine artery remodeling and by an increase in prostacyclin and NO synthesis (33). Estradiol also plays an important role in lowering uterine vasculature resistance through the key nitric oxide (NO) molecule, its endothelial NO synthase enzyme (eNOS) and prostacycline (34). It has been demonstrated that NOS inhibitors decrease estrogen-induced uterine blood flow (35). The E2-mediated NO and prostacyclin upregulation are partially under VEGF signaling pathway and in turn NO promotes VEGF synthesis (3). Other estrogens such as estrone, estriol, and catecholestrogens have vasodilator effects on the uterine arteries, through upregulation of prostacyclin synthesis and calcium channel activities of vascular endothelial cells (3). Uterine blood flow is thus under maternal but also fetal control since estriol has a fetal origin.

Estrogens and P play an active role in the systemic vasodilation which occurs as early as five weeks of gestation and which results in reduced blood pressure in a normal pregnancy. E2 and its metabolites act through genomic and non-genomic signaling to induce uterine and systemic artery vasodilation (3), thus reducing systemic and uterine vessels resistance despite the activation of the renin-angiotensin-aldosterone system during pregnancy. Specifically, estradiol upregulates hydroxysteroid dehydrogenase 11B2 (HSD11B2), which converts active cortisol into inactive cortisone (36).

5.7 Neuroestrogens

Estrogens have effects on the maternal and fetal brains as demonstrated by the fact that several brain sites exhibit ER-alpha ER-beta and GPER (37). They are implicated in cognition, behavior, and sexual dimorphism. They have numerous cellular and molecular effects (37). Besides circulating estrogens, there is also a local estrogen source and several types of brain cells express the required enzymes for estrogen biosynthesis from cholesterol or DHEA (3). Moreover, local estrogen biosynthesis increases the concentration of specific neurosteroids (allopregnanolone) in preclinical models, suggesting the critical role of estrogens for the maternal brain adaptation during pregnancy and the development of the fetal brain. E2 promotes myelinization, axonal growth as well as proliferation and differentiation of oligodendrocytes. However, in hypoxic conditions E2 can cause brain damage via an excess release of GABA (38). Allopregnanolone is brain protective during complications of pregnancy, such as pre-term delivery or intrauterine growth restriction (IUGR), reducing the impact of hypoxia, and excitotoxic brain damage. Negative behavioral consequences of altered estrogens/allopregnanolone ratio for maternal brain adaptation have been also hypothesized in the post-partum.

5.8 Estrogens and Preeclampsia

Preeclampsia is a worldwide disease complicating 3–7 percent of pregnancies and is characterized by new onset high blood pressure and proteinuria or organ dysfunction.

Placental dysfunction is the cornerstone of preeclampsia, with changes in gene and enzyme expression and/or activity associated with low maternofetal exchanges. The first studies that assessed estrogen levels during preeclampsia displayed contradictory results which were affected by the technical limits of the tests used. ELISA and RIA techniques do not separate some estrogens and therefore do not provide reliable measures. In the last decade, the development of liquid or gas chromatography (LC or GC) coupled with mass spectrometry (MS) or MS/MS techniques has improved the accuracy of the results and allowed for concomitant measurement of estrogen concentrations, enabling the calculation of estrogen product and substrate ratio.

Recent studies using LC or GC/MS or MS/MS found significant lower E2 levels associated with pre-eclampsia (13,39) suggestive of an aromatization reduced activity/expression. Using a pregnant-rabbit model of placental hypoxia, Perez et al concluded that the aromatization deficiency is attributable to placenta hypoxia (40). Specific microRNAs (miRNAs) working as transcriptional inhibitors of aromatase gene expression in trophoblasts cells, (miRNA-19b and miRNA-106a), are displayed in higher levels in pre-eclamptic placentas compared to controls (41). Other transcriptional factors and certain aromatase gene polymorphisms which inhibit aromatase activity or expression have also been observed in association with pre-eclampsia (42). Only one study found an increase in aromatase activity in women under chronic hypoxic conditions, but this was obtained in a very specific population and these results cannot be extrapolated to the general population (43). As an approach to evaluating aromatase expression and/or activity, E1/delta-4 androstenedione ratio was used and a significantly lower ratio was found in pre-eclamptic women several weeks before the development of clinical signs (44).

Besides aromatase, COMT involvement in PE has also been considered. COMT knockout mice have low 2-ME2 levels and present with a mild PE-like syndrome. Authors have postulated that low 2-ME2 promotes shallow implantation and abnormal placenta development which in turn leads to low estradiol levels (45). In addition, placental weight and clinical signs of PE improve when 2-ME2 treatments are introduced. However, this model remains different to human PE, and the association between COMT polymorphisms with low COMT activity, and PE remains conflicting (3).

Finally, changes in expression of HSD17B1, the enzyme converting E1 into E2, and its involvement in PE have been assessed. HSD17B1 is found in trophoblast cells such as STs and CTs but also invasive CTs (10,34). Higher expression of miRNAs post-transcriptionally dysregulating HSD17B1 have been observed in placenta from preeclampsia compared with controls (46). Moreover, lower plasmatic concentrations of HSD17B1 circulating protein have been found in women with PE compared to those with normal pregnancies (47). However, the implication of HSD17B1 changes in PE is still debated as

Berkane et al. using the E2/E1 ratio did not find any difference in HSD17B1 activity at 26 weeks in women who later developed PE compared with controls (44).

Diseases with constitutively very low levels of estrogens such as genetic aromatase deficiency (i.e., CYP19 mutations) should be associated with pregnancies complicated by hypertension; however, this is not the case. During pregnancy, aromatase deficiency, which is an autosomic recessive genetic disease, induces an excess of circulating androstenedione which cannot be converted into estrogens and will therefore be converted into efficient androgens (testosterone, etc) (48), giving rise to maternal and fetal virilization. This may seem surprising because androgens are known to negatively regulate placental oxygenation (49). However, androgens may stimulate VEGF through androgen receptors (50). We hypothesize that in the absence of estrogen, androgen receptor expression raises and allows androgen-mediated VEGF synthesis. X-linked placental steroid sulfatase deficiency is also a condition with very low estrogen levels and is characterized by normal or slightly increased testosterone levels with (51).

5.9 Parturition and Estrogens

The mechanisms underpinning the parturition process are still debated, but estrogens and progesterone are undoubtedly involved. While progesterone decreases at the end of pregnancy, estradiol and estriol increase throughout pregnancy. However, unlike other mammalians, humans do not exhibit a sharp increase in circulating estrogens immediately before parturition (52). During pregnancy, there is a need for a no-contractile uterus to protect the fetoplacental unit and promote its development. Just before labor, an influx of inflammatory cells in the myometrium is observed (53). Progesterone plays a key role in maintaining a quiescent uterus, through inhibition of pro-inflammatory transcription factor NF-$_\kappa$B and by enhancing the synthesis of inhibitory factors which suppress gene expression of oxytocin receptor and the gap junction protein connexin 43 (COX 43) (53). Conversely, estrogens increase uterine development and increase oxytocin receptors and synthesis of prostaglandins (PgE2 and Pg F2a) along with modulation of membrane calcium channels. Estrogens control the synchrony of uterine contractions through cellular communications enhancing COX 43 expression (53). Besides uterine contractility, there is a decrease in cervical estrogen receptors to allow for cervical ripening (54).

Several hypotheses have been proposed to explain the role of estrogens in uterine contractility including changes in E2/E3 balance or an increase in E3 at the end of pregnancy as well as in the weeks before premature delivery. The E3 hypothesis highlights the potential fetal trigger for parturition as E3 is mainly derived from fetal 16-OH-DHEAS.

5.10 Conclusion

Estrogens are essential during pregnancy, and their importance stems from their role in the development and maturation of trophoblast cells.

They are also involved in the remodeling process of the uterine arteries, through the spreading and migration of invasive CTs. Estradiol-mediated angiogenesis and the lowering of uterine vasculature resistance are essential to the maintenance of pregnancy and the promotion of placental development. Together with progestogens, they exert tight control over the processes involved in maternal adaptations to pregnancy. Finally, estrogens are also involved in normal parturition at the end of pregnancy. Dysregulation of estrogen synthesis may lead to some pathological conditions of pregnancy such as pre-eclampsia or pre-term labor. Besides estrogen concentrations, estrogens act through different receptors whose presence and modulation remain relatively unknown in human pregnancy to date. Moreover, the role of neuroestrogens is a largely unknown and remains a field to be explored.

References

1. Abbassi-Ghanavati M, Greer LG, and Cunningham FG. Pregnancy and laboratory studies: A reference table for clinicians. *Obstet Gynecol.* 2009, 114 (6):1326–1331.

2. Devroey P, Camus M, Palermo G, et al. Placental production of estradiol and progesterone after oocyte donation in patients with primary ovarian failure. *Am J Obstet Gynecol.* 1990, 162(1): 66–70.

3. Berkane N, Liere P, Oudinet JP, et al. From pregnancy to preeclampsia: A key role for estrogens. *Endocr Rev.* 2017, 38:123–144.

4. N, Osawa Y. Purification of human placental aromatase cytochrome P-450 with monoclonal antibody and its characterization. *Biochemistry.* 1991, 30(12):3003–3010.

5. Pepe GJ, and Albrecht ED. Actions of placental and fetal adrenal steroid hormones in primate pregnancy. *Endocr Rev.* 1995, 16(5): 608–648.

6. Siiteri PK. The continuing saga of dehydroepiandrosterone (DHEA). *J Clin Endocrinol Metab.* 2005, 90(6): 3795–3796.

7. Kragie L. Aromatase in primate pregnancy: A review. *Endocr Res.* 2002, 28(3):121–128.

8. Fournet-Dulguerov N, MacLusky NJ, Leranth CZ, et al. Immunohistochemical localization of aromatase cytochrome P-450 and estradiol dehydrogenase in the syncytiotrophoblast of the human placenta. *J Clin Endocrinol Metab.* 1987, 65 (4):757–764.

9. Kumar P, Kamat A, and Mendelson CR. Estrogen receptor alpha (Eralpha) mediates stimulatory effects of estrogen on aromatase (CYP19) gene expression in human placenta. *Mol Endocrinol.* 2009, 23 (6):784–793.

10. Calzada-Mendoza CC, Sa´ nchez EC, Campos RR, et al. Differential aromatase (CYP19) expression in human arteries from normal and neoplasic uterus: An immuno-histochemical and in situ hybridization study. *Front Biosci.* 2006, 11:389–393.

11. Zbella EA, Ilekis J, Scommegna A, et al. Competitive studies with dehydroepiandrosterone sulfate and 16 alpha- hydroxyde-hydroepiandrosterone sulfate in cultured human choriocarcinoma JEG-3 cells: Effect on estrone, 17 beta-estradiol, and estriol secretion. *J Clin Endocrinol Metab.* 1986, 63 (3):751–757.

12. Milewich L, MacDonald PC, and Carr BR. Estrogen 16 alpha-hydroxylase activity in human fetal tissues. *J Clin Endocrinol Metab.* 1986, 63 (2):404–406.

13. Jobe SO, Tyler CT, and Magness RR. Aberrant synthesis, metabolism, and plasma accumulation of circulating estrogens and estrogen metabolites in preeclampsia implications for vascular dysfunction. *Hypertension.* 2013, 61(2):480–487.

14. Holinka CF, Diczfalusy E, and Coelingh Bennink HJT. Estetrol: A unique steroid in human pregnancy. *J Steroid Biochem Mol Biol.* 2008, 110 (1–2):138–143.

15. Pluchino N, Santoro AN, Casarosa E, et al. Effect of

estetrol administration on brain and serum allopregnanolone in intact and ovariectomized rats. *J Steroid Biochem Mol Biol.* 2014, 143: 285–290.

16. Jobe SO, Ramadoss J, Koch JM, et al. Estradiol-17beta and its cytochrome P450- and catechol-O-methyltransferase-derived metabolites stimulate proliferation in uterine artery endothelial cells: Role of estrogen receptor-alpha versus estrogen receptor-beta. *Hypertension.* 2010, 55(4): 1005–1011.

17. Aitio A. UDPglucuronosyltransferase of the human placenta. *Biochem Pharmacol.* 1974, 23 (15):2203–2205.

18. Gamage N, Barnett A, Hempel N, et al. Human sulfotransferases and their role in chemical metabolism. *Toxicol Sci.* 2006, 90(1):5–22.

19. Falany CN, Wheeler J, Oh TS, et al. Steroid sulfation by expressed human cytosolic sulfotransferases. *J Steroid Biochem Mol Biol.* 1994, 48 (4):369–375.

20. Tong MH, Jiang H, Liu P, et al. Spontaneous fetal loss caused by placental thrombosis in estrogen sulfotransferase-deficient mice. *Nat Med.* 2005, 11(2):153–159.

21. Pepe GJ, Burch MG,and Albrecht E. Estroge regulates 11ß-hydroxysteroid dehydrogenase-1 and -2 localization in placental syncytiotrophoblast in the second half of primate pregnancy. *Endocrinology.* 2001, 142.4496–4503.

22. Hu W, Weng X, Dong M, et al. Alteration in methylation level at 11ß-hydroxysteroid dehydrogenase type 2 gene promoter in infants born to preeclamptic women. *BMC Genetics.* 2014, 15:96.

23. Dao B, VanageG, MA, Bardin CW, et al. Anti-implantation activity of antiestrogens and mifepristone. *Contraception.* 1996, 54: 253–258.

24. Bukovsky A, Cekanova M, Caudle MR, et al. Expression and localization of estrogen receptor-alpha protein in normal and abnormal term placentae and stimulation of trophoblast differentiation by estradiol. *Reprod Biol Endocrinol.* 2003, 1:13.

25. Bukovsky A, Caudle MR, Cekanova M, et al. Placental expression of estrogen receptor beta and its hormone binding variant – Comparison with estrogen receptor alpha and a role for estrogen receptors in asymmetric division and differentiation of estrogen-dependent cells. *Reprod Biol Endocrinol.* 2003, 1:36.

26. Pijnenborg R, Vercruysse L, and Hanssens M. The uterine spiral arteries in human pregnancy: Facts and controversies. *Placenta.* 2006, 27(9–10):939–958.

27. Liu LX, Lu H, Luo Y, et al. Stabilization of vascular endothelial growth factor mRNA by hypoxia-inducible factor 1. *Biochem Biophys Res Commun.* 2002, 291 (4):908–914.

28. Losordo DW, and Isner JM. Estrogen and angiogenesis: A review. *Arterioscler Thromb Vasc Biol.* 2001, 21(1):6–12.

29. CE, ZM, Bucak K, Chu S, et al. 17Beta-estradiol up-regulates vascular endothelial growth factor receptor-2 expression in human myometrial microvascular endothelial cells: Role of estrogen receptor-alpha and -beta. *J Clin Endocrinol Metab.* 2002, 87(9):4341–4349.

30. Fotsis T, Zhang Y, Pepper MS, et al. The endogenous oestrogen metabolite 2-methoxyoestradiol inhibits angiogenesis and suppresses tumour growth. *Nature.* 1994, 368(6468):237–239.

31. Thaler I, Manor D, Itskovitz J, et al. Changes in uterine blood flow during human pregnancy. *Am J Obstet Gynecol.* 1990, 162 (1):121–125.

32. Mabie WC, DiSessa TG, Crocker LG, et al. A longitudinal study of cardiac output in normal human pregnancy. *Am J Obstet Gynecol.* 1994, 170(3):849–856.

33. Dubey RK, and Jackson EK. Potential vascular actions of 2-methoxyestradiol. *Trends Endocrinol Metab.* 2009,20 (8):374–379.

34. Rupnow HL, Phernetton TM, Shaw CE, et al. Endothelial vasodilator production by uterine and systemic arteries. VII. Estrogen and progesterone effects on eNOS. *Am J Physiol Heart Circ Physiol.* 2001, 280 (4):H1699–H1705.

35. Miller SL, Jenkin G, and Walker DW. Effect of nitric oxide synthase inhibition on the uterine vasculature of the late-pregnant ewe. *Am J Obstet Gynecol.* 1999, 180 (5):1138–1145.

36. Baggia S, Albrecht ED, and Pepe GJ. Regulation of 11 beta-hydroxysteroid dehydrogenase activity in the baboon placenta by estrogen. *Endocrinology.* 1990, 126(5):2742–2748.

37. Almey A, Milner TA, and Brake W. Estrogen receptors in the central nervous system and their implication for dopamine-dependent cognition in females. *Horm Behav.* 2015, 74:125–138.

38. Baud O, Berkane N. Hormonal changes associated with intra-uterine growth restriction: Impact on the developing brain and future neurodevelopment. *Front Endocrinol.* 2019, 10:179.

39. Hertig A, Liere P, Chabbert-Buffet N, et al. Steroid profiling in preeclamptic women: Evidence for aromatase deficiency. *Am J Obstet*

Gynecol. 2010, 203(5):477. e1–477.e9.

40. Perez-Sepulveda A, Monteiro LJ, Dobierzewska A, et al. Placental aromatase is deficient in placental ischemia and preeclampsia. *PLoS ONE.* 2015, 10(10):e0139682.

41. Kumar P, Luo Y, Tudela C, et al. The c-Myc-regulated microRNA-17~92 (miR-17~92) and miR- 106a~363 clusters target hCYP19A1 and hGCM1 to inhibit human trophoblast differentiation. *Mol Cell Biol.* 2013, 33(9): 1782–1796.

42. Ma CX, Adjei AA, Salavaggione OE, et al. Human aromatase: Gene resequencing and functional genomics. *Cancer Res.* 2005, 65(23):11071–11082.

43. Charles SM, Julian CG, Vargas E, et al. Higher estrogen levels during pregnancy in Andean than European residents of high altitude suggest differences in aromatase activity. *J Clin Endocrinol Metab.* 2014, 99(8):2908–2916.

44. Berkane N, Liere P, Lefevre G, et al. Abnormal steroidogenesis and aromatase activity and the risk of preeclampsia. *Placenta.* 2018, 69:40–49.

45. Kanasaki K, Palmsten K, Sugimoto H, et al. Deficiency in catechol-O-methyltransferase and 2-methoxyoestradiol is associated with pre-eclampsia. *Nature.* 2008, 453(7198):1117–1121.

46. Ishibashi O, Ohkuchi A, Ali MM, et al. Hydroxysteroid (17-b) dehydrogenase 1 is dysregulated by miR-210 and miR-518c that are aberrantly expressed in preeclamptic placentas: a novel marker for predicting pre-eclampsia. *Hypertension.* 2012, 59 (2):265–273.

47. Ohkuchi A, Ishibashi O, Hirashima C, et al. Plasma level of hydroxysteroid (17-b) dehydrogenase 1 in the second trimester is an independent risk factor for predicting preeclampsia after adjusting for the effects of mean blood pressure, bilateral notching and plasma level of soluble fms-like tyrosine kinase 1/ placental growth factor ratio. *Hypertens Res.* 2012, 35 (12):1152–1158.

48. Ludwikowski B, Heger S, Datz N, et al. Aromatase deficiency: Rare cause of virilization. *Eur J Pediatr Surg.* 2013, 23 (5):418–422.

49. Maliqueo M, Echiburú, B, and Crisosto N. Sex steroids modulate uterine-placental vasculature: Implications for obstetrics and neonatal outcomes. *Front Physiol.* 2016, 7:152.

50. Salih SM, Salama SA, Fadl AA, et al. Expression and cyclic variations of catechol-O-methyl transferase in human endometrial stroma. *Fertil Steril.* 2008, 90(3):789–797.

51. Rabe T, Hösch R, and Runnebaum B. Sulfatase deficiency in the human placenta: Clinical findings. *Biol Res Pregnancy Perinatol.* 1983, 4(3):95–102.

52 Young I, Renfree M, Mesiano S, et al. The comparative physiology of parturition in mammals: Hormones and parturition in mammals. 2011, 5:95–116.

53. Renthal NE, Williams KC, Montalbano AP, et al. Molecular regulation of parturition: A myometrial perspective. *Cold Spring Harb Perspect Med.* 2015, 5:a023069.

54. Weiss G. Clinical review 118. Endocrinology of parturition. *J Clin Endocrinol Metab.* 2000, 85:4421–4425.

Chapter

The Role of Progesterone in Pregnancy

6

Sam Mesiano

6.1 Introduction

Pregnancy is a remarkable physiologic state in which the female retains the conceptus in her uterus for a specific amount of time during which it grows and develops and is eventually expelled by the process of parturition as a live offspring. Intrauterine retention of the conceptus involves coordination between the uterine tissues, especially the endometrium, and the early embryo. The endometrium must be receptive to an embryo with the capacity to implant into the uterine wall and establish a physical and biochemical link with the maternal compartment to establish pregnancy. During pregnancy maternal physiology is altered such that the uterus accommodates the conceptus, and maternal metabolism changes to favor supplying the conceptus with

nutrients and oxygen. Multiple hormones, most of which are produced by the conceptus, induce the specific maternal adaptations necessary for pregnancy. One of the most important is the steroid hormone progesterone (P4) (Figure 6.1). As its name implies, P4 is "pro-gestational." It acts on the uterus to promote the establishment and maintenance of pregnancy. This chapter considers P4 from the perspective of evolutionary biology of viviparity and past and recent advances in research to elucidate its role and mechanism of actions in the hormonal control of pregnancy. Understanding the pro-gestation actions of P4 at the molecular, cell, and organism levels will be critical for the development of strategies to prevent adverse pregnancy outcomes, especially preterm birth.

Progesterone

17α-Hydroxyprogesterone

RU-486

17α-Hydroxyprogesterone caproate

Figure 6.1 Structure of progesterone, 17α-hydroxyprogesterone, 17α-hydroxyprogesterone caproate and RU-486.

6.2 Evolutionary Perspective

Embryo retention is the hallmark trait of viviparity (birth of live offspring after internal development). This highly successful reproductive strategy evolved from oviparity (egg laying and embryo development externally). Typically, the oviparous egg is endowed with a large amount of yolk and is expelled from the female soon after fertilization. The embryo then develops in the external environment using yolk as a principal nutrient. In contrast, the viviparous embryo lacking yolk has the capacity to implant into the uterine wall where it continues its development program for a specific gestation time. In eutherian species, specialized trophoblast cells in the embryo form a placenta through which oxygen and nutrients are extracted from the maternal compartment.

A common characteristic of all viviparous species is that a single hormone, P4 – produced by the maternal ovary – induces a uterine phenotype that is conducive for embryo survival and receptive for embryo implantation, retention, and gestation. In all vertebrate species, P4 is produced by the developing follicle during the pre-ovulatory period. In oviparous species, P4 levels decline immediately after ovulation (1). In contrast, in the ovary of viviparous species, the remnants of the ovulated follicle forms a distinct endocrine organ – the corpus luteum (CL) – that produces P4, that in turn acts on the reproductive tract to promotes egg retention. This effect of P4 is evolutionarily ancient. The endocrinologist and evolutionary biologist Fredrick Hisaw (2) proposed that the endocrine function of P4 to retain the conceptus is derived from "the old reptilian custom of carrying ova in the uterus until a favorable time and place was found to lay the whole clutch at once." Comparisons of oviparous and viviparous reptiles show strong correlation between the duration of egg retention after ovulation and existence and longevity of the CL (2), and administration of P4 to chickens during the post ovulatory period delays oviposition by slowing the passage of the ovulated egg through the reproductive tract (3). Thus, in the evolution of viviparity, natural selection likely favored formation and longevity of a P4-producing CL.

Hormone action is dependent on target cell receptivity and the role of P4 in the evolution of viviparity requires appropriate action of P4 in uterine cells. Actions of P4 to promote pregnancy are mediated by P4 receptors (PRs). The human PR exists as 2 isoforms – the full length PR-B and the truncated (by 164 N-terminal amino acids) PR-A that are encoded by a single gene, *PGR* (Figure 6.2). Phylogenetic and genome mapping analyses suggest that *PGR* evolved from duplication of *ERS1*, which encodes the estrogen receptor (4). This implies that estrogenic actions in vertebrate reproduction preceded P4/PR activity. Interestingly, estrogenic activity is important for egg development and sexual dimorphism in all vertebrates (oviparous and viviparous), whereas P4/PR activity is critical for pregnancy in viviparous species. Thus, P4/PR action on the female

Figure 6.2 Structure of the human PR isoforms, PR-A and PR-B. The PRs are encoded by a single gene, *PGR*, under the control of two promoters, that produces two mRNA transcripts encoding two proteins, the full- length PR-B and the truncated (by 164 amino acids) PR-A. The PRs have structures typical of steroid hormone receptors with a ligand-binding domain (LBD), a DNA-binding domain (DBD), and a nuclear localization signal (NLS), regulatory region that is highly phosphorylated, and in PR-B the B-upstream segment (BUS). PR-A and PR-B induce the expression of distinct and overlapping gene sets, and PR-A inhibits the expression (transrepression) of some PR-B-responsive genes. Response to progesterone (P4) is ultimately determined by ligand-dependent PR transcriptional activity that is affected by cell type-specific serine phosphorylation that occurs on multiple residues in both isoforms.

reproductive tract was likely critical in the constellation of traits leading to the evolution of viviparity.

6.3 History of Progesterone Discovery

The discovery of P4 (5–9) originates with the work of anatomists and histologists in the sixteenth and seventeenth centuries studying the female reproductive system. The CL was first described by the Italian anatomist Gabriele Falloppio in the mid 1500s. A role for the CL in pregnancy was suggested by the French physician and anatomist Regnier de Graaf, who in the late 1600s noted that in cows, the presence of a CL on the maternal ovaries is closely associated with pregnancy. In the next 200 years, studies of the function of multiple organs – using techniques of ablation, transplantation, and treatment with organ tissue extracts – suggested the existence of "internal secretions" as a means by which tissues in distant parts of the body communicate. This led Emil Knauer, an Austrian gynecologist and obstetrician working at the University of Vienna in the late 1800s, to perform a series of studies in rabbits that demonstrated hormonal communication between the CL and the uterus. The rabbit was an ideal model for this purpose because in this species ovulation and formation of the CL is induced by copulation and implantation occurs typically seven days later, providing a convenient window to observe and perform experiments on the post ovulatory changes in the uterine function and the process of implantation. Knauer found that embryo implantation did not occur if the ovaries were removed soon after copulation. Importantly, he found that implantation occurs normally if ovaries containing CL were retransplanted into ovariectomized animals. He also found that ovariectomy abolished the characteristic post-ovulatory thickening of the endometrium, which was also restored by CL transplantation. At around the same time, the German anatomist and microscopist Johannes Sobotta described the ultrastructure of the mouse CL as typical of a ductless gland with a robust blood supply. Studies by Gustave Born, a German experimental embryologist, who found that implantation in rabbits was prevented by post-coital removal of

the CL by cauterization, leaving the remainder of the ovary intact. At the same time, similar outcomes were reported by Auguste Prénant, a French histologist studying the cyclic changes in the endometrium. Thus, in the early 1900s it was clear that the CL, via internal secretion mediated by the blood stream, induces thickening of the endometrium, and is essential for the establishment of pregnancy in rabbits.

This set a path to isolate and characterize the pro-pregnancy CL substance; a task that was taken up by George Corner and Willard Allen at the University of Rochester in the 1920s. Corner and Allen produced extracts of porcine CL and used the rabbit bioassay to isolate and characterize the CL substance that promotes thickening of the endometrium. They found that the CL substance, which they referred to as "progestin," partitioned exclusively in alcohol extracts of CL. They subsequently reported a highly enriched progestin with an empirical formula: $C_{21}H_{30}O_2$. In 1934, crystalline forms of progestin from porcine CL were isolated (10–13) and, as its structure was determined to be a delta-4-3-ketosteroid (11) (Figure 6.1), it was aptly renamed "progesterone" (14). The term "progestin" continues to be used to describe natural or synthetic compounds with pro-gestational activity.

In the following decades innovative strategies to synthesize P4 were developed and sufficient pure hormone became available for basic and clinical research. Multiple groups confirmed that P4 thickens the endometrium and induces an intrauterine state that is receptive for embryo implantation. In the 1940s and 50s, P4 derivative and other steroids with progestin activity were synthesized. A champion of this effort was Karl Junkmann at the pharmaceutical company Schering, AG, who examined multiple compounds, and in 1958 reported that the caproic acid salt of 7α-hydroxyprogesterone (17HPC) (Figure 6.1) has potent progestin activity in animal models. Clinical studies of various compounds in estrogen-primed castrated women confirmed that 17HPC is more potent and longer-acting than pure P4 (15). Those studies paved the way for clinical trials of 17HPC for the prevention of pre-term birth (discussed below).

By the mid 1950s it was clear from animal studies that P4 produced by the CL is essential for embryo implantation and the maintenance of pregnancy. However, understanding of P4 in human pregnancy was scant. A major problem was the inability to accurately measure circulating levels of P4 during pregnancy. A solution to the problem came in 1936 when Elenor Venning and J. S. L. Browne (16,17) found that P4 is metabolized to pregnanediol and excreted as urinary pregnanediol-3α-glucuronide. Importantly, they developed a relatively simple (compared with the rabbit endometrium bioassay) gravimetric method to measure urinary pregnanediol glucuronidate, and thus provided a convenient assay, albeit indirect, for circulating P4. Multiple studies using that assay found that the level of circulating total P4 in women during pregnancy is high relative to levels in nonpregnant women and remains elevated during parturition, decreasing only after delivery of the placenta.

Those studies suggested that the placenta is the source of P4 in human pregnancy. This was inconsistent with animal studies at the time showing that the CL is the exclusive source of P4 during pregnancy. Nonetheless, a role for P4 produced by the CL in human pregnancy was suspected from earlier clinical studies in the 1930s showing that miscarriage is common in pregnancies with ovarian abnormalities, especially those affecting the CL (18). In the 1960s, Arpad Csapo, an obstetrician and research biochemist working at Johns Hopkins University, explored the source of P4 in human pregnancy as part of a clinical trial of oophorectomy in women seeking pregnancy termination. He found that removal of the ovaries caused miscarriage. However, this effect occurred only if the ovaries were removed sometime before weeks seven to ten of pregnancy. Miscarriage did not occur if oophorectomy was performed after the tenth week (19). The studies showed the maternal CL is the exclusive source of P4 prior to approximately week ten weeks of pregnancy, and after that time the placenta becomes an additional site of P4 production. Csapo referred to the initiation of placental P4 production as the luteo-placental shift (20). It is now clear that P4 required for the establishment of human pregnancy is provided by the CL and that the prolonged longevity of the CL – which usually regresses in the latter half of the luteal phase – and its continued production of P4 is induced by chorionic gonadotropin (CG) secreted by trophoblast cells in the embryo. At around the end of the

first trimester the placenta also produces P4, which continues for the remainder of pregnancy.

6.4 Mechanism of P4 Action

The mechanism by which P4 affect uterine cells was unknown until the mid-1960s. The basic principals were set by Elwood Jensen who first identified estrogen receptors (ERs) by tracking the tissue uptake of radiolabeled estradiol (E2) injected into castrated rats. He found specific uptake of labelled E2 into the uterus and vagina. At around the same time Bert O'Malley and colleagues found that P4 induces gene expression in chicken oviduct (21,22). In 1970, Etienne-Emile Baulieu and colleagues (23), using the same methods as Jensen, injected radiolabeled P4 into castrated and E2-treated guinea pigs and identified a high affinity binding protein in the cytosol of uterus. The putative PR was detected only in the uterus, and its level was increased by E2. Subsequent studies found that the PR accumulates and is retained in the nucleus of uterine cells. The nuclear localization was consistent with O'Malley's finding that P4 affects gene expression. Several years later O'Malley and colleagues isolated and characterized the human PR (24) and confirmed that it functions primarily as a ligand-activated transcription factor. They went on to identify some key co-regulatory factors that qualitatively and quantitatively modulate P4/PR transcriptional activity in a cell type and gene promoter specific manner. It is now well-established that P4 affects cell function primarily by binding to the PR isoforms, PR-A and PR-B (encoded by *PGR*) that each function as ligand activated transcription factors to affect the expression of specific genes whose products cause the response to P4. The pleiotropic actions of P4 can be explained by the fact that PR function is affected by cell type, physiologic state, and gene promoter region. Transcriptional activity of PRs is also modulated by transcription co-regulators (repressors and activators) and by the interaction of PRs with other transcription factors (e.g. AP-1, NF-kB) and signaling molecules (e.g. Src). In addition cell-type specific PR function is affected by post-translational modifications, such as site-specific phosphorylation and sumoylation.

Ligand structure also affects PR transcriptional activity, which has led to the development of selective PR modulators (SPRMs). A well characterized SPRM is RU-486, a steroidal compound (Figure 6.1) that binds the PR with high affinity but fails to activate its transcriptional activity. RU-486 also binds the glucocorticoid receptor (GR), albeit with lower affinity. As RU-486 predominantly binds to the PRs (25) it is considered to act primarily in the reproductive systems as a competitive PR antagonist. RU-486 is a potent abortifacient that ends pregnancy by either miscarriage or parturition at all stages of pregnancy and in all species examined so far. This reflects the fundamental role for P4/PR signaling in the establishment and maintenance of pregnancy.

6.5 Establishment of Pregnancy

To establish pregnancy, P4 produced by the CL acts via PRs on uterine endometrial cells to induce an endometrial phenotype conducive for embryo implantation. In a typical ovarian cycle (estrus or menstrual), P4 is produced initially by granulosa cells of the pre-ovulatory ovarian follicle and then by luteinized granulosa cells in the CL. P4 production by the CL is stimulated by luteinizing hormone (LH) secreted by the anterior lobe of the pituitary gland. The cells also produced E2, albeit to a lesser extent than P4. Consequently, during the post-ovulatory luteal phase, the CL produces P4 and E2 in response to LH. The production of E2 is important because it sensitizes uterine cells to P4 by inducing expression of *PGR*.

P4/PR signaling induces the stratum functionalis layer of the endometrium to transform into a glandular, secretory, and highly vascularized tissue that is receptive for embryo implantation, especially between days 20 and 24 of the menstrual cycle (i.e. 6 to 10 days after ovulation). This is considered to be the optimum time window for implantation. After this time the endometrial stromal cells, in response to P4, undergo morphologic change by a process referred to as decidualization. Decidualization occurs in all cycles (fertile and nonfertile) and involves the proliferation and hypertrophy of stromal fibroblasts, the formation of dense extracellular matrix between stromal cells, and shrinkage and altered secretory activity of glandular epithelium (26). Decidualization facilitates embryo implantation. However, once established, the dense extracellular matrix of the decidualized endometrium restricts

de novo embryo implantation, effectively closing the implantation window.

In nonfertile cycles, beginning in the latter third of the luteal phase, the CL gradually regresses, leading to a decrease in P4 production. Withdrawal of P4 support causes tissue-level inflammation and necrosis in the decidualized endometrium, leading to its shedding by menstruation. A new receptive endometrium is then regenerated in response to rising levels of E2 in the follicular phase of the following cycle. In a fertile cycle, CG produced by trophoblast cells in the embryo prevents CL regression, leading to sustained P4 production. The prolonged longevity of the CL and its continued production of P4 maintains the decidualized endometrium, which is crucial for the establishment of pregnancy. Under the influence of P4, the decidualized endometrium, referred to as the decidua, persists for the remainder of pregnancy and sheds with the placenta and fetal membranes at parturition.

The decidua is composed of decidual stromal cells and resident maternal immune cells that together form the maternal component of the physical maternal-fetal interface. As the adjacent fetal cell (cytotrophoblast cells in the chorion membrane, the syncytiotrophoblast of the placental villus, and invading trophoblast cells) are immunologically foreign, resident immune cells in the decidua must be in a tolerogenic state to avoid immune rejection of the semi-allogeneic conceptus. P4 is thought to promote immune tolerance by inducing cytokines and chemokines in the decidual cells that recruit and enrich leukocytes to the maternal-fetal interface with attenuated cytotoxic activity and increased immunosuppressive activity (27). Loss of P4-induced immune tolerance is thought to create a tissue-level inflammatory state that causes labor.

6.6 Maintenance of Pregnancy

In 1956, Arpad Csapo proposed that P4 maintains pregnancy by blocking labor. This implies that the uterus is poised to expel or resorb the conceptus throughout pregnancy were it not for the blocking actions of P4/PR. Indeed, in all animals examined to date, specific removal of the P4/PR block by ablating the source of P4 (e.g. by ovariectomy) or inhibiting PR activity (e.g. by treating with RU-486) induces resorption or parturition. A leading hypothesis to explain how P4/PR blocks labor is that it inhibits expression of genes encoding pro-labor factors, referred to collectively as contraction-associated proteins (CAPs). For example, Renthal et al. (28) found that in myometrial cells, P4/PR increases the transcription factor ZEB1, which inhibits expression of two important CAP genes: *GJA1*, which encodes connexin-43 that forms gap junctions to electrically couple myometrial cells, and *OXTR*, which encodes the receptor for oxytocin, a potent stimulator of uterine contraction.

P4/PR also maintains uterine quiescence by inhibiting responsiveness of uterine cells to pro-labor/pro-inflammatory stimuli (i.e. an anti-inflammatory action). In the 1970s, Pentti Siiteri and colleagues proposed that P4 blocks labor by immunosuppressive and anti-inflammatory actions (29). This hypothesis was supported by more recent in vitro studies showing that in myometrial cells, P4/PR inhibits responsiveness to inflammatory cytokines associated with the onset of labor (30). Anti-inflammatory action of P4/PR are important because parturition is considered to be an inflammatory event characterized by activated neutrophil infiltration, edema, and expression of pro-inflammatory cytokines and chemokines in the myometrium, cervix, and decidua (31,32). Tissue-level inflammation is thought to increase local production of prostaglandins that induce myometrial contraction, cervical ripening, and membrane rupture (i.e. labor).

6.7 Parturition and P4 Withdrawal

The success of viviparity requires that pregnancy ends with a viable neonate and a healthy mother. Withdrawal of the P4 block to parturition is a core event in the constellation of physiologic signals to end pregnancy. In most animals (e.g. mouse, rat, rabbit, sheep) this occurs by a prepartum systemic decrease in maternal P4 levels caused by CL regression (e.g. mouse, rat, rabbit) or changes in placental P4 metabolism (e.g. sheep), and in all animals ablation of P4 production or disruption of PR signaling with RU-486 induces parturition. Human parturition occurs without a decrease in maternal blood P4 levels. Instead, uterine cells are exposed to high levels of P4 before and during parturition. Nonetheless, interruption of PR activity with RU-486 increases myometrial contractility and promotes softening of the cervix, and generally induces the full parturition cascade all stages of pregnancy. This suggests that human parturition is triggered by changes in P4/PR activity in uterine cells such that the P4/PR block to labor is functionally withdrawn.

Several mechanisms for functional P4/PR withdrawal have been proposed. The PR-A/PR-B hypothesis posits opposing actions of the PR isoforms in uterine cells whereby PR-B mediates labor-blocking actions of P4, whereas PR-A opposes those actions (33). In this scenario, labor is induced by a switch from PR-B to PR-dominance. In vitro studies show that in myometrial cells, PR-A inhibits the transcriptional activity of PR-B and that this occurs when the level of PR-A is greater than that of PR-B (34). Studies of term myometrium show that the onset of labor is associated with an increase in the abundance of PR-A relative to PR-B (35) and that this may be induced by epigenetic modification of the *PGR* promotor region controlling PR-A expression (36). Studies of the molecular biology PR isoform activity in human myometrial cells show that phosphorylation of PR-A at serine residues 344 and 345 (pSer[344/345]-PRA; numbering relative to amino acid 1 in PR-B) induces its inhibitory activity on P4/PR-B anti-inflammatory activity (37). Importantly, parallel analyses showed that in term, myometrium pSer[344/345]-PRA was present exclusively in the nucleus of myometrial cells, and its abundance increased in association with the onset of labor. P4/PR transcriptional activity in term myometrium also could be inhibited by a decrease in the level of PR co-activators and reduced histone acetylation (impedes transcription by increasing chromatin condensation) in the promoters of PR target genes (38).

An intracrine mechanism for localized P4 withdrawal also may affect PR transcriptional activity. In this model, increased 20α hydroxysteroid dehydrogenase (20αHSD) activity in uterine cells converts P4 to an inactive form that cannot activate PR, thus decreasing intracellular P4 activity (39). In vitro data suggest that this produces ligand-free PR-A with transcriptional activity that increases expression of stimulatory pro-labor CAP genes, such as *GJA1* (40,41).

Taken together, the data suggest that for most of pregnancy, P4 via PR-B in uterine effector cells blocks labor by inhibiting the response to pro-labor/pro-inflammatory stimuli. Functional withdrawal of P4/PR-B anti-inflammatory could be

Figure 6.3 Mechanisms for P4/PR-B withdrawal to initiate human parturition. This could occur by increased PR-A trans-repressive activity via increased abundance of PR-A relative to PR-B and/or phosphorylation of PR-A, metabolism of P4 to an inactive form and the formation of unliganded PR-A, and direct inhibition of PR-B transcriptional activity by a decreases in co-activators or an increase on co-repressors [from (49)].

mediated by increased trans-repressive activity of PR-A, decreased transcriptional activity of the PRs at promoters of specific target genes, and/or localized intracellular P4 withdrawal leading to altered PR-A activity. The net effect is to allow tissue-level inflammation that transforms the uterus to the laboring state (Figure 6.3).

The finding that P4/PR withdrawal occurs by multiple pathways, some of which are linked to stress/inflammation, is consistent with the diversity in the timing of term parturition across viviparous species. Progestin activity of P4/PR is highly conserved whereas diversity exists in mechanisms by which the P4 block to labor is withdrawn to trigger parturition. The timing of term birth would have been under strong selective pressure to match other traits in the reproductive cycle, such as seasonal versus continuous fertility; polytocous versus singleton pregnancy; postpartum estrus versus lactation-associated infertility; level of social structure; extent of fetal encephalization relative to the size of the pelvic outlet (i.e. the obstetric dilemma); and the capacity to supply sufficient energy for fetal brain growth. Natural selection would have favored birth timing traits that optimize pregnancy outcome and overall reproductive efficiency. In this contexts it is plausible that natural selection favored multiple redundant mechanisms to end pregnancy via

P4/PR withdrawal. A major influence was likely the survival risks conferred by pregnancy and parturition to the female and her offspring. In this scenario the interests of the female and her future pregnancies would be favored over the current pregnancy. Although pregnancy should ideally end with a healthy neonate and mother, it should at least end with a healthy female capable of future pregnancies. Therefore, signaling pathways likely evolved to link P4/PR withdrawal with exposure of the uterine tissues to stress-related inflammatory stimuli. This system is likely threshold-limited such that P4/PR withdrawal occurs only when the stress/inflammatory load on the uterine tissues exceeds a certain level. One hypothesis is that the stress/inflammatory load on the uterine tissues increases with advancing gestation with a trajectory that usually reaches the threshold at term. The inflammatory load trajectory could be affected by intrinsic (e.g. uterine wall distention; fetal development) and extrinsic (e.g. intrauterine infection; maternal stress) factors, and under pathologic high-stress conditions could be shifted to the left leading to pre-term birth (Figure 6.4). Based on this model therapies to control birth timing, and especially prevent pre-term birth, may involve targeting the inflammatory load trajectory, and the mechanism by which inflammation induces P4/PR withdrawal.

6.8 Progestin Therapy to Prevent Pre-term Birth

In the mid-1950s, increased availability of pure P4 led to clinical trials of its effectiveness to prevent threatened and recurrent early pregnancy loss and pre-term birth. It was found that P4 therapy promoted and sustained pregnancy only in conditions of endogenous P4 deficiency due to CL insufficiency, if the CL was surgically removed, or in cases of fetal/placental demise (42). Although it was clear that P4 therapy was effective only in cases where it corrects endogenous P4 deficiency, in the 1960s clinical trials were performed to explore the capacity for P4 to suppress labor. Early studies examined the tocolytic effects of P4 administered as an intravenous or intra-amniotic bolus in laboring women. It was concluded that acute P4 (up to 1g P4 was injected in some studies) therapy is not effective as a tocolytic (43). Thus, once labor begins it cannot be stopped by exogenous P4. Another series of clinical studies

Figure 6.4 Model linking stress/inflammation to P4 withdrawal. Cells of the gravid uterus are exposed to inflammatory stress from multiple intrinsic (e.g. uterine wall over-distention) and extrinsic (e.g. maternal environmental stress; intrauterine infection) sources that impart a net inflammatory load. The inflammatory load increases with advancing gestation, and the trajectory of increase can be affected by pathologic and environmental conditions. At a specific inflammatory load threshold pathways are activated by stress stimuli that induce P4/PR-B withdrawal. Upon loss of P4/PR-B anti-inflammatory activity, a positive feedback proinflammatory state occurs in the uterine tissues leading to the onset of labor.

examined the effect of progestin prophylaxis with 17HPC. Although clinical trials of 17HPC prophylaxis produced mixed outcomes and were generally underpowered, meta-analysis of the data suggested that 17HPC prophylaxis decreased the incidence of pre-term birth (44). This provided the justification of larger trials that examined the effect of progestin therapy beginning at mid-gestation with micronized P4 administered by vaginal suppository daily (45) or 17HPC administered by intramuscular injection weekly (46). Both treatments decreased the incidence of pre-term birth. 17HPC appeared effective in women with elevated risk due to a history of pre-term birth, and vaginal micronized P4 was affective in women with a short cervix detected at mid gestation by ultrasound. Those findings led to the widespread use of progestin prophylaxis in the form of 17HPC or micronized P4 to reduce the risk for pre-term birth in women with specific risk factors. However, recent larger clinical trials showed that neither therapy decreases the risk for pre-term birth regardless of predisposing risk (47,48). Progestin prophylaxis for pre-term birth prevention is currently an area of controversy among clinicians, and the mechanism(s) by which the therapies may prevent PTB in some women remains unknown. However, from a purely physiologic perspective the negative outcomes are expected because there is no evidence

that pre-term birth is caused by P4 deficiency that can be corrected by supplementation. Nonetheless, the potent progestin activity of P4/PR is unequivocal, and exploiting this action is a biologically plausible approach to control the timing of birth. The next generation of P4/PR-based therapies will likely come from ongoing advances in understanding the molecular biology of P4/PR signaling in human uterine cells and how it is controlled to cause P4/PR withdrawal (49).

6.9 Conclusion

Aptly referred to as the hormone of pregnancy, P4 is essential for the establishment and maintenance of pregnancy, and the physiologic control of its withdrawal, whether actual or functional, is the principal trigger for parturition. Research leading to the discovery of P4 was performed by leaders in the fields of anatomy, histology, reproductive biology, biochemistry, and clinical endocrinology. The concept of the CL as an "organ of internal secretion" was prescient, occurring a decade before Baylis and Starling reported their discovery of the hormonal actions of the pancreases that heralded the field of endocrinology. Since its discovery in 1934, major advances in understanding the role and mechanism of action of P4 in the control of

57

pregnancy and parturition have led to the current consensus that progestin actions of P4 to maintain pregnancy are mediated by transcriptional activity of the nuclear PRs in uterine myometrial, decidual and cervical cells. Importantly, parturition in women involves changes in PR transcriptional activity that removes the P4/PR block to labor. Current advances in understanding the molecular biology of P4/PR signaling in uterine cells, especially in the context of human pregnancy and parturition, will likely reveal novel therapeutic strategies to effectively boost the progestin activity of P4 to prevent adverse pregnancy outcomes, especially pre-term birth.

Acknowledgments

Supported by funding from the Eunice Kennedy Shriver National Institute of Child Health and Human Development, and March of Dimes.

References

1. Callard IP, Fileti LA, Perez LE, et al. Role of the corpus luteum and progesterone in the evolution of vertebrate viviparity. *Am. Zool.* 1992, 32:264–275.

2. Hisaw FL. Endocrine adaptations of the mammalian estrous cycle and gestation. In: Gorbman A, ed. *Comparative Endocrinology.* 1959; 533–552. New York.: John Wiley & Sons.

3. Wilson SC, andSharp PJ. The effects of progesterone on oviposition and ovulation in the domestic fowl (Gallus domesticus). *Br Poult Sci.* 1976, 17:163–173.

4. Thornton JW. Evolution of vertebrate steroid receptors from an ancestral estrogen receptor by ligand exploitation and serial genome expansions. *Proc Natl Acad Sci USA.* 2001, 98:5671–5676.

5. Corner GW. *The Hormones in Human Reproduction.* London: Princeton University Press.

6. Allen WM. Recollections of my life with progesterone. *Gynecol Invest.* 1974, 5:142–182.

7. Corner GW, Sr. The early history of progesterone. *Gynecol Invest.* 1974, 5:106–112.

8. Medvei VC. A History of Clinical Endocrinology. New York: The Parthenon Publishing Group.

9. Frobenius W. Ludwig Fraenkel: 'Spiritus rector' of the early progesterone research. *Eur J Obstet Gynecol Reprod Biol.* 1999, 83:115–119.

10. Allen WM, and Wintersteiner O. Crystalline progestin. *Science.* 1934, 80:190–191.

11. Butenandt A, andWestphal U. Zur Isolierung und Characterisierung des Corpus-luteum-Hormons. *Ber Chem Ges.* 1934, 67:1440–1442.

12. Hartmann M, and Wettstein A. Ein krystallisiertes Hormon aus Corpus luteum. *Helv Chim Acta.* 1934, 17:878–882.

13. Slotta K, Ruschig H, and Fels E. Reindarstellung der Hormone aus dem Corpus luteum. *Ber Chem Ges.* 1934, 67:1270–1273.

14. Allen WM, Butenandt A, Corner GW, et al. Nomenclature of corpus luteum hormone. *Science.* 1935, 82:153.

15. Davis ME, and Wied GL. 17-alpha-hydroxyprogesterone-caproate: A new substance with prolonged progestational activity: A comparison with chemically pure progesterone. *J Clin Endocrinol Metabol.* 1955, 15:923–930.

16. Venning EH, and Browne JSL. Isolation of a water-soluble pregnandiol complex from human pregnancy urine. *Proc Soc Exper Biol and Med.* 1936, 34:729.

17. Venning EH. Gravimetric method for the determination of sodium pregnandiol glucuronidate (an excretion product of progesterone). *J Biol Chem.* 1937, 119:473.

18. Wilson KM, and Rochester NY. Pregnancy complicated by ovarian and paraovarian tumors. *Am J Ob/Gyn.* 1937, 34:977–986.

19. Csapo AI, Pulkkinen MO, Ruttner B, et al. The significance of the human corpus luteum in pregnancy maintenance. I. Preliminary studies. *Am J Obstet Gynecol.* 1972, 112:1061–1067.

20. Csapo A. The luteo-placental shift, the guardian of pre-natal life. *Postgrad Med J.* 1969, 45:57–64.

21. O'Malley BW. In vitro hormonal induction of a specific protein (avidin) in chick oviduct. *Biochemistry.* 1967, 6:2546–2551.

22. O'Malley BW, and Korenman SG. Studies on the mechanism of hormone induction of a specific protein. Immunological identity and kinetic studies of avidin synthesized in vitro by the chick oviduct. *Life Sci.* 1967, 6:1953–1959.

23. Milgrom E, Atger M, and Baulieu EE. Progesterone in uterus and plasma. IV. Progesterone receptor(s) in guinea pig uterus cytosol. *Steroids.* 1970, 16:741–754.

24. Smith RG, Iramain CA, Buttram VC, Jr., et al.

Purification of human uterine progesterone receptor. *Nature*. 1975, 253:271–272.

25. Heikinheimo O, Kontula K, Croxatto H, et al. Plasma concentrations and receptor binding of RU 486 and its metabolites in humans. *J Steroid Biochem*. 1987, 26:279–284.

26. Gellersen B, Brosens IA, and Brosens JJ. Decidualization of the human endometrium: mechanisms, functions, and clinical perspectives. *Sem Reprod Med*. 2007, 25:445–453.

27. Mao G, Wang J, Kang Y, et al. Progesterone increases systemic and local uterine proportions of CD4+CD25+ Treg cells during midterm pregnancy in mice. *Endocrinology*. 2010, 151:5477–5488.

28. Renthal NE, Chen CC, Williams KC, et al. miR-200 family and targets, ZEB1 and ZEB2, modulate uterine quiescence and contractility during pregnancy and labor. *Proc Natl Acad Sci USA*. 2010, 107:20828–20833.

29. Siiteri PK, Febres F, Clemens LE, et al. Progesterone and maintenance of pregnancy: is progesterone nature's immunosuppressant? *Ann NY Acad Sci*. 1977, 286:384–397.

30. Hardy DB, Janowski BA, Corey DR, et al. Progesterone receptor plays a major antiinflammatory role in human myometrial cells by antagonism of nuclear factor-kappaB activation of cyclooxygenase 2 expression. *Mol Endocrinol*. 2006, 20:2724–2733.

31. Thomson AJ, Telfer JF, Young A, et al. Leukocytes infiltrate the myometrium during human parturition: further evidence that labour is an inflammatory process. *Hum Reprod*. 1999, 14:229–236.

32. Osman I, Young A, Jordan F, et al. Leukocyte density and proinflammatory mediator expression in regional human fetal membranes and decidua before and during labor at term. *J Soc Gynecol Invest*. 2006, 13:97–103.

33. Mesiano S, Chan EC, Fitter JT, et al. Progesterone withdrawal and estrogen activation in human parturition are coordinated by progesterone receptor A expression in the myometrium. *J Clin Endocrinol Metabol*. 2002, 87:2924–2930.

34. Tan H, Yi L, Rote NS, et al. Progesterone receptor-A and -B have opposite effects on proinflammatory gene expression in human myometrial cells: Implications for progesterone actions in human pregnancy and parturition. *J Clin Endocrinol Metabol*. 2012, 97:E719–730.

35. Merlino AA, Welsh TN, Tan H, et al. Nuclear progesterone receptors in the human pregnancy myometrium: evidence that parturition involves functional progesterone withdrawal mediated by increased expression of progesterone receptor-A. *J Clin Endocrinol Metabol*. 2007, 92:1927–1933.

36. Chai SY, Smith R, Fitter JT, et al. Increased progesterone receptor A expression in labouring human myometrium is associated with decreased promoter occupancy by the histone demethylase JARID1A. *Mol Hum Reprod*. 2014, 20:442–453.

37. Amini P, Michniuk D, Kuo K, et al. Human parturition involves phosphorylation of progesterone receptor-A at serine-345 in myometrial cells. *Endocrinology*. 2016, 157:4434–4445.

38. Condon JC, Jeyasuria P, Faust JM, et al. A decline in the levels of progesterone receptor coactivators in the pregnant uterus at term may antagonize progesterone receptor function and contribute to the initiation of parturition. *Proc Natl Acad Sci USA*. 2003, 100:9518–9523.

39. Mahendroo MS, Porter A, Russell DW, et al. The parturition defect in steroid 5alpha-reductase type 1 knockout mice is due to impaired cervical ripening. *Mol Endocrinol*. 1999, 13:981–992.

40. Nadeem L, Shynlova O, Matysiak-Zablocki E, et al. Molecular evidence of functional progesterone withdrawal in human myometrium. *Nat Commun*. 2016, 7:11565.

41. Nadeem L, Shynlova O, Mesiano S, et al. Progesterone via its type-A receptor promotes myometrial gap junction coupling. *Sci Rep*. 2017, 7:13357.

42. Bengtsson LP. The Effect of Progesterone on the Maintenance of Early Pregnancy. Paper presented at: Brook Lodge Symposium: Progesterone 1961; Augusta, MI.

43. Pinto RM, Montuori E, Lerner U, et al. Effect of progesterone on the oxytocic action of estradiol-17-beta. *Am J Obstet Gynecol*. 1965, 91:1084–1089.

44. Keirse MJ. Progestogen administration in pregnancy may prevent preterm delivery. *Br J Obstet Gynaecol*. 1990, 97:149–154.

45. da Fonseca EB, Bittar RE, Carvalho MH, et al. Prophylactic administration of progesterone by vaginal suppository to reduce the incidence of spontaneous preterm birth in women at increased risk: a randomized placebo-controlled double-blind study. *Am J Obstet Gynecol*. 2003, 188: 419–424.

59

46. Meis PJ, Klebanoff M, Thom E, et al. Prevention of recurrent preterm delivery by 17 alpha-hydroxyprogesterone caproate. *N Engl J Med.* 2003, 348:2379–2385.

47. Norman JE, Marlow N, Messow CM, et al. Vaginal progesterone prophylaxis for preterm birth (the OPPTIMUM study): A multicentre, randomised, double-blind trial. *Lancet.* 2016, 387:2106–2116.

48. Blackwell SC, Gyamfi-Bannerman C, Biggio JR, Jr., et al. 17-OHPC to prevent recurrent preterm birth in singleton gestations (PROLONG Study): A multicenter, international. *Randomized Double-Blind Trial. Am J Perinatol.* 2020, 37:127–136.

49. Weatherborn M, and Mesiano S. Rationale for current and future progestin-based therapies to prevent preterm birth. *Best Prac Res Clin Obstet Gynaecol.* 2018, 52:114–125.

Chapter

7

Hormones and Cardiovascular Systems in Pregnancy

Daniele Farsetti and Herbert Valensise

7.1 Introduction

Maternal cardiovascular adaptation to pregnancy is expected to create optimal conditions for growth and development of the fetus. Several studies have demonstrated progressive structural and functional changes in maternal cardiovascular and volume regulatory systems. Conversely, inadequate cardiac adaptation is related to several gestational disorders and to the inability to support fetal growth.

Many studies suggest that the driver mechanism of these changes is linked to endocrine system, leading to vasodilation and decreasing responsiveness to vasoconstrictor stimuli.

Different mechanisms are related to the decreasing systemic vascular resistance (SVR) during pregnancy. The role of vasodilator factors – such as estrogen, progesterone, prostaglandin, nitric oxide (NO), and relaxin – and the contribution of the uteroplacental unit's low resistance have been studied extensively.

This chapter aims to explore the role of hormonal system in the cardiovascular changes during pregnancy.

7.2 Cardiovascular Changes

Cardiovascular changes during pregnancy are so intense that they are even greater than those observed in athletes after several years of exercise. These profound changes aim to create optimal conditions for the growth and development of the fetus without compromising maternal health.

During the early phase of pregnancy, the SVR suddenly drops, probably as a consequence of the hormonally driven opening of microcirculatory arteriovenous shunts (1). Arterial blood pressure later decreases and that's detected by baroreceptors. Then, the activation of autonomic and hormonal systems leads to two main compensatory mechanisms: the rise of sympathetic tone, and the activation

of renin-angiotensin-aldosterone system (RAAS). Cardiac sympathetic tone increases heart rate (HR) and stroke volume (SV) in order to increase cardiac output (CO) to comply arterial demands.

The first response of the cardiovascular system is to compensate for arterial demands using the blood volume reserve of the venous system; subsequently, the RAAS produces an increment in plasma volume to balance loss in venous reserve.

7.2.1 Plasma Volume

As just described, plasma volume starts to increase in the early phase of pregnancy. It gradually increases throughout gestation, reaching the maximum expansion (about 50 percent) during the last weeks (Table 7.1). This increment is related to the size and the number of fetuses. In fact, it is progressively higher in twins, triplets, and quadruplets. Plasma volume increases more than red blood cell mass causing a "physiological anemia." After pregnancy, it returns to normal value in about three months.

Plasma volume expansion is the result of sodium and water retention which is caused by the compensatory systems to vascular underfilling described in previous section. These systems modify the volume homeostasis and compensate for water dissipation mechanisms: The renal blood flow is increased, as well as the renal hyperfiltration, and the progesterone has a competing action with aldosterone for binding receptors in distal tubules. On the other hand, increased antidiuretic hormone (ADH) secretion and drinking result in increased water retention and consequently plasma osmolality is reduced despite sodium retention.

About two thirds of plasma volume is usually contained in the venous system. This reserve is used by the organism to compensate for increased arterial demands, as it happens in early pregnancy. The venous compartment and plasma volume depend on several determinants, such as body composition, daily exercise level, and renal function, but also the birth weight centile. Women who were born Small for Gestational Age (SGA) are predisposed for low plasma volume in adult life, and they also have an increased risk of developing hypertension during pregnancy and during their life in general. It has been demonstrated that birth weight centile is associated with adult plasma volume regardless of body composition, smoking, blood pressure, physical activity, cardiac performance, lipid levels, glucose metabolism, renal function, and levels of sex hormones (2). Plasma volume also relates with sympathetic tone and venous system function. The venous system function is the capacity to modify the venous compartment tone in response to external changes. This function can be reduced by structural and functional changes like increased smooth muscle contraction and collagen mass, secondary to an increased sympathetic tone.

All the described conditions could result in low plasma volume, which could be present even before pregnancy. It predisposes to early-pregnancy circulatory maladaptation and subsequent development of hypertensive disorders. In pregnant women with hypertensive disorders or fetal growth restriction (FGR), plasma volume is consistently lower throughout the gestation compared to healthy pregnancies, long before clinical manifestations of these conditions.

7.2.2 Hemodynamic Changes

Maternal hemodynamics change in order to meet the increased metabolic demands of the mother and the fetus and to ensure adequate uteroplacental perfusion.

Cardiovascular system modifications begin during the first weeks of pregnancy, prior to complete placentation. The CO is the volume of blood that heart pumps per minute. It is defined as the product between SV and HR. It starts to increase by the fifth week throughout the first trimester (3), and reaches a peak at the beginning of the third trimester that is approximately 30 to 50 percent higher than nonpregnant women's values (Table 7.1).

The rise of CO in the early phase of pregnancy is mediated by the increment of SV, which remains stable during the second and third trimesters. The HR, that gradually increases by 15 to 25 percent during pregnancy, mainly contributes

to the CO changing after the end of the second trimester (4). After delivery the CO decreases and returns to pre-pregnancy values in four to six months.

SVR is the steady component of afterload which is the force against which the heart has to pump to open the aortic valve ejecting blood. As described above, the systemic vasodilation is the result of the action of several hormones, such as progesterone, estradiol, and relaxin, and of simultaneous set-point resetting of various systems that regulates vascular tone and intravascular volume.

During pregnancy, the vasodilation leads to a reduction of SVR that begins in fifth week and progressively decreases to the nadir (35 to 50 percent) during the second trimester. SVR slightly increases at the end of pregnancy, and after the delivery it gradually returns to pre-pregnancy levels.

Arterial blood pressure decreases during pregnancy. In particular, diastolic blood pressure reduces more than systolic blood pressure. Blood pressure starts reducing in early pregnancy. By the sixth week, it has already fallen by about 3 to 5 mmHg relative to pre-pregnancy values. It reaches the nadir during the second trimester and slightly increases until the end of pregnancy to reach pre-pregnancy values near the term (Table 7.1). Recently some authors have talked about "first-trimester blood pressure dip" instead of "mid-pregnancy dip." As a matter of fact, they affirm that the nadir is in the first trimester, and at the beginning of the second trimester blood pressure starts to increase slightly.

Twin pregnancies present more profound hemodynamic changes compared to singleton: The CO is 15 percent higher, and there is higher volume overload and larger left atrial diameter.

The hemodynamic assessment in pregnancy is performed by using noninvasive techniques. The echocardiography is the gold standard for this kind of evaluation, and it is important to follow some rules to obtain reliable measurements. For example, the position of the woman during the exam is crucial: She should lie down in the left lateral decubitus position in order to avoid aortocaval compression that could reduce the cardiac output.

7.2.3 Cardiac Changes

During pregnancy, the cardiac volume overload, secondary to increased blood volume, leads the heart to develop a physiological eccentric hypertrophy which is characterized by chamber enlargement and proportional change in wall thickness (Table 7.1). This hypertrophy occurs as a response to the raised cardiac work, overload volume, and hormonal changes. It is reversible, and the signaling pathway activated to lead this modification is similar to the exercise-induced hypertrophy. A pregnant heart is protected from cardiac fibrosis, and it is accompanied by upregulation of vascular endothelial growth factor (VEGF) and an increased angiogenesis. The postpartum resolution of the cardiac hypertrophy seems to take longer than the rest of the cardiovascular changes.

The pregnancy-induced hypertrophy is similar to exercise-induced hypertrophy, but there are some differences. The signaling pathways induced by exercise are different from those induced in pathological models. In particular the PI3K/Akt signaling pathway has been implicated in exercise-induced cardiac hypertrophy, while the pathological cardiac adaptation is mediated by Gαq pathway (5). The major downstream signaling cascade of PI3K is Akt and GSK3β. The downstream targets of Gαq are calcium-dependent molecule calcineurin and mitogen-activated protein kinases (MAPK) as ERK1/2. However, there is a cross-talk between the two signaling pathways. Pregnancy-induced cardiac hypertrophy is mediated by Akt and its downstream targets, like exercise-induced hypertrophy. However, unlike exercise-induced hypertrophy, in mid-pregnancy there is an increased phosphorylation of ERK1/2 and dephosphorylation of p38. Estradiol action is implicated in p38 phosphorylation decrease, while progesterone treatment seems to induce myocyte hypertrophy and phosphorylation of ERK1/2.

Calcineurin activity is historically implicated in pathological hypertrophy and heart disease. Recently it has been shown that calcineurin activity is required for pregnancy-induced cardiac hypertrophy. In fact, it initiates the pathways responsible for the development of physiological hypertrophy. Unlike pathological hypertrophy, the calcineurin level is not constantly elevated during pregnancy, but shows an increase in early pregnancy and a significant decrease in late pregnancy (5).

Exercise and pregnancy-induced cardiac hypertrophy are considered physiological. Pregnancy-induced cardiac hypertrophy is unique

and, as described above, it differs from the one induced by exercise training. The hormonal changes during pregnancy play a key role in cardiac adaptation and in the regulation of the described signaling pathways. In particular, progesterone appears to trigger the hypertrophic signaling cascade during early pregnancy, while estradiol, in late pregnancy, appears to start the cardiac remodeling of postpartum.

The dimensions of both atria increase during pregnancy. The left ventricular end-diastolic (LVED) and end-systolic (LVES) diameters and volumes increase from the twelfth week, reach a plateau (by about 20 percent) at the beginning of third trimester, and remain stable until term. The left ventricular mass (LVM) increases by approximately 50 percent, with a peak in the third trimester, and normalizes around 6 to 12 months after the delivery. Besides, in pregnancy it is possible to observe a right ventricular dilatation (by about 18 percent).

Cardiac metabolism also deeply changes during pregnancy in order to support an increased cardiac work and to satisfy fetal needs. The metabolic shift observed during pregnancy consists in a decreased glucose utilization and an increased fatty acid oxidation that becomes almost the only resource to produce energy. Estrogen, progesterone, prolactin, and placental hormones are crucial to induce the metabolic shift and to provide fatty acids to the heart. On the contrary, the pathological heart shows a shift from lipid to glucose metabolism due to the expression of fetal genes in response to noxa (5).

The cardiac efficiency, defined as the ratio between cardiac work and myocardial oxygen consumption, increases during pregnancy. This is because the volume expansion and the subsequent rise in preload provide more blood to the heart enabling Frank-Starling mechanism to eject a larger stroke volume. This step is crucial to ensure all the cardiovascular changes that will sustain normal pregnancy development (6).

7.2.4 Maternal Cardiovascular Involvement in Preeclampsia

Several authors affirm that the cardiovascular system derangement is the primary cause of preeclamptic syndrome, instead of a secondary effect. In preeclamptic women has been described altered hemodynamics with increased SVR, abnormal ventricular hypertrophy, impaired

Table 7.1. Hemodynamic changes during pregnancy

	1st trimester	2nd trimester	3rd trimester
Systemic vascular resistance	↓	↓	↑
Cardiac output	↑	↑	↑/=
Stroke volume	↑	=	=
Heart rate	↑	↑	↑
Systolic blood pressure	↓	=	=
Diastolic blood pressure	↓	=	=
Plasma volume	↑	↑	↑
Osmolality	↓	=/↓	=
Left ventricular mass	↑	↑	↑
Left ventricular dimension	↑	↑	↑

myocardial relaxation, diastolic dysfunction and, in some cases, systolic dysfunction.

Some cardiovascular alterations are present before the clinic manifestation of preeclampsia. For this reason, the early identification of abnormal cardiovascular and volume adaptation allows to identify women at risk of developing preeclampsia. These alterations are often already present in the first trimester because they are the manifestation of a cardiovascular system that fails to adapt to pregnancy demands. A hemodynamic checkup in a woman that is planning a pregnancy could be a promising test to identify limited reserve capacity of her cardiovascular system.

7.3 Hormonal Change

Pregnancy is accompanied by significant changes in the activity of all endocrinal glands and by the development of a new endocrinal organ: the fetoplacental unit. Hormones produced have a crucial role in physiological adaptations of all organ systems and especially of cardiovascular system. During the gestation, the level of the different hormones is dynamic and leads to various cardiovascular changes.

7.3.1 Estrogen

Estrogen levels progressively increase during pregnancy reaching a peak in the last trimester. They are produced by ovaries during the first 10 weeks of gestation and by placenta during the rest of the pregnancy.

Placenta lacks 17-hydroxylase 17-20 desmolase enzyme activity, and therefore it is unable to produce estrogens from cholesterol or progestogens. For this reason, placenta relies on dehydroisoandrosterone sulfate (DHA), produced by fetal adrenal glands, to synthesize estrogens.

There are three main types of estrogen:

- Estradiol (E2) is the predominant form. It is synthesized by the aromatization of testosterone in granulosa cells of ovary and during the first five to six weeks the corpus luteum is the exclusive source of estradiol. After the first trimester the placenta becomes the major producer of circulating 17β-estradiol which gradually increases during pregnancy to a range of 6–30 ng/mL at term.
- Estrone (E1) is synthesized by the aromatization of delta-4 androstenedione. It is the predominant form in post-menopausal period, and it has a weaker activity compared to estradiol. During early pregnancy it is produced by ovaries, adrenals, or peripheral conversion. Later the placenta becomes the major source of estrone and its production increases reaching a range of 2–30 ng/ml at term.
- Estriol (E3) is the least prevalent hormone. It is synthesized by the placenta from estrone through 16α-hydroxylation and is detectable in maternal serum at nine weeks of gestation. Estriol levels are undetectable in nonpregnant women, they increase during pregnancy and are approximately 10–30 ng/ml at term (7).

7.3.1.1 Mechanism of Action

Estrogen receptors (ER) are present in two different forms, ERα and ERβ. They are expressed in several tissues. Endothelium, epithelium, muscle, bone, cartilage, hematopoietic cells, neurons, and glia have ER with different mechanisms of action. ERα is mostly expressed in mammalian and uterine cells, while ERβ is expressed in bone and vascular tissue.

After binding to steroid hormone in cytoplasm, ERα and ERβ enter into the nucleus and act as transcription factors. They bind estrogen response elements (ERE) in the promoter of target gene, regulating the expression of several genes.

Nevertheless, a nongenomic estrogenic mechanism has also been described. It consists in the activation of a G-protein estrogen receptor, that is probably expressed on cytoplasmatic membrane, and the subsequent activation of MAPK and PI3K, the generation of cyclic adenosine monophosphate (cAMP), and calcium mobilization. This mechanism explains the rapid estrogenic effect on cardiovascular system.

7.3.1.2 Effect on Cardiovascular System

Estrogens have important effects on cardiovascular system by regulating vascular function, inflammatory response, metabolism, insulin sensitivity, cardiomyocyte survival, mitochondrial function, development of cardiac hypertrophy, and cardiac protection (8).

Estrogens play a key role to maintain sufficient perfusion of the feto-placental unit, supporting the maternal vascular adaptations during all phases of pregnancy (Table 7.2). Current knowledge about these effects on cardiovascular system is based on several studies conducted in vitro or in vivo animal model (9). Estrogens produced *de novo* by uterus during embryo implantation are crucial in stromal differentiation and angiogenesis in order to maintain pregnancy (10).

In vitro studies revealed that estrogenic activity on blood vessels consists in vasorelaxation and reduction of vasoconstrictor response. As matter of fact, estrogen has a direct effect on endothelial and smooth-muscle cells activating rapid signaling pathways and genomic mechanisms described above. It reduces vascular smooth muscle cell proliferation and calcium influx, while it increases endothelial Nitric Oxide Synthase (eNOS) activity and prostacyclin (PGI2) production (11,12).

Among the several protective effects on cardiovascular systems, there is the activation of COX-2, mediated by ERα, that stimulates PGI2 production. PGI2 is an effective vasodilator, and inhibits platelet activation and the vascular smooth muscle cells proliferation. In addition, estrogen has anti-inflammatory and antioxidant effects that promote repair and regeneration of endothelium (13,14).

During pregnancy, estradiol is primary produced by the feto-placental unit and secreted in utero-placental bed. Its local vasodilatory action results in an increased uterine blood flow. The estrogenic activity also increases uterine artery angiogenesis (15), amplifying the effect of VEGF in uterine circulation (16).

There are contrasting studies regarding the estrogenic role in cardiac hypertrophy. In vitro studies show that estrogenic effects depend on hormonal concentration: A lower concentration reveals a hypertrophic effect and a higher concentration shows an anti-hypertrophic effect. Some authors have described an anti-hypertrophic action of estradiol in mice; in particular, it attenuates the hypertrophic response to pressure overload (17). Anti-hypertrophic effect seems to be mediated by calcineurin degradation, control of p38 MAPK pathways, and the regulation of histone deacetylases (8). Conversely, hypertrophic effect is mediated by ERK activation (8,18). In addition, estrogen improves the defense against oxidative stress in cardiomyocytes, contrasts apoptosis, and protects cardiac function (19,20).

In vivo studies conducted in ERβ knock out mice, and identify alterations in vascular smooth muscle function, systolic and diastolic blood pressure increment, and heart failure (21). Estrogen supplementation, increasing VEGF, angiogenesis, and eNOS production, protect the cardiovascular system from pressure overload and vessel injury (19).

Exogenous administration of estradiol to nonpregnant female pinea pigs shows haemodynamic modifications similar to pregnancy as increased CO, SV, and blood volume. In addition, it contributes to downregulation of cardiac Kv4.3 channel gene expression that implies reduction in transient outward K+ currents and prolongation of the QT interval in pregnancy (22).

7.3.2 Progesterone

Progesterone is a steroid hormone with 21 atoms of carbonium. During the first 8–10 weeks of

65

Table 7.2. Estrogen action during pregnancy

Estrogen action

- Angiogenesis in embryo-implantation site
- Systemic Vasorelaxation
- Increased CO and blood volume
- Increased uterine blood flow volume
- Endothelium repairment and regeneration
- Myocardial remodeling
- Inhibits cardiac fibrosis
- Protection against oxidative stress
- Protection from apoptosis in cardiomyocyte and endothelial cells
- Anti-inflammatory effects

pregnancy, it is produced by the corpus luteum and is essential for supporting the pregnancy development during the early stages. Then the placenta takes over progesterone production which will gradually increase until the end of pregnancy, as proof of the progressive growth of the placental tissue. Cholesterol is the principal precursor for the biosynthesis of progesterone by the placenta and it comes from maternal low-density lipoprotein (LDL). The fetal contribution to progesterone production is negligible and, in fact, fetal demise doesn't affect progesterone levels (7).

During follicular phase, progesterone concentration is less than 1 ng/mL, but it rapidly increases after LH surge to a plateau of 10–35 ng/mL. It remains stable during the first 10 weeks and progressively increases, reaching a concentration of 100–300 ng/mL at term of pregnancy (7).

7.3.2.1 Effect on Cardiovascular System

Progesterone also plays physiological protective effects on cardiovascular system, and these effects are independent from estrogenic activity (Table 7.3). Before pregnancy the cyclic changes in blood pressure during the menstrual cycle correlate with progesterone levels and not with estrogen concentrations (23).

Progesterone induces vasodilation mediated by NO synthesis in endothelial cells. This effect is mediated by PI3k/Akt pathways, causing the phosphorylation and activation of eNOS which produces NO. This molecule is an important regulator of vasodilation, acting on vascular smooth muscle cells surrounding endothelial cells and promoting vasorelaxation. Progesterone treatment causes a rapid increase in the activity of eNOS in human endothelial cells (24). However, it has also

been described as a direct action of progesterone in vascular smooth muscle: It causes a rapid decrease of intracellular calcium concentrations in myometrial cells and smooth muscle cells.

Progesterone enhances the action of eNOS (25), it decreases arterial blood pressure and protects against intimal proliferation in response to vessel injury (26). *In vivo* model showed that progesterone treatment during pregnancy mitigates the pressure response to AT-II and norepinephrine as well as other protective effects.

All the effects described above could explain the capacity of progesterone treatment to reduce blood pressure in pregnancy-induced hypertension. In addition, serum concentrations of progesterone in early stages of pregnancy are related to mean systolic blood pressures in the second and third trimesters. This relation has not been observed for estrogen levels (27).

Furthermore, progesterone seems to promote the physiological cardiac hypertrophy during pregnancy, and it partly mediates the metabolic shift of cardiomyocyte inhibiting pyruvate dehydrogenase (28). Progesterone administration in nonpregnant mice induces a nonpathological cardiac hypertrophy since it is not associated with cardiac dysfunction, pathological cardiac gene expression, and pro-fibrotic anti-angiogenic gene expression (29).

As described in the previous section, calcineurin plays a role in the development of physiological hypertrophy in early pregnancy. Calcineurin dephosphorylates NFAT and induces hypertrophic gene expression, and its regulation in early pregnancy is mediated by increased progesterone levels.

Progesterone hypertrophic effect is also mediated by activation of ERK 1/2 signaling pathway. Several studies demonstrated that calcineurin and ERK 1/2 signaling pathways are interdependent (29).

Progesterone seems to protect cardiomyocytes from apoptosis: It induces the expression of anti-apoptotic gene and the transcription of genes with cytoprotective effects (30).

7.3.2.2 Mechanism of Action

Progesterone has two different mechanisms of action that mediate effects on cardiovascular system. Genomic mechanism is mediated by nuclear receptors that are bound by progesterone which diffuses into cytoplasm. There are two main isoforms of the nuclear progesterone receptor (PR): PRA and PRB. There is also a third isoform

Table 7.3. Progesterone action during pregnancy

Progesterone Action

- Vasodilation
- Vascular protective effects
- Cardiac hypertrophy
- Protection against cardiomyocite apoptosis
- Metabolic shift in cardiomyocite
- Reduces blood pressure
- Regulates hydroelectrolytic balance
- Increases blood volume

(PRC) with an inhibitory action, and it is more present in myometrium. The levels of PRA and PRB can change in different tissues and in various conditions. Progesterone binds the nuclear receptors forming homo- and heterodimers which enter into the nucleus and bind progesterone response elements (PRE) located on target genes.

It has also been described as a nongenomic mechanism mediated by membrane-bound PR, that plays an important role in the rapid cardiovascular protective effects of progesterone.

These receptors are expressed in endothelial and vascular smooth muscle cells and are involved in the rapid activation of different signaling pathways. In particular they promote the activation of MAPK and cAMP pathways, regulating the Ca2+ intracellular level.

7.3.3 Prolactin

Prolactin is a protein hormone secreted by the lactotroph cells of the anterior pituitary gland. Its main role is to promote milk production in mammals, but it is a multifunctional hormone that influences multiple physiological processes. During pregnancy prolactin level gradually increases after the sixth week and reaches a peak in the late phase (10–20 times higher than nonpregnant levels). The activation of specific neurons in the arcuate nucleus regulates the prolactin production and its daily surges.

Prolactin has several functions, and its receptors are expressed in almost all organs, regulating multiple processes; during gestation, it acts on corpus luteum, stimulating progesterone secretion that is crucial to maintain pregnancy in early stages.

7.3.3.1 Mechanism of Action

Prolactin receptor (PRLR) is a type I cytokine transmembrane receptor, and it is expressed in

several tissues including the cardiovascular system. There are three different isoforms: the full-length activating receptor-long form (PRLR LF), and the isoforms derived from proteolytic digestion of full-length form (PRLR short and intermediate).

Second messenger cascades of this receptor include several transduction pathways. The predominant pathway employed by PRL is JAK-STAT pathway. Other pathways, such as the PI3K/AKT/mTOR pathway and Ras-Raf-MAPK, are also activated. The final effect is the modulation of several genes involved in cellular differentiation and proliferation.

7.3.3.2 Cardiovascular Effects

Prolactin acts on endothelial cells and promotes angiogenic process. Furthermore, it protects cardiomyocytes against intermittent hypoxia-induced cell damage by the modulation of signaling pathways related to cardiac hypertrophy and proliferation (Table 7.4) (31).

In a recent study it has been proved that prolactin family hormones, including growth hormone (GH), human placental lactogen (hPL), and PRL, regulate angiogenesis and endothelium-dependent vessel dilation. GH and hPL activate eNOS that produces NO which spreads to smooth-muscle cells and induces NO-dependent relaxation. On the other hand, PRL induces NO-independent and endothelial-dependent vasodilation, which is partly mediated by prostaciclyns (Table 7.4) (32).

7.3.3.3 Vasoinhibin

Prolactin is a 23 kDa single chain protein of 199 amino acids. Proteolytic cleavage of the 23 kDa protein generates smaller prolactin variants. The 16 kDa variant containing N-terminal region of PRL is a product of cleavage by cathepsin D or matrix metalloproteinase. This peptide is also known as vasoinhibin for its local and blood-borne action on endothelial cells (Table 7.4).

Vasoinhibin has several effects on endothelial cells binding a specific receptor on cellular membrane:

- induces PAI-1 expression and inhibits cell migration,
- stimulates apoptosis via Bcl-Xs and NFkB,
- inhibits vasodilation by blocking eNOS, and
- contrasts VEGF mediated vasodilation and cell proliferation.

67

Table 7.4. Prolactin and Vasoinhibin action during pregnancy

PRL action	Vasoinhibin action
• Promotes angiogenesis • Protects cardiomyocites from apoptosis • Vasodilation	• Contrasts endothelial cell migration, proliferation, differentiation and survival • Development of PPCM

PPCM: peripartum cardiomyopathy

In addition, vasoinhibin is implicated in the pathogenesis of postpartum cardiomyopathy (PPCM). The increased oxidative stress induces a detrimental conversion of the full-length 23-kDA PRL into its antiangiogenic 16 kDa variant. This peptide, acting on the coronary microvasculature, promotes myocardial hypoxia, apoptopsis, and subsequent development of PPCM. This evidence supports the therapeutic effect of bromocriptine which is a PRL antagonist.

7.3.4 Relaxin

Relaxin is a peptide hormone predominantly produced by the corpus luteum and placenta, undetectable in nonpregnant women and with high circulating levels during pregnancy. It reaches a peak of about 1 ng/ml at the end of the first trimester and subsequently settles down to an intermediate value of 0.5 ng/ml during the rest of pregnancy.

In pregnant women relaxin stimulates the tissue remodeling in different organs. In particular, it plays a key role in remodeling the reproductive tract with different effects on extracellular matrix (ECM) and collagen turnover. In fact, studies on pregnant relaxin-deficient mice showed an abnormal ECM remodeling in the entire reproductive system. The pubic ligament presents a more condensed collagen and poor water content. Vaginal and cervical epithelium remained relatively atrophic. Furthermore, in relaxin-deficient mice collagen density increases and water content decreases as a result of a reduced glycosaminoglycan hyaluronan concentration. Moreover, this hormone has an endothelium-dependent vasodilatory role in pregnancy that can reduce arterial resistance vessels and support the maternal hemodynamic changes (Table 7.5).

7.3.4.1 Mechanism of Action
Relaxin peptide receptors (RXFP) belong to G-protein coupled receptors family. There are four types of RXFP, and type 1 has been localized in several nonreproductive tissues as gastrointestinal tract, central nervous system and cardiovascular system. In particular, RXFP1 has been localized in endothelial and vascular smooth muscle cells of blood vessels and mediates the cardiovascular effects of relaxin.

RXPF interacts with a G-protein to increase cAMP and activates PI3K and PKC. The final effect of these proteins is to increase the activity of eNOS in order to produce NO. Moreover, relaxin upregulates MMP-2 which activates endothelin-1, resulting in the activation of endothelin-B receptor and subsequent NO production. The activation of this receptor is also involved in the increment of renal blood flow during pregnancy (33).

7.3.4.2 Cardiovascular Effects
The pattern of relaxin level during pregnancy is similar to the trend of systemic vasodilation, suggesting its hemodynamic effects. Relaxin administration in nonpregnant female or male rats reduces SVR by about 25 percent and increases CO, without modifying the MAP. These hemodynamic changes are very similar to those occurring during pregnancy, when relaxin impacts vascular structure, leading to a decreased SVR and an increased arterial compliance by 25 percent.

In humans, higher concentrations of progesterone and relaxin in early pregnancy are significantly associated with lower mean SBP in the second and third trimesters. Moreover, women with a DBP higher than 90 mmHg had lower relaxin values in early pregnancy compared to women without hypertension (34).

Relaxin has antifibrotic properties in cardiac tissue by modulating MMP activity and fibroblast collagen synthesis. It has also a crucial role in renal function, regulating the renal plasma flow, the glomerular filtration rate, and plasma volume. The intravenous infusion of relaxin in nonpregnant women, with a dosage that was chosen to sustain serum concentrations that are comparable to early pregnancy, increased the renal plasma flow of about 60 percent (35).

Relaxin increases eNOS and COX-2 activity, and the expression of PGI2 receptor, and consequently enhances endothelial vasodilator

Table 7.5. Relaxin action during pregnancy

Relaxin action

- Vasodilation
- Increases arterial compliance
- Attenuates vasoconstrictor effect
- Increases CO
- Contrasts cardiac fibrosis
- Increases renal plasma flow
- Regulates uterine artery remodeling

function. It has been proved that relaxin treatment attenuates endothelium-derived vasoconstriction in arteries isolated from hypertensive rats (36).

Studies on animal models treated with monoclonal antibody against relaxin have revealed the effects of this hormone during pregnancy. Relaxin increases arterial compliance, reduces SVR, and regulates the uterine artery remodeling, reducing uterine artery myogenic tone; therefore, it is crucial to uteroplacental perfusion and fetal growth. The vasodilator action of this hormone is not restricted to uteroplacental circulation, but it has also been observed in mesenteric arteries, where relaxin attenuates the angiotensin-II vasoconstrictor effect. Considering its beneficial cardiovascular effects and its protective actions on macrovasculature and microvasculature, relaxin has been studied to improve the clinical course of heart failure patients with promising results.

7.3.5 Renin-Angiotensin-Aldosterone System

The renin-angiotensin-aldosterone system (RAAS) regulates blood pressure, blood volume, and vascular smooth muscle tone. This system is activated by several factors: decreased blood pressure, beta-adrenergic activation, or decreased sodium load in the distal convoluted tubule (detected by macula densa cells). These factors can activate the juxtaglomerular cells to secrete renin in the bloodstream. Renin cleaves angiotensinogen into angiotensin I, the precursor of angiotensin II. The angiotensin converting enzyme (ACE) is the enzyme that converts angiotensin I to angiotensin II; it is present in vascular endothelium of lungs and kidneys. Angiotensin II has a vasoconstrictive action and stimulates the secretion of aldosterone from adrenal gland. Aldosterone increases sodium and water reabsorption and potassium excretion in the distal tubule and collecting duct of the nephron.

During early pregnancy there is an activation of this system that leads to a plasma volume increase that rises progressively until the thirtieth week. Since the early stages of pregnancy, estrogen leads to increased angiotensinogen levels and activation of RAAS. This is crucial to respond to underfilled circulation caused by systemic and renal vasodilation, maintaining blood pressure, and retaining sodium and water. The sodium retention progressively increases during the second and third trimesters and so does the plasma volume. Moreover, relaxin stimulates ADH secretion contributing to water retention. Progesterone, as an aldosterone antagonist, acts on the mineralocorticoid receptor to prevent sodium retention and contrast hypokalemia. On the contrary, estrogens stimulate liver production of angiotensinogen with subsequent increased levels of aldosterone. Plasma levels of aldosterone correlate with those of estrogens and rise progressively during pregnancy (37).

In preeclamptic syndrome there is a condition of hypovolemia with lower aldosterone levels. Furthermore, some authors have studied this correlation identifying a direct action of this hormone to increase placental growth (38).

References

1. Spaanderman, M, and Staelens, A (2018). Plasma volume changes in pregnancy. In: C. Lees & W. Gyselaers (Eds.), *Mater Hemodyn*. Cambridge: Cambridge University Press. https://doi.org/10.1017/9781316661925.

2. Scholten RR, Oyen WJ, Van der Vlugt MJ, et al. Impaired fetal growth and low plasma volume in adult life. *Obstet Gynecol*. 2011, 118 (6):1314–1322. https://doi.org/10.1097/AOG.0b013e3182383781. PMID: 22105261.

3. Sanghavi M, and Rutherford JD. Cardiovascular physiology of pregnancy. *Circulation*. 2014, 130(12):1003–1008. https://doi.org/10.1161/CIRCULATIONAHA.114.009029. PMID: 25223771.

4. Ouzounian JG, and Elkayam U. Physiologic changes during normal pregnancy and delivery. *Cardiol Clin*. 2012, 30 (3):317–329. https://doi.org/10.1016/j.ccl.2012.05.004. Epub 2012. PMID: 22813360.

5. Chung E, and Leinwand LA. Pregnancy as a cardiac stress

69

model. *Cardiovasc Res.* 2014, 101(4):561–570. https://doi .org/10.1093/cvr/cvu013. Epub 201. PMID: 24448313; PMCID: PMC3941597.

6. Peeters, L. Cardiovascular and volume regulatory functions in pregnancy: An overview. In C. Lees & W. Gyselaers (Eds.), *Maternal Hemodynamics.* 2018; 13–23. Cambridge: Cambridge University Press. https://doi .org/10.1017/9781316661925 .002.

7. Tal R, Taylor HS, Burney RO, et al. Endocrinology of Pregnancy. In Feingold KR, Anawalt B, Boyce A, Chrousos G, de Herder WW, Dungan K, Grossman A, Hershman JM, Hofland J, Kaltsas G, Koch C, Kopp P, Korbonits M, McLachlan R, Morley JE, New M, Purnell J, Singer F, Stratakis CA, Trence DL, Wilson DP, (Eds). 2000. South Dartmouth, MA: MDText.com, Inc..

8. Kodogo V, Azibani F, and Sliwa K. Role of pregnancy hormones and hormonal interaction on the maternal cardiovascular system: A literature review. *Clin Res Cardiol.* 2019, 108(8):831–846. https://doi.org/10.1007/s00392- 019-01441-x. Epub 2019. PMID: 30806769.

9. Napso T, Yong HEJ, Lopez-Tello J, et al. The role of placental hormones in mediating maternal adaptations to support pregnancy and lactation. *Front Physiol.* 2018, 9:1091. https:// doi.org/10.3389/fphys.2018 .01091. PMID: 30174608; PMCID: PMC6108594.

10. Das A, Mantena SR, Kannan A, *et al. De novo* synthesis of estrogen in pregnant uterus is critical for stromal decidualization and angiogenesis. *Proc Natl Acad Sci USA.* 2009, 106 (30):12542–12547. https://doi .org/10.1073/pnas .0901647106.

11. Takahashi K, Ohmichi M, Yoshida M, *et al.* Both estrogen and raloxifene cause G1 arrest of vascular smooth muscle cells. *J Endocrinol.* 2003, 178 (2):319–329. https://doi.org/10 .1677/joe.0.1780319. PMID: 12904179.

12. Castardo-de-Paula JC, de Campos BH, Amorim EDT, et al. Cardiovascular risk and the effect of nitric oxide synthase inhibition in female rats: The role of estrogen. *Exp Gerontol.* 2017, 97:38–48. https://doi.org/10.1016/j.exger .2017.07.016. Epub 2017. PMID: 28757113.

13. Favre J, Gao J, Henry J-P, et al. Endothelial estrogen receptor {alpha} plays an essential role in the coronary and myocardial protective effects of estradiol in ischemia/reperfusion. *Arterioscler Thromb Vasc Biol.* 2010, 30:2562–2567.

14. Fortini F, Dalla Sega FV, Caliceti C, et al. Estrogen receptor β-dependent Notch1 activation protects vascular endothelium against tumor necrosis factor α (TNFα)-induced apoptosis. *J Biol Chem.* 2017, 292:18178–18191.

15. Jobe SO, Ramadoss J, Koch JM, et al. Estradiol-17beta and its cytochrome P450- and catechol-O-methyltransferase-derived metabolites stimulate proliferation in uterine artery endothelial cells: Role of estrogen receptor-alpha versus estrogen receptor-beta. *Hypertension.* 2010, 55(4):1005–1011. https://doi .org/10.1161/ HYPERTENSIONAHA.109 .146399. Epub 2010. PMID: 20212268; PMCID: PMC2876348.

16. Storment JM, Meyer M, and Osol G. Estrogen augments the vasodilatory effects of vascular endothelial growth factor in the uterine circulation of the rat. *Am J Obstet Gynecol.* 2000, 183 (2):449–453. https://doi.org/10

.1067/mob.2000.105910. PMID: 10942485.

17. van Eickels M, Grohé C, Cleutjens JP, et al. 17beta-estradiol attenuates the development of pressure-overload hypertrophy. *Circulation.* 2001, 104 (12):1419–1423. https://doi .org/10.1161/hc3601.095577. PMID: 11560859.

18. Bueno OF, De Windt LJ, Lim HW, et al. The dual-specificity phosphatase MKP-1 limits the cardiac hypertrophic response in vitro and in vivo. *Circ Res.* 2001, 88(1):88–96. https://doi .org/10.1161/01.res.88.1.88. PMID: 11139479.

19. Fliegner D, Schubert C, Penkalla A, et al. Female sex and estrogen receptor-beta attenuate cardiac remodeling and apoptosis in pressure overload. *Am J Physiol Regul Integr Comp Physiol.* 2010, 298 (6):R1597–606. https://doi.org/ 10.1152/ajpregu.00825. 2009. Epub 2010.

20. Liou C-M, Yang A-L, Kuo C-H, et al. E ects of 17 Beta-estradiol on cardiac apoptosis in overiectomized rats. *Cell Biochem Funct.* 2010, 28:521–528. https://doi.org/10 .1016/j.numecd.2011.11.002.

21. Zhu Y, Bian Z, Lu P, et al. Abnormal vascular function and hypertension in mice deficient in estrogen receptor beta. *Science.* 2002, 295 (5554):505–508. https://doi .org/10.1126/science.1065250. PMID: 11799247.

22. Eghbali M, Deva R, Alioua A, et al. Molecular and functional signature of heart hypertrophy during pregnancy. *Circ Res.* 2005, 96(11):1208–1216. https://doi.org/10.1161/01.RES .0000170652.71414.16. Epub 2005. PMID: 15905459.

23. Karpanou EA, Vyssoulis GP, Georgoudi DG, et al. Ambulatory blood pressure changes in the menstrual cycle of hypertensive women.

Significance of plasma renin activity values. *Am J Hypertens.* 1993, 6(8):654–659. https://doi.org/10.1093/ajh/6.8.654. PMID: 8217027.

24. Simoncini T, Fu XD, Caruso A, et al. Drospirenone increases endothelial nitric oxide synthesis via a combined action on progesterone and mineralocorticoid receptors. *Hum Reprod.* 2007, 22 (8):2325–2334. https://doi.org/10.1093/humrep/dem109. Epub 2007. PMID: 17545686.

25. Simoncini T, Mannella P, Fornari L, et al. Differential signal transduction of progesterone and medroxyprogesterone acetate in human endothelial cells. *Endocrinology.* 2004, 145 (12):5745–5756. https://doi.org/10.1210/en.2004-0510. Epub 2004. PMID: 15358673.

26. Zhang L, Fishman MC, and Huang PL. Estrogen mediates the protective effects of pregnancy and chorionic gonadotropin in a mouse model of vascular injury. *Arterioscler Thromb Vasc Biol.* 1999, 19(9):2059–2065. https://doi.org/10.1161/01.atv.19.9.2059. PMID: 10479646.

27. Thomas P, and Pang Y. Protective actions of progesterone in the cardiovascular system: potential role of membrane progesterone receptors (mPRs) in mediating rapid effects. *Steroids.* 2013, 78(6):583–588. https://doi.org/10.1016/j.steroids.2013.01.003. Epub 2013. PMID: 23357432.

28. Liu LX, Rowe GC, Yang S, et al. PDK4 Inhibits Cardiac

Pyruvate Oxidation in Late Pregnancy. *Circ Res.* 2017, 121 (12):1370–1378. https://doi.org/10.1161/CIRCRESAHA.117.311456. Epub 2017. PMID: 28928113; PMCID: PMC5722682.

29. Chung E, Yeung F, and Leinwand LA. Calcineurin activity is required for cardiac remodelling in pregnancy. *Cardiovasc Res.* 2013, 100 (3):402–410. https://doi.org/10.1093/cvr/cvt208. Epub 2013. PMID: 23985902; PMCID: PMC3826703.

30. Morrissy S, Xu B, Aguilar D, et al. Inhibition of apoptosis by progesterone in cardiomyocytes. *Aging Cell.* 2010, 9(5):799–809. https://doi.org/10.1111/j.1474-9726.2010.00619.x. PMID: 20726854; PMCID: PMC4133411.

31. Hsieh DJ, Huang CY, Pai P, et al. Prolactin protects cardiomyocytes against intermittent hypoxia-induced cell damage by the modulation of signaling pathways related to cardiac hypertrophy and proliferation. *Int J Cardiol.* 2015, 181:255–266. https://doi.org/10.1016/j.ijcard.2014.11.154. Epub 2014. PMID: 25531577.

32. Gonzalez C, Rosas-Hernandez H, Jurado-Manzano B, et al. The prolactin family hormones regulate vascular tone through NO and prostacyclin production in isolated rat aortic rings. *Acta Pharmacol Sin.* 2015, 36(5):572–586. https://doi.org/10.1038/aps.2014.159. Epub 2015. PMID: 25891087; PMCID: PMC4422941.

33. Zamani P, and Greenberg BH. Novel vasodilators in heart

failure. *Curr Heart Fail Rep.* 2013, 10(1):1–11. https://doi.org/10.1007/s11897-012-0126-4. PMID: 23299783.

34. Kristiansson P, and Wang JX. Reproductive hormones and blood pressure during pregnancy. *Hum Reprod.* 2001, 16(1):13–17. https://doi.org/10.1093/humrep/16.1.13. PMID: 11139529.

35. Smith MC, Danielson LA, Conrad KP, et al. Influence of recombinant human relaxin on renal hemodynamics in healthy volunteers. *J Am Soc Nephrol.* 2006, 17 (11):3192–3197. https://doi.org/10.1681/ASN.2005090950. Epub 2006. PMID: 17035617.

36. Leo CH, Ng HH, Marshall SA, et al. Relaxin reduces endothelium-derived vasoconstriction in hypertension: Revealing new therapeutic insights. *Br J Pharmacol.* 2020, 177 (1):217–233. https://doi.org/10.1111/bph.14858. Epub 2019. PMID: 31479151; PMCID: PMC6976785.

37. Soma-Pillay P, Nelson-Piercy C, Tolppanen H, et al. Physiological changes in pregnancy. *Cardiovasc J Afr.* 2016, 27(2):89–94. https://doi.org/10.5830/CVJA-2016-021. PMID: 27213856; PMCID: PMC4928162.

38. Gennari-Moser C, Khankin EV, Schüller S, et al. Regulation of placental growth by aldosterone and cortisol. *Endocrinology.* 2011, 152 (1):263–271. https://doi.org/10.1210/en.2010-0525. Epub 2010. PMID: 21068161.

Chapter

8

Prolactin, Prolactinoma, and Pregnancy

Dominique Maiter and Philippe Chanson

8.1 Introduction

Prolactin (PRL) is mainly synthesized and secreted by the pituitary gland, but also by extra-pituitary sites such as the mammary gland, placenta, uterus, and T lymphocytes (1–4). The hormone is a key player in human reproduction and is essential for the perpetuation of mammalian species as it drives the development of the mammary gland and stimulates milk synthesis and secretion (1–5). However, as opposed to what is observed in rodents, the presence of functional PRL and PRL receptors is not critical to ensure fertility in humans (6,7). PRL might support pregnancy and lactation through actions on nonreproductive tissues, as it has been shown to induce proliferation of islet beta cells during metabolic adaptation in such conditions (3,5).

On the contrary, high prolactin concentrations negatively affect the gonadotropic axis in both men and women, and this inhibition occurs at multiple levels and irrespective of the cause (2,8). The main well-known effect of hyperprolactinemia is to suppress pulsatile GnRH secretion through inhibition of hypothalamic kisspeptin neurons and possibly other GnRH afferent neurons (9,10). Excessive PRL might also directly suppress LH and FSH secretion at the pituitary level as well as the positive feedback of estradiol on gonadotropin release at mid-cycle. Although its hypothalamic-pituitary effects are predominant, PRL may also inhibit granulosa cell aromatase activity, as well as progesterone and estrogen secretion from human ovaries (11,12). Thus, although low amounts of PRL (<20 µg/L) seem to be requested for progesterone production by granulosa cell cultures, high concentrations of the hormone will suppress it (13) and a shortened luteal phase may be the earliest abnormality in the menstrual cycle caused by hyperprolactinemia (14).

Among the several causes of hyperprolactinemia, the presence of a prolactinoma is expected to be present in every 500 women of reproductive age (15–17). It is usually associated with anovulation and infertility as a result of the above-mentioned inhibitory effects of hyperprolactinemia on the female hypothalamic-pituitary-gonadal axis. Besides, hyperprolactinemia and prolactinoma are frequent causes of female infertility, and a prolactinoma should always be ruled out whenever a true hyperprolactinemia of unclear etiology is confirmed in such circumstances (18).

In men, the prevalence of both hyperprolactinemia and prolactinoma are about 10-fold lower than in women, and the sensitivity of the male gonadotropic axis appears to be less lower than in the female counterpart (19). Nevertheless, PRL excess must also be ruled out in any man presenting with signs of hypogonadism and/or infertility (20).

In this chapter, we will review the physiology of prolactin secretion during pregnancy and lactation, the effects of hyperprolactinemia on female and male gonadal steroid production and fertility, as well as current recommendations on the management of prolactinomas from the desire of conception to the post-breastfeeding period.

8.2 The Physiology of Prolactin Secretion during Normal Pregnancy and Breastfeeding

In normal conditions, dopamine is the major PRL regulating hormone (21). Tubero-infundibular (TI) dopamine is released into the hypothalamic-pituitary portal vessels in the median eminence, reaches the pituitary gland, and has direct action on it (22) via D2 dopamine receptors located on the surface of lactotroph cells. Conversely, PRL provides negative feedback on its own secretion, by stimulating hypothalamic dopamine secretion via PRL receptors located on TI dopaminergic (TIDA) membranes (23). Estrogens affect the secretion of PRL both indirectly as they modify the activity of the TIDA neurons and block partially the secretion of dopamine, and directly at the level of pituitary lactotrophs where they control PRL gene expression. This may be largely due to the direct action of estrogens on the estrogen response element located in the PRL gene promoter, but also to a change in sensitivity of lactotrophs to dopamine (2,3,23). Moreover, estrogens are presumably responsible for the differentiation of lactotrophs from a pluripotent pool of somatotrophs and mammosomatotrophs (24).

A estrogen dependent lactotroph hyperplasia is observed during pregnancy (25). The size of the normal pituitary gland increases by more than 100 percent during pregnancy, and pituitary height attains maximal values of up to 10 mm in late pregnancy and 12 mm in the early postpartum period as demonstrated by magnetic resonance imaging (MRI) (26,27). Estrogens are also responsible for the increased PRL release (25). The profile of PRL release during pregnancy in humans involves three independently regulated compartments: maternal, fetal, and decidual (3,28). Maternal serum PRL levels starting from the 6th to 8th week on gradually increase during the remaining period of pregnancy to reach 200–300 μg/L at term (29,30) (Figure 8.1). PRL also comparable in the fetal circulation to reach levels to maternal serum PRL. The decidua produces very large amounts of PRL, which accumulate in the amniotic fluid, attaining very high levels (4,000–5,000 μg/L) between 16 to 22 weeks' gestation and then decrease to attain 400–500 μg/L at term (3,28). Despite such profound changes in PRL in the fetal compartment, its role in fetal physiology is unknown. The high PRL levels reached at term prepare the breast for lactation.

During the four to six weeks following delivery, PRL levels stay high in lactating women, and each suckling episode triggers a rapid release of PRL resulting in a three- to five-fold increase in serum levels, peaking about 10 minutes after the end of suckling (3,28). Then PRL levels gradually decrease to reach pre-nursing concentrations in a few hours. Over the next four to 12 weeks, basal PRL levels gradually fall to normal and the PRL

Figure 8.1 Evolution of PRL concentrations and pituitary gland height during normal pregnancy. Adapted from reference (88) with permission. Pituitary height values, in mm, are derived from reference (26).

stimulation produced by each suckling episode decreases, as a result of decreased breastfeeding. Eventually there is little or no rise in PRL with suckling, despite continued milk production. However, intense nursing (80 minutes of daily nursing with at least six nursing episodes) is able to maintain elevated serum PRL levels and postpartum amenorrhea (3). Moreover, the loss of sensitivity of the short-loop feedback system during late pregnancy and lactation allows the persistence of hyperprolactinemia during lactation, and thus the promotion of milk production (31).

8.3 Effects of Hyperprolactinemia on the Gonadotropic Axis and Fertility in Women

Prevalence of hyperprolactinemia in infertile women is variable according to studies. In a study of the World Health Organization (WHO) on 8500 infertile couples (32), hyperprolactinemia was reported to account for about 7 percent of the female causes. A similar prevalence (5.2 percent) was found in a group of 1328 infertile women with regular menses and no galactorrhea (18). In this study, PRL concentrations were only mildly elevated (31.8 ± 13.2 µg/L) and the overall prevalence of hyperprolactinemia did not differ with the infertility diagnosis or the presence or absence of menstrual irregularities. Although rather low, such a prevalence of 5–7 percent is 30 times higher than that found in the general population of similar sex and age (175/100,000) (33) and 100 times higher than the reported prevalence of prolactinomas (25–63/100,000) (17), suggesting that PRL should be measured in all women presenting for a first evaluation of infertility, whether or not they have other symptoms suggestive of hyperprolactinemia. Of note, short-lasting hyperprolactinemia during the menstrual cycle has also been documented in some infertile women, and these women may respond to dopamine agonists with an increase in progesterone level during the luteal phase and an improvement in fertility (34). On the other hand, when other symptoms are present such as oligo- or amenorrhea and/or galactorrhea, the probability becomes much higher. Thus in a compilation of 367 symptomatic women with infertility, up to one third had hyperprolactinemia (35). In other studies, after having excluded pregnancy, nearly 15 percent of women who had secondary amenorrhea or oligomenorrhea showed hyperprolactinemia (36,37).

In such populations, all known causes of hyperprolactinemia may be found, and prolactinoma is by far not the most frequent. Among a group of 590 unselected women seeking medically assisted reproduction in our center in 2010, 70 (12 percent) had a mild PRL elevation (range 21–89 µg/L) at their first hormonal evaluation. However, only half of them had a confirmed hyperprolactinemia at a second control and only a minority of them (n = 6) had a final diagnosis of prolactinoma (our unpublished data). Physiological causes such as stress, a protein-rich meal, ovulation, or a naturally occurring hormonal pulse are likely responsible for frequent mild PRL elevations which are not confirmed on a subsequent fasting determination. Clinicians have also to consider the possibility of an artifact, particularly the presence of macroprolactin. If the clinical picture is not typical (i.e. if amenorrhea and galactorrhea are not present), the increased

PRL levels must be confirmed by reassaying the serum after PEG precipitation (38). Indeed, significant amounts of macroprolactin (related to the presence of multimeric complexes of several molecules of prolactin and one molecule of IgG) should always be ruled out, as it may represent 15–30 percent of all hyperprolactinemic serum, depending on the selected cohort and type of assay used (38,39).

When true hyperprolactinaemia is confirmed on several occasions, pituitary MRI may be advised to rule out a prolactin-secreting pituitary tumor or other hypothalamic-pituitary diseases. This issue is still a matter of debate as the probability to find a significant pituitary abnormality is rather low in this population (20 percent) and must be compared with the incidence of pituitary incidentaloma (10 percent). The prevalence seems, however, to be independent of the level of hyperprolactinemia (18) and no clear cut-off for imaging has emerged. Other main causes include drug-induced hyperprolactinemia, primary hypothyroidism (which must always be ruled out before pregnancy), polycystic ovary syndrome (although the link with hyperprolactinemia is debated), or idiopathic hyperprolactinemia (16).

Any confirmed hyperprolactinemia should be treated in a young woman who wishes to become pregnant, as it may cause infertility even in the presence of normal cycles (due to luteal insufficiency). In some cases, the cause of excessive prolactin can be withdrawn or treated (drug-induced hyperprolactinemia, primary hypothyroidism). If this is not possible, a dopamine agonist (DA) must be initiated at the lowest possible dose to restore normal ovulatory pattern and fertility in most cases, in particular in non-tumoral hyperprolactinemia. We give preference to cabergoline over other DA as it has shown better efficacy and tolerability, as well as a good safety profile in pregnant women (8,15,16).

The issue whether a woman with mild hyperprolactinemia going through assisted reproductive technology (ART) must be treated or not with a DA remains currently unsettled. The same is true for a woman with high prolactin levels related to the presence of macroprolactin. Although this condition seems to be associated with a higher prevalence of infertility (40), this association might be the result of an ascertainment bias.

8.4 Effects of Hyperprolactinemia on the Gonadotropic Axis and Fertility in Men

Except for the notable exception of (macro)prolactinomas, hyperprolactinemia in men is a largely overlooked research area. Basically, most of the causes and effects of hyperprolactinemia observed in women can be observed in men (16,19). However, regardless of the etiology, hyperprolactinemia is a much less frequent finding in males than in females, as confirmed in a recent Scottish epidemiology study (33). Moreover, male PRL concentrations are usually lower than female ones in most causes of hyperprolactinemia other than prolactinomas. As an example, the maximal level of hyperprolactinemia related to a pituitary stalk effect caused by a non-lactotroph tumor of the sellar region is lower in men than in women (41).

Overall, endocrine disorders (including hyperprolactinemia) are a rare etiology of infertility in men, accounting for only 2–4 percent of cases, whereas primary testicular defects in spermatogenesis are largely predominant (75 percent). In a recent review of 3,101 men presenting for initial fertility evaluation at a tertiary care, 65 (2.1 percent) had hyperprolactinemia (likely including cases of hyperprolactinemia related to the presence of macroprolactin) and only 11 (0.35 percent) were diagnosed with a prolactinoma. These men showed lower testosterone concentrations and a significant proportion of them had oligospermia (20). Thus, it is not surprising (though questionable) that some European guidelines do not include assessment of serum PRL levels during evaluation of male infertility (42). Another concern lies in the fact that the degree of infertility is often relative and men with endocrine disorders and subnormal semen parameters are still capable of reproduction (43).

In addition, the male gonadotropic axis is much less sensitive to the effects of high – and even very high – PRL concentrations, as shown in men with macroprolactinoma who can still retain normal testosterone concentrations and normal fertility (44,45). Likewise, semen quality is significantly altered in only half of men with prolactinomas and nearly all of them retain some sperm production capacity (46–48). The reasons for this differential sensitivity of the male reproductive axis are not fully elucidated.

Regarding prolactinoma in men, symptoms of male hypogonadism and procreation difficulties – though often present – stay unrecognized for a long period of time and often attributed to other causes such as aging, drugs, or depression (19). In a series of 65 men with prolactinoma (including 50 with a macroprolactinoma), 46 (71 percent) had testosterone deficiency and 16 (25 percent) had been referred for infertility (47). Several alterations of semen quality were found in a subset of these patients, such as a total sperm count $\leq 40 \times 10^6$/volume of ejaculate in 43 percent, a sperm forward progression <25 percent in 71 percent and a live spermatozoa count <75 percent in 83 percent. Importantly, the prevalence of altered semen quality was similar in the patients with macro- and microprolactinomas.

As in women, restoring normal or near normal PRL concentrations with a DA in hypogonadal men with prolactinoma usually allows the re-establishment of normal testosterone concentrations and normal semen quality (45–47). Symptomatic hypogonadism may however persist in a significant subset of these patients, even when PRL levels are normalized (49).

Other non-tumoral causes of chronic hyperprolactinemia in men may also be responsible for hypogonadism and infertility but there are no robust data regarding prevalence, severity, and effects of PRL normalization. It seems however wise to treat with a DA any male infertile patient with significant and confirmed hyperprolactinemia, whether or not he is symptomatic or has low testosterone levels.

8.5 Management of Prolactinoma before Pregnancy

When a prolactinoma has been diagnosed in a young woman who wishes to be pregnant, normalizing PRL concentrations and – in the case of a macroprolactinoma – reducing tumor size before conception are key goals to allow a safe and spontaneous pregnancy (8,15,50). As already mentioned, treatment is also recommended in those women with mild hyperprolactinemia and apparently regular normal cycles, as elevated PRL concentrations may only affect progesterone secretion and lead to luteal phase insufficiency and inadequate embryo implantation (14,15).

In this regard, DAs are highly effective in restoring fertility in women with either a micro- or a macroprolactinoma and thus represent the first choice treatment (8,50–53). As both bromocriptine and cabergoline have shown great efficacy and a good safety profile for both the mother and child, medical treatment should not be preventively withdrawn in a woman wishing to become pregnant. Nowadays Cabergoline is the most used DA as it is better tolerated and shows a higher efficacy in normalizing PRL levels than bromocriptine (54,55). However, few studies have directly compared both drugs in their efficacy to achieve gestation, showing only a slight advantage in favor of cabergoline (56). In a series of 85 infertile women with prolactinoma (31 BRC-resistant, 32 BRC-intolerant, and 22 drug-naïve patients), up-titrated doses of cabergoline restored ovulatory cycles in all and allowed pregnancy in 80 (94 percent) (57) of cases. In a Belgian study of 455 hyperprolactinemic women treated with cabergoline, PRL was normalized in >90 percent of patients with a microprolactinoma and in 77 percent of those with a macroadenoma (58). Several studies have also indicated a higher frequency of significant pituitary tumor shrinkage with cabergoline (rev in [16]), which may represent a valuable advantage in case of a woman with a large macroprolactinoma seeking to get pregnant in the short term. Treatment with cabergoline should be pursued until a diagnosis of pregnancy is confirmed, which means that in most women, the drug will be administered for the first six to eight weeks of gestation. The safety issues regarding this treatment for the mother and the baby are discussed in Chapter 7.

Trans-sphenoidal selective adenomectomy may be an option option in selected cases, such as in women with a recent diagnosis of macroprolactinoma and an immediate desire of conception or a late age to conceive (59). Surgery is considered less efficient than medical therapy, achieving in expert hands an immediate normalization of PRL levels in 70–80 percent of microadenomas, but in only 30–40 percent of macroadenomas (16,60,61). Moreover, surgery may entail some morbidity, in particular postoperative pituitary hormone deficits. As in every patient with prolactinoma, pituitary surgery should also be proposed to women who cannot tolerate DAs, who are not responsive to maximally tolerated doses of Das, or those who choose to undergo surgery for personal reasons, such as poor compliance to drug therapy (8,16,52).

Patients with large macroprolactinomas may sometimes require high doses of cabergoline and may also be good candidates for surgery, even though tumor resection is incomplete. Surgical debulking not only improves subsequent hormonal control under medical treatment (62), but also reduces a subsequent risk of tumor enlargement during pregnancy (8).

The patients who do not respond to previous treatment modalities may need additional hormonal maneuvers to facilitate ovulation, such as clomiphene citrate, gonadotropin stimulation (63), or in vitro fertilization (IVF). Noticeably, the mean age of prolactinoma women at first conception is older than in the general population (32 years versus 30 years, respectively) and the need for ART is more frequent (64).

8.6 Management of Prolactinoma during Pregnancy

DAs cross the placental barrier and, although the use of bromocriptine and cabergoline has not been associated with increased teratogenicity, it is preferred to limit any drug exposure to the embryo as much as possible (52,65). In most cases, DA may be stopped as soon as pregnancy is confirmed, so the exposure time from ovulation to drug withdrawal will be limited to three to four weeks. It is important to warn patients that restoration of ovulation and fertility may be immediate when they start DA treatment (even before normal menses return and even if amenorrhea was long-lasting...!).

While the probability of tumor-related complications appears to be very low – between 2 and 7 percent – in case of microprolactinomas or when the tumor had been operated irradiated, or has shrunk on prolonged DA therapy before pregnancy, a significantly higher risk of symptomatic tumor growth during pregnancy – ranging between 15 and 30 percent – has been reported in women with untreated macroprolactinomas. A typical example of macroprolactinoma growth during pregnancy is illustrated in Figure 8.2. The main studies published before 2017 have been summarized in recent reviews (50,71). We have completed these reviews with additional data collected from the few studies published after 2017 (68–70,72–75) and found an overall prevalence of symptomatic tumor growth during pregnancy of 2.5 percent, 15.5

Figure 8.2 Typical evolution of a macroprolactinoma diagnosed in a 24-year-old woman complaining of recurrent headaches and secondary amenorrhea with a wish of pregnancy. Prolactin (PRL) concentration was increased at 132 µg/L (normal values: 5–23 µg/L). Coronal sections in the same plane are shown from serial magnetic resonance imaging (MRI) of the pituitary gland. The prolactinoma is indicated on each figure by the white arrow.

[A] Contrast-enhanced T1-weighed (T1W) MRI performed at diagnosis and showing a macroadenoma located on the left side and measuring 10x9 mm. Treatment with cabergoline 0.5 mg 2x/week was started. [B] Contrast-enhanced T1W MRI performed 6 months after diagnosis. A marked reduction in tumor size is noted (7x6 mm) while PRL level is normal at 7.9 µg/L. Soon after, the patient became pregnant and cabergoline was discontinued at 6 weeks of gestation. [C] Non-enhanced T1W MRI performed at 6.5 months of pregnancy as the patient suddenly complained from severe headaches. There was a clear increase in the size of the adenoma (12x14 mm) which was now abutting the optic chiasm. Cabergoline was reintroduced (0.5 mg 2x/week) with a rapid improvement of symptoms. Delivery was uneventful but the patient could not breastfeed on continued cabergoline treatment.

[D] Contrast-enhanced T1W MRI performed 4 months after delivery. The prolactinoma has shrunk to a 7x4mm residue located next to the left cavernous sinus. Prolactin concentration was normal (5.4 µg/L). [E] Non-enhanced T1W MRI performed at 7.5 months of a second pregnancy occurring two years later. Cabergoline had been withdrawn at the diagnosis of pregnancy and the patient remained asymptomatic. MRI was performed for safety reasons after informed discussion with the patient. No treatment was initiated and the patient had a normal et term delivery and could breastfeed for 4 months. After weaning, prolactin remained elevated at 60 µg/L and cabergoline was resumed at 0.25 mg 2x/week.

[F] Contrast-enhanced T1W MRI performed 5 years after the second pregnancy, showing a small devascularized tumor residue (3x4 mm). Prolactin was normal at 17 µg/L on cabergoline 0.25 mg/week. A trial of treatment withdrawal had been made but was unsuccessful with rapid recurrence of moderate hyperprolactinemia (35 µg/L) and irregular cycles.

percent, and 6.6 percent in patients with microprolactinomas, macroprolactinomas, and macroprolactinomas previously treated with surgery and/or radiotherapy, respectively (Table 8.1).

In a recent Brazilian multicenter study, Sant'Anna et al. reported that symptoms of tumor growth (headaches and/or visual defects) occurred in 6 percent of untreated pregnant women with a microprolactinoma, in 17 percent of those with a macroprolactinoma previously treated with DA only and in 33 percent (3/9) of women with a macroprolactinoma treated with DA and (incomplete) surgery (68). Lambert

et al. performed a prospective and observational study including 49 macroprolactinomas diagnosed before or during pregnancy. Six patients (12 percent) had tumor growth during pregnancy (69). Very recently, Barraud and colleagues reviewed the data on 85 viable pregnancies in 46 patients with a macroprolactinoma. They observed tumor growth-related symptoms during 12 pregnancies in nine patients (19.6 percent) including three cases of pituitary apoplexy (70).

Based on these data, careful follow-up with regular clinical and visual field testing is recommended in pregnant women with a

Table 8.1. Documented symptomatic tumor growth of prolactinomas during pregnancy

1st author, year, ref.	Microprolactinomas		Macroprolactinomas		Macroprolactinomas with previous R/[*]	
	Total	Nb. with growth	Total	Nb. with growth	Total	Nb. with growth
Molitch, 2019 [50][§]	764	18	304	50	148	7
Lambert K, 2017 [69]	–	–	46	6	3	0
Karaca Z, 2018 [89]	50	0	25	2	NR	NR
Sant'Anna, 2020 [68]	69	4	95	16	9	3
Barraud, 2020 [70]	–	–	79	11	6	1
Overall numbers	**883**	**22 (2.5%)**	**549**	**85 (15.5%)**	**166**	**11 (6.6%)**

§ This review [50] summarizes data from 15 studies published before 2017.
* R/ means macroprolactinomas previously treated by surgery and/or radiotherapy
Nb.: number; NR: not reported

macroadenoma, while no particular surveillance (except for usual clinical monitoring) is advised for patients with a microprolactinoma. Pituitary MRI without gadolinium injection, although not harmful (66), should be reserved for patients with symptoms of tumor enlargement, visual field defects or in those where the tumor is judged by the clinician of critical size at the time of pregnancy. Unfortunately, longitudinal prospective studies are lacking to support an evidence-based algorithm to perform imaging during pregnancy and lactation and the decision should be based on the risk/benefit ratio, taking into account patient's safety, quality of care, and outcomes [67].

A quite similar PRL secretory pattern is usually seen in pregnant women with prolactinoma compared to normal pregnancies (8,76). Moreover, in some prolactinoma patients, serum PRL levels may not increase as much during pregnancy and PRL is not considered as a reliable marker of tumor progression (8,77). Therefore, it is not recommended to measure PRL levels during pregnancy in women with a prolactinoma.

In case of symptomatic growth of a prolactinoma during pregnancy, reinitiation of DA is the first treatment option and will be successful in the majority of cases. A high efficacy of either BRC or cabergoline was demonstrated in this setting in several reports (64,68,69,74,75). Cabergoline appears to be slightly preferable in terms of side effects compared to BRC, and efficient doses in pregnant women with prolactinoma are similar to those used in non-pregnant women.

Continuation of DA therapy throughout the pregnancy may be considered as an option in women bearing large macroprolactinomas close to or abutting the optic chiasm at the time of conception and without prior medical or surgical tumor reduction. In the few reported cases where DA was continued throughout pregnancy, no symptomatic tumor growth was reported, except for two exceptional cases of apoplexy requiring surgery (53,78). In several cases where DAs were required during pregnancy, the drug was successfully discontinued a few weeks before delivery in order to allow breastfeeding. Whether this is a safe and effective option remains to be confirmed.

Trans-sphenoidal surgery should be recommended only in case of failure of medical treatment to rapidly relieve severe visual impairment or intractable headache due to tumor growth in a pregnant woman. It may be safely performed during the second trimester or the early third trimester of pregnancy (79). Close to term, labor induction is also an option worth dicussion with the patient.

Pituitary apoplexy is an uncommon cause of sudden and severe headache, visual defects or ophthalmoplegia during pregnancy (80,81) (Figure 8.3). It may occur both in patients treated with DAs (78) and in untreated pregnant women with prolactinoma (70) and will often require decompressive surgery (70). However, hemorrhagic necrosis of a macroprolactinoma during pregnancy may also be asymptomatic, thus not requiring surgery and having a favorable outcome without any treatment (15,82).

Figure 8.3 Magnetic resonance imaging (MRI) showing acute apoplexy of a macroprolactinoma diagnosed in a 31-year-old woman complaining of severe headaches, visual disturbances, nausea, vomiting, and confusion at week 29 of a first pregnancy. The diagnosis of a 12x9x9mm macroprolactinoma had been made 10 months earlier and a treatment with cabergoline was started (0.5 mg 2x/week) but rapidly stopped after 3 months for ongoing pregnancy. Apoplexy was first treated with dopamine agonists and hormonal replacement with hydrocortisone and thyroxine, but worsening of symptoms required neurosurgical resection at week 30, without complications for the mother or the fetus. The patient suffered also at the same time from eclampsia and pre-term delivery was performed by cesarean section at week 33.
[A] Non-enhanced T1W coronal section showing a large 21x17 mm hemorrhagic macroadenoma with a suprasellar extension compressing the optic chiasm. The hyperintense signal is due to the presence of methemoglobin. **[B]** Non-enhanced T2W coronal section showing the same hemorrhagic tumor with a hypointense signal in the posterior part which is due to the presence of deoxyhemoglobin. **[C]** Non-enhanced T2W sagittal section showing a liquid-liquid level separating a protein-rich liquid at the top (left part of the tumor indicated by the asterisk) and a blood cells and fibrin-rich sediment at the bottom (right part of the tumor, indicated by the white circle).

8.7 Safety of DA Treatment for the Mother and Child

Bromocriptine has gained a very large safety record in pregnancy. Data recorded from a database of over 6200 pregnancies initiated on teratment have shown rates of spontaneous abortion (10 percent), ectopic pregnancy (0.5 percent), pre-term delivery (12.5 percent), multiple births (1.9 percent), as well as fetal or congenital malformations (2.5 percent) compared to the general population (8,83).

Cabergoline is equally safe in this context as now indicated by several studies and reviews (50,71). We further expanded these data by reviewing data from additional recent studies performed in hyperprolactinemic women (most of them with a prolactinoma) having started their pregnancy while treated with cabergoline and overall results collected from 1395 pregnancies are shown in Table 8.2. The observed rates of spontaneous miscarriage (8.3 percent), termination of pregnancy for malformation (1.1 percent), ectopic pregnancies (0.2 percent), pre-term delivery (10.2 percent), stillbirths (1.1 percent) and neonatal malformations (2.5 percent) are similar to those quoted for pregnancies initiated on BRC or those reported in a normal age-matched population. Moreover, follow-up studies of the children up to 12 years after fetal exposure to cabergoline did not show any physical or developmental abnormalities in more than 230 children (50,64,68).

Regarding the use of quinagolide, in a review of 176 pregnancies, in which this drug was given for a median duration of 7 weeks, Webster reported 24 spontaneous abortions, one stillbirth and nine fetal malformations (54). Thus, quinagolide appears to be less safe during pregnancy, although the number of available data remains so far limited and no definitive conclusion can really be made.

Limited safety data are also available regarding the use of bromocriptine and cabergoline throughout gestation, which indicate no increased risk of fetal or congenital malformation (50,53,68). These drugs might therefore be continued in case of large, visual-threatening macroprolactinomas.

8.8 Breastfeeding and Management of Prolactinoma after Pregnancy

Breastfeeding is successful and safe in the vast majority of women with a prolactinoma, in particular in those who could successfully cease DA treatment at the beginning of or during

Table 8.2. Pregnancy outcomes for women who became pregnant while taking cabergoline, compared to what is expected in the normal population

First author, year, reference	Molitch$ 2019 [50]	Araujo et al. 2017 [72]	Galvao et al. 2017 [73]	Lambert et al. 2017 [69]	Karaca et al. 2018 [74]	O'Sullivan et al. 2020 [75]	Sant'Anna et al. 2020 [68]	Barraud et al. 2020 [70]	Overall (%)	Normal Values (%)$
Number of pregnancies	1016	6	4	32	45	41	221#	30	1395	–
Miscarriages	77	0	0	NR	5	3	26	NR	111/1333 (8.3%)	10–15
Termination for malformation	14	0	0	0	1	0	0	NR	15/1365 (1,1%)	1.0–2.5
Ectopic (%)	3	0	0	NR	0	0	0	NR	3/1333 (0.2%)	1.0–1.5
Preterm* (% of deliveries)	74/746	1/6	0/4	2/32	NA	6/41	23/197	2/30	108/1055 (10.2%)	12.5
Stilbirths* (% of deliveries)	7/746	0/6	0/4	0/32	1/40	1/41	3/197	0/30	12/1096 (1.1%)	0.9
Neonatal malformation* (% of living babies)	21/863	0/6	0/4	0/32	1/38	1/40	7/195	0/30	30/1208 (2.5%)	3.0

$ This review [50] summarizes data from 16 studies published before 2017, most of them were included in a previous publication (8).
* The indicated numbers concern deliveries and babies with known details.
# Not taking into account 10 ongoing pregnancies.
$ Normal values reproduced from reference (50).
NR: not reported

pregnancy. Although PRL secretion is physiologically stimulated by suckling and breast stimulation, there is no evidence that sustained lactation results in tumor growth. It is also considered safe to withhold DA treatment as long as breastfeeding is desired (15,84). For example, in the study reported by Auriemma et al. there was no difference in PRL levels of those who breastfed or not (84). In addition, the remission rate of prolactinoma after pregnancy is not affected by lactation (84,85). An old study, prior to the era of modern endoscopic surgery, suggested that patients after trans-sphenoidal surgery had lower PRL values and were less likely to have sufficient milk production (86). However, no recent post-surgical data support this finding

8.9 Management of Prolactinoma after Pregnancy and Breastfeeding

There is a large subset of prolactinomas that will involute during the pregnancy and lactation period (the exact timing is not known)

(Figure 8.2), and some will sustain remission for a substantial number of months. In various recent studies, including mostly women with microprolactinomas and using mainly cabergoline at the time of conception, these percentages ranged from 11 to 68 percent, with an average remission rate of 40 percent for a median time of 30 months (Table 8.3). Factors predicting remission after pregnancy are usually a lower PRL level at diagnosis and postpartum and a smaller tumor size at diagnosis and before pregnancy. There is a higher number of remission for microprolactinomas (46 percent) than macroprolactinomas (26 percent). Biochemical remission may coincide with disappearance of the tumor but small remnant tissue may also persist (68,85).

It is therefore recommended to re-evaluate the status of the prolactinoma after each pregnancy and lactation period, providing clinical assessment, PRL measurement, and pituitary MRI (the lack of visible tumor being associated with a higher chance of prolonged remission). In case of remission, clinical and hormonal follow-up is

Table 8.3. Main outcomes of prolactinoma after pregnancy and breast-feeding in recent series published after 2010

First author, year, ref	Total Nb. of women	Nb. with prolactinoma (m/M)	Previous DA treatment	Nb. with breastfeeding (%)	Nb. with remission* (%)	Median length of follow-up (months)
Huda, 2010 [90]	16	16 (16/0)	BRC	NR	4/16 (25%)	58
Lebbe, 2010 [64]	72	60 (45/15)	CAB	62	20/72 (38%)	12
Auriemma, 2013 [84]	91	86 (76/10)	CAB	88	62/91 (68%)	60
Domingue, 2014 [85]	73	73 (54/19)	CAB	59	39/73 (40%)	22
Karaca, 2018 [74]	60	60 (36/17)[§]	BRC (24) - CAB (33)	NR	5/46 (11%)	12
Araujo, 2017 [72]	29	29 (23/5)[§]	BRC (24) - CAB (5)	NR	3/25 (12%)	10
O'Sullivan, 2020 [75]	47	47 (36/11)	BRC (12) - CAB (35)	31 (65%)[#]	13/41 (32%)	31
Overall	**388**	**371 (286/77)[§]**	**BRC (76) - CAB (303)**	**240/293 (85%)**	**146/364 (40%)**	**30**

[*] Numbers of women with a normal prolactin concentration at the last follow-up visit related to the total numbers of patients with available follow-up.
[#] Number of women breastfeeding for more than 3 months.
[§] Information on initial tumor size missing in some patients.
Nb.: number; m: microadenoma; M: macroadenoma; BRC: bromocriptine; CAB: cabergoline; NR: not reported

recommended after six months and yearly thereafter since recurrence may occur in a significant proportion of cases within five years. In case of recurrence of symptomatic hyperprolactinemia, in particular in the context of a wish of new pregnancy, DA should be reinitiated, usually at a similar or even lower dose than that used at the end of the last treatment period.

8.10 Conclusions

PRL is intimately connected with the normal physiology and pathophysiology of pregnancy in animals and humans and, for example, the antigonadal effects are the most broadly conserved physiological actions of PRL across all vertebrates including fishes, amphibians, reptiles, birds, and mammals (87). Although not indispensable to achieve normal gestation in humans (as opposed to rodents), PRL is essential for the development of the mammary gland and for lactation.

Hyperprolactinemia is a frequent finding in young women with infertility and PRL determination is warranted in these patients, whether or not they have other symptoms suggestive of excessive PRL such as galactorrhea or menstrual cycle disturbances. Whatever the cause, any confirmed hyperprolactinemia should be treated in a young woman who wishes to become pregnant, and we give preference to cabergoline at the lowest possible doses which will normalize PRL and restore fertility in the vast majority of these women. Data are much less robust in men in whom PRL concentrations are less prone to increase and the reproductive axis less sensitive to the effects of hyperprolactinemia. Nevertheless, chronic and significant hyperprolactinemia in men may also cause hypogonadism and infertility and must be treated as in women.

Most women of reproductive age with a prolactinoma may nowadays become pregnant with current modern therapies, mainly DAs (plus surgery and medically-assisted reproduction techniques if necessary). Cabergoline seems to be more efficient than bromocriptine to restore fertility and is better tolerated. Both drugs are safe to use during early gestation, although there is a larger safety record for bromocriptine. Symptomatic tumor growth is a rare event in microprolactinomas (2–3 percent) but more frequent in the case of a macroprolactinoma without previous ablative therapy (15–20 percent). Early withdrawal of the DA is usually warranted without complication for the mother but close surveillance is needed for large adenomas. Symptomatic tumor enlargement should be treated with resumption of a DA, while surgery is rarely necessary. Breastfeeding is not contra-indicated in such conditions. In addition pregnancy may have a beneficial role on the size and secretion of the prolactinoma and might induce remission in about 40 percent of these women.

The authors declare that they have no conflict of interest regarding this review.

References

1. Bachelot A, and Binart N. Reproductive role of prolactin. *Reproduction*. 2007, 133 (2):361–369.

2. Bernard V, Young J, Chanson P, et al. New insights in prolactin: Pathological implications. *Nat Rev Endocrinol*. 2015, 11 (5):265–275.

3. Binart N. Prolactin. In: Melmed S, editor. *The Pituitary*. 2017; 129–161. London: Elsevier.

4. Bernard V, Young J, and Binart N. Prolactin – A pleiotropic factor in health and disease. *Nat Rev Endocrinol*. 2019, 15 (6):356–365.

5. Horseman ND. Physiological actions and receptors. In: Tritos NA, Klibanski A, editors. Prolactin disorders from basic science to clinical management. 2019; 79–94. Springer Nature Switzerland AG: Humana Press.

6. Newey PJ, Gorvin CM, and Thakker RV. Mutant prolactin receptor and familial hyperprolactinemia. *N Engl J Med*. 2014, 370(10): 977–978.

7. Kobayashi T, Usui H, Tanaka H, et al. Variant prolactin receptor in agalactia and hyperprolactinemia. *N Engl J Med*. 2018, 379 (23):2230–2236.

8. Molitch ME. Endocrinology in pregnancy: Management of the pregnant patient with a prolactinoma. *Eur J Endocrinol*. 2015, 172(5): R205–13.

9. Kaiser UB. Hyperprolactinemia and infertility: New insights. *J Clin Invest*. 2012, 122 (10):3467–3468.

10. Sonigo C, Bouilly J, Carre N, et al. Hyperprolactinemia-induced ovarian acyclicity is reversed by kisspeptin administration. *J Clin Invest*. 2012, 122(10):3791–3795.

11. Demura R, Ono M, Demura H, et al. Prolactin directly inhibits basal as well as gonadotropin-stimulated secretion of progesterone and 17 beta-estradiol in the human ovary. *J Clin Endocrinol Metab.* 1982, 54(6):1246–1250.

12. Dorrington JH, and Gore-Langton RE. Antigonadal action of prolactin: Further studies on the mechanism of inhibition of follicle-stimulating hormone-induced aromatase activity in rat granulosa cell cultures. *Endocrinology.* 1982, 110 (5):1701–1707.

13. McNatty KP. Relationship between plasma prolactin and the endocrine microenvironment of the developing human antral follicle. *Fertil Steril.* 1979, 32 (4):433–438.

14. Seppala M, Ranta T, and Hirvonen E. Hyperprolactinaemia and luteal insufficiency. *Lancet.* 1976, 1(7953):229–230.

15. Maiter D. Prolactinoma and pregnancy: From the wish of conception to lactation. *Ann Endocrinol (Paris).* 2016, 77 (2):128–134.

16. Chanson P, and Maiter D. Prolactinoma. In: Melmed S, editor. *The Pituitary.* 4th ed. 2017; 467–514. London: Elsevier.

17. Chanson P, and Maiter D. The epidemiology, diagnosis and treatment of prolactinomas: The old and the new. *Best Pract Res Clin Endocrinol Metab.* 2019:101290.

18. Souter I, Baltagi LM, Toth TL, et al. Prevalence of hyperprolactinemia and abnormal magnetic resonance imaging findings in a population with infertility. *Acta Obstet Gynecol Scand.* 2010, 94(3):1159–1162.

19. Maiter D. Prolactinomas in men. In: Tritos NA, Klibanski A, editors. *Prolactin Disorders from Basic Science to Clinical Management.* 2019; 189–204. Springer Nature Switzerland AG: Humana Press.

20. Ambulkar SS, Darves-Bornoz AL, Fantus RJ, et al. Prevalence of hyperprolactinemia and clinically apparent prolactinomas in men undergoing fertility evaluation. *Urology.* 2021.

21. Ben-Jonathan N, and Hnasko R. Dopamine as a prolactin (PRL) inhibitor. *Endocr Rev.* 2001, 22(6):724–763.

22. Schuff KG, Hentges ST, Kelly MA, et al. Lack of prolactin receptor signaling in mice results in lactotroph proliferation and prolactinomas by dopamine-dependent and -independent mechanisms. *J Clin Invest.* 2002, 110(7):973–981.

23. Freeman ME, Kanyicska B, Lerant A, et al. Prolactin: Structure, function, and regulation of secretion. *Physiol Rev.* 2000;80(4):1523–1631.

24. Boockfor FR, Hoeffler JP, and Frawley LS. Estradiol induces a shift in cultured cells that release prolactin or growth hormone. *Am J Physiol.* 1986, 250(1 Pt 1):E103–105.

25. Ben-Jonathan N, LaPensee CR, and LaPensee EW. What can we learn from rodents about prolactin in humans? *Endocr Rev.* 2008, 29(1):1–41.

26. Dinc H, Esen F, Demirci A, et al. Pituitary dimensions and volume measurements in pregnancy and post partum. *MR assessment. Acta Radiol.* 1998, 39(1):64–69.

27. Gonzalez JG, Elizondo G, Saldivar D, et al. Pituitary gland growth during normal pregnancy: An in vivo study using magnetic resonance imaging. *Am J Med.* 1988, 85 (2):217–220.

28. Knuth UA, and Friesen HG. Prolactin and pregnancy. *In:* Martini L, James VHT, editors. *Current Topics in Experimental Endocrinology.* 1983. 69–96. 4: Elsevier.

29. Biswas S. Prolactin in amniotic fluid: Its correlation with maternal plasma prolactin. *Clin Chim Acta.* 1976, 73(2):363–367.

30. Rigg LA, Lein A, and Yen SS. Pattern of increase in circulating prolactin levels during human gestation. *Am J Obstet Gynecol.* 1977, 129 (4):454–456.

31. Grattan DR, and Kokay IC. Prolactin: A pleiotropic neuroendocrine hormone. *J Neuroendocrinol.* 2008, 20 (6):752–763.

32. Recent advances in medically assisted conception. Report of a WHO Scientific Group. 1992, 820:1-. Geneva: WHO; 1992.

33. Soto-Pedre E, Newey PJ, Bevan JS, et al. The epidemiology of hyperprolactinaemia over 20 years in the Tayside region of Scotland: The Prolactin Epidemiology, Audit and Research Study (PROLEARS). *Clin Endocrinol.* 2017, 86 (1):60–67.

34. Huang KE, Bonfiglio TA, and Muechler EK. Transient hyperprolactinemia in infertile women with luteal phase deficiency. *Obstet Gynecol.* 1991, 78(4):651–655.

35. Molitch ME, and Reichlin S. Hyperprolactinemic disorders. *Dis Mon.* 1982, 28(9):1–58.

36. Touraine P, Plu-Bureau G, Beji C, et al. Long-term follow-up of 246 hyperprolactinemic patients. *Acta Obstet Gynecol Scand.* 2001, 80(2):162–168.

37. Lee DY, Oh YK, Yoon BK, et al. Prevalence of hyperprolactinemia in adolescents and young women with menstruation-related problems. *Am J Obstet Gynecol.* 2012, 206(3):213 e1–5.

38. Binart N, Young J, and Chanson P. Prolactin assays

and regulation of secretion: animal and human data. In: Tritos NA, Klibanski A (Eds.) *Prolactin Disorders from Basic Science to Clinical Management.* Contemporary Endocrinology 2019; 55–78. Springer Nature Switzerland AG: Humana Press.

39. Fahie-Wilson M, and Smith TP. Determination of prolactin: The macroprolactin problem. *Best Pract Res Clin Endocrinol Metab.* 2013, 27 (5):725–742.

40. Kalsi AK, Halder A, Jain M, et al. Prevalence and reproductive manifestations of macroprolactinemia. *Endocrine.* 2019, 63 (2):332–340.

41. Karavitaki N, Thanabalasingham G, Shore HC, et al. Do the limits of serum prolactin in disconnection hyperprolactinaemia need re-definition? A study of 226 patients with histologically verified non-functioning pituitary macroadenoma. *Clin Endocrinol (Oxf).* 2006, 65 (4):524–529.

42. Dohle GR, Colpi GM, Hargreave TB, et al. EAU guidelines on male infertility. *Eur Urol.* 2005, 48(5):703–711.

43. Patel DP, Chandrapal JC, and Hotaling JM. Hormone-Based Treatments in Subfertile Males. *Curr Urol Rep.* 2016, 17(8):56.

44. Iglesias P, Bernal C, Villabona C, et al. Prolactinomas in men: A multicentre and retrospective analysis of treatment outcome. *Clin Endocrinol (Oxf).* 2012, 77 (2):281–287.

45. Shimon I, and Benbassat C. Male prolactinomas presenting with normal testosterone levels. *Pituitary.* 2014;17(3):246–250.

46. Colao A, Vitale G, Cappabianca P, et al. Outcome of cabergoline treatment in men with prolactinoma: effects of a 24-month treatment on prolactin levels, tumor mass, recovery of pituitary function, and semen analysis. *J Clin Endocrinol Metab.* 2004, 89 (4):1704–1711.

47. De Rosa M, Ciccarelli A, Zarrilli S, et al. The treatment with cabergoline for 24 month normalizes the quality of seminal fluid in hyperprolactinaemic males. *Clin Endocrinol (Oxf).* 2006, 64 (3):307–313.

48. De Rosa M, Zarrilli S, Di Sarno A, et al. Hyperprolactinemia in men: clinical and biochemical features and response to treatment. *Endocrine.* 2003, 20 (1-2):75–82.

49. Pinzone JJ, Katznelson L, Danila DC, et al. Primary medical therapy of micro- and macroprolactinomas in men. *J Clin Endocrinol Metab.* 2000, 85(9):3053–3057.

50. Molitch M. Prolactin and pregnancy. In: Tritos NA, Klibanski A (Eds.), *Prolactin Disorders from Basic Science to Clinical Management.* Contemporary Endocrinology. 2019; 161–174. Springer Nature Switzerland AG: Humana Press.

51. Gillam MP, Molitch ME, Lombardi G, et al. Advances in the treatment of prolactinomas. *Endocr Rev.* 2006, 27 (5):485–534.

52. Melmed S, Casanueva FF, Hoffman AR, et al. Diagnosis and treatment of hyperprolactinemia: an Endocrine Society clinical practice guideline. *J Clin Endocrinol Metab.* 2011, 96 (2):273–288.

53. Glezer A, and Bronstein MD. Prolactinomas, cabergoline, and pregnancy. *Endocrine.* 2014, 47(1):64–69.

54. Webster J. A comparative review of the tolerability profiles of dopamine agonists in the treatment of hyperprolactinaemia and inhibition of lactation. *Drug Saf.* 1996, 14(4):228–238.

55. Webster J, Piscitelli G, Polli A, et al. A comparison of cabergoline and bromocriptine in the treatment of hyperprolactinemic amenorrhea. Cabergoline Comparative Study Group (see comments). *N Engl J Med.* 1994, 331(14):904–909.

56. Wang AT, Mullan RJ, Lane MA, et al. Treatment of hyperprolactinemia: a systematic review and meta-analysis. *Syst Rev.* 2012, 1:33.

57. Ono M, Miki N, Amano K, et al. Individualized high-dose cabergoline therapy for hyperprolactinemic infertility in women with micro- and macroprolactinomas. *J Clin Endocrinol Metab.* 2010.

58. Verhelst J, Abs R, Maiter D, et al. Cabergoline in the treatment of hyperprolactinemia: a study in 455 patients. *J Clin Endocrinol Metab.* 1999, 84(7):2518–2522.

59. Laws ER, Jr., Fode NC, Randall RV, et al. Pregnancy following transsphenoidal resection of prolactin-secreting pituitary tumors. *J Neurosurg.* 1983, 58 (5):685–688.

60. Buchfelder M, Zhao Y, and Schlaffer SM. Surgery for prolactinomas to date. *Neuroendocrinology.* 2019.

61. Zamanipoor Najafabadi AH, Zandbergen IM, de Vries F, et al. Surgery as a viable alternative first-line treatment for prolactinoma patients. A systematic review and meta-analysis. *J Clin Endocrinol Metab.* 2020, 105(3).

62. Primeau V, Raftopoulos C, and Maiter D. Outcomes of transsphenoidal surgery in prolactinomas: improvement of hormonal control in dopamine agonist-resistant patients. *Eur J Endocrinol.* 2012, 166(5):779–786.

63. McGarrigle HH, Sarris S, Little V, et al. Induction of ovulation with clomiphene and human chorionic gonadotrophin in women with hyperprolactinaemic amenorrhoea. *Br J Obstet Gynaecol.* 1978, 85(9):692–697.

64. Lebbe M, Hubinont C, Bernard P, et al. Outcome of 100 pregnancies initiated under treatment with cabergoline in hyperprolactinaemic women. *Clin Endocrinol (Oxf).* 2010, 73 (2):236–242.

65. Casanueva FF, Molitch ME, Schlechte JA, et al. Guidelines of the pituitary society for the diagnosis and management of prolactinomas. *Clin Endocrinol (Oxf).* 2006, 65(2):265–273.

66. Ray JG, Vermeulen MJ, Bharatha A, et al. Association between MRI exposure during pregnancy and fetal and childhood outcomes. *JAMA.* 2016, 316(9):952–961.

67. Proenca F, Guerreiro C, Sa G, et al Neuroimaging safety during pregnancy and lactation: a review. *Neuroradiology.* 2021.

68. Sant' Anna BG, Musolino NRC, Gadelha MR, et al. A Brazilian multicentre study evaluating pregnancies induced by cabergoline in patients harboring prolactinomas. *Pituitary.* 2020, 23(2): 120–128.

69. Lambert K, Rees K, Seed PT, et al. Macroprolactinomas and nonfunctioning pituitary adenomas and pregnancy outcomes. *Obstet Gynecol.* 2017, 129(1):185–194.

70. Barraud S, Guedra L, Delemer B, et al. Evolution of macroprolactinomas during pregnancy: A cohort study of 85 pregnancies. *Clin Endocrinol (Oxf).* 2020, 92(5):421–427.

71. Huang W, and Molitch ME. Pituitary tumors in pregnancy. *Endocrinol Metab Clin North Am.* 2019, 48(3):569–581.

72. Araujo B, Belo S, and Carvalho D. Pregnancy and tumor outcomes in women with prolactinoma. *Exp Clin Endocrinol Diabetes.* 2017, 125 (10):642–648.

73. Galvao A, Goncalves D, Moreira M, et al. Prolactinoma and pregnancy – A series of cases including pituitary apoplexy. *J Obstet Gynaecol.* 2017;37(3):284–287.

74. Karaca Z, Yarman S, Ozbas I, et al. How does pregnancy affect the patients with pituitary adenomas: a study on 113 pregnancies from Turkey. *J Endocrinol Invest.* 2018, 41 (1):129–141.

75. O'Sullivan SM, Farrant MT, Ogilvie CM, et al. An observational study of pregnancy and post-partum outcomes in women with prolactinoma treated with dopamine agonists. *Aust N Z J Obstet Gynaecol.* 2020, 60 (3):405–411.

76. Schlechte JA. Clinical practice. *Prolactinoma. N Engl J Med.* 2003, 349 (21):2035–2041.

77. Divers WA, Jr., and Yen SS. Prolactin-producing microadenomas in pregnancy. *Obstet Gynecol.* 1983, 62 (4):425–429.

78. Rastogi A, Bhansali A, Dutta P, et al. A comparison between intensive and conventional cabergoline treatment of newly diagnosed patients with macroprolactinoma. *Clin Endocrinol (Oxf).* 2013, 79 (3):409–415.

79. Graillon T, Cuny T, Castinetti F, et al. Surgical indications for pituitary tumors during pregnancy: a literature review. *Pituitary.* 2020, 23(2):189–199.

80. Grand'Maison S, Weber F, Bedard MJ, et al. Pituitary apoplexy in pregnancy: A case series and literature review. *Obstet Med.* 2015, 8 (4):177–183.

81. Kuhn E, Weinreich AA, Biermasz NR, et al. Apoplexy of microprolactinomas during pregnancy. *Eur J Endocrinol.* 2021.

82. Bronstein MD. Prolactinomas and pregnancy. *Pituitary.* 2005, 8(1):31–38.

83. Molitch ME. Prolactinoma in pregnancy. *Best Pract Res Clin Endocrinol Metab.* 2011, 25 (6):885–896.

84. Auriemma RS, Perone Y, Di Sarno A, Grasso LF, Guerra E, Gasperi M, et al. Results of a single-center observational 10-year survey study on recurrence of hyperprolactinemia after pregnancy and lactation. *J Clin Endocrinol Metab.* 2013, 98 (1):372–379.

85. Domingue ME, Devuyst F, Alexopoulou O, et al. Outcome of prolactinoma after pregnancy and lactation: a study on 73 patients. *Clin Endocrinol (Oxf).* 2014, 80(5):642–648.

86. Ikegami H, Aono T, Koizumi K, et al. Relationship between the methods of treatment for prolactinomas and the puerperal lactation. *Fertil Steril.* 1987, 47(5):867–869.

87. Bern HA, and Nicoll CS. The comparative endocrinology of prolactin. *Recent Prog Horm Res.* 1968, 24:681–720.

88. Biswas S, and Rodeck CH. Plasma prolactin levels during pregnancy. *Br J Obstet Gynaecol.* 1976, 83(9):683–687.

89. Karunakaran S, Page RC, and Wass JA. The effect of the menopause on prolactin levels in patients with hyperprolactinaemia. *Clin Endocrinol (Oxf).* 2001, 54 (3):295–300.

90. Huda MS, Athauda NB, Teh MM, et al. Factors determining the remission of microprolactinomas after dopamine agonist withdrawal. *Clin Endocrinol (Oxf).* 2010, 72 (4):507–511.

Chapter

9

Growth Hormone Disorders in Pregnancy

Marie Helene Schernthaner-Reiter, Greisa Vila, Peter Wolf, and Anton Luger

9.1 Introduction

In normal pregnancy, the placenta starts to produce a Growth Hormones (GH) variant (hPGH) that differs from pituitary GH by 13 amino acids in the first gestational weeks. Maximal human Placental Growth Hormone (hPGH) levels comparable to those in acromegaly of 20–40 ng/mL are reached around week 37 (1) (Figure 9.1). In contrast to the pulsatory pituitary GH release, hPGH is secreted continuously, without peaks. Pituitary GH decreases in parallel to the rise of hPGH to undetectable concentrations after week 24. Insulin-like growth factor 1 (IGF-1) concentrations decline between week 5 and 12 of gestation and increase thereafter to maximal concentrations that are above the age specific reference range for nonpregnant women in the third trimester (2,3).

9.2 GH and Fertility

The role of growth hormone therapy in women without GH deficiency during ovarian stimulation in In Vitro Fertilization/Intracytoplasmic Sperm Injection (IVF/ICSI) treatment is controversial. Several reports and animal models suggest that GH can stimulate the secretion of IGF-1 not only in the liver but also in the ovary and enhance the follicular response to gonadotropin stimulation (4). In addition, a randomized controlled study in 158 women with poor embryonic development found that GH supplementation improved live birth rate during in vitro fertilization (5). However, a recent meta-analysis of studies investigating growth hormone co-treatment in poor responders undergoing in vitro fertilization cycles showed that while GH supplementation increased clinical pregnancy rate, number of oocytes retrieved, number of Methaphase II (MII) oocytes, and number of embryos available to transfer, it had no effect on the live birth rate (4,6). A recently published guideline of the European Society of Human Reproduction and Embryology (ESHRE) included a conditional recommendation "that the use of adjuvant GH before and/or during ovarian stimulation is probably not recommended" (7).

9.3 Growth Hormone Deficiency (GHD)

There is evidence that growth hormone deficiency is associated with decreased fertility (8,9). Apart

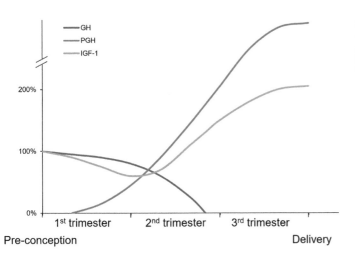

Figure 9.1 Schematic diagram of serum concentrations of growth hormone (GH), placental growth hormone (PGH), and insulin-like growth factor-1 (IGF-1) in healthy women during pregnancy.

from the effect of estrogen, GH determines uterus size, enhances the follicular response to gonadotropin stimulation, and affects maturation of the follicle and gamete (4,10). In addition, IGF-1 potentiates Follicle stimulating Hormone (FSH) actions on granulosa cells and stimulates proliferation and differentiation of granulosa and theca cells (11).

There is no clear evidence how GH-substitution therapy should be handled in Growth Hormone Deficiency (GHD) patients on GH replacement therapy before and after conception (12). Apart from case reports and small series, the largest series of pregnancies in GHD women has been reported using data retrieved from a prospective pharmacoepidemiologic surveillance study (9,13). Of the 173 pregnancies observed in 144 women, 39 percent had childhood onset GHD, and 90 percent had additional pituitary deficiencies (13). Spontaneous conception was reported in 36 percent of cases. In almost half of the women, GH therapy was stopped either before conception or at confirmation of pregnancy, whereas it was partially continued in 25 percent. However, in 28 percent of the women, GHRT was continued throughout pregnancy according to the women's preference and in agreement with the treating physician despite the physiological increase of hPGH production by the syncytiotrophoblast from week 5 on. Pregnancy outcomes including malformations appeared to be unaffected whether GH substitution was continued throughout pregnancy or stopped at any time during pregnancy. There was no association between live births and GH dose at conception, IGF-1 Social defeat stress before conception, or GHRT use during pregnancy. Whereas it would appear logical to mimic nature as closely as possible and gradually decrease the GH dose during the first trimester and stop it in the second trimester, there is no clear evidence to support this approach.

9.4 Growth Hormone Excess (Acromegaly)

If acromegaly is diagnosed in fertile women with or without current wish for pregnancy, careful evaluation of the adenoma size, disease activity, comorbidities, and pituitary functions should be performed (14). These women should be treated in a Pituitary Center of Excellence (15) or reference center with adequate experience and prerequisites for optimal counseling and treatment.

Gonadal dysfunction is common in women with acromegaly and might be related to a size effect of the tumor suppressing gonadotropic function, co-secretion of prolactin, or direct GH effects (16). In women with a microadenoma and mildly active disease, no comorbidities, and regular ovulatory cycles, pregnancy is considered safe and surgical or medical treatment can be postponed until after delivery (14). Usually GH producing adenomas do not increase in size during pregnancy, serum IGF-1 concentrations decrease, and GH levels remain stable (16). However, women with macroadenomas compromising the optic chiasm or with tumors in close vicinity to it, as well as those with very active disease causing serious comorbidities or impaired gonadotroph function, should be informed about the option of transsphenoidal surgery aiming at removal or debulking of the adenoma and biochemical cure (14). In many cases gonadotroph function can be restored by surgery, although women should be informed that impairment of gonadotroph function can be caused by surgery also in those with preoperatively normal ovulatory cycles (14,17).

Women wishing to conceive – including those who have not been cured by surgery and therefore are being treated with the long-acting first-generation somatostatin analogs octreotide (Sandostatin LAR®) or lanreotide (Somatuline Autogel®) or, in the case of mild postoperative GH excess, with the dopamine agonist cabergoline (Dostinex®) – should be informed to discontinue medical therapy when pregnancy is confirmed. Whereas the 2014 Endocrine Society Clinical Practice Guideline recommended that women on treatment with long-acting first-generation somatostatin analogs should discontinue them two months before attempting to conceive and be switched to short-acting somatostatin analogs, a recent Clinical Guideline of the European Society of Endocrinology suggested that it is safe to continue them until confirmation of pregnancy (14,18). No data on the second-generation somatostatin analog pasireotide (Signifor®) and very limited data on the GH antagonist pegvisomant (Somavert®) are available (19). Therefore they should not be used in women wishing to conceive or during pregnancy.

During pregnancy, GH and IGF-1 concentrations do not provide any useful information about activity or size changes of an adenoma and therefore should not be measured (14,18). Women should be monitored clinically, and in case of symptoms that might be related to tumor enlargement – such as impairment of visual fields, visual acuity, any other nerve palsy, or severe headache a neuro-ophthalmologic – evaluation including optical coherence tomography to evaluate retinal nerve fiber layer and ganglion cell complex should be performed (14). Routine Magnetic Resonance imaging (MRI) monitoring during pregnancy is not recommended. MRI should be performed only depending on the results of the neuro-ophthalmological examination and the severity of the symptoms (14). An MRI should be done without gadolinium since the required information is usually obtained by an MRI without contrast media (14,20).

If there is evidence of symptomatic tumor growth during pregnancy, therapy with first-generation somatostatin analogs might be initiated. Lanreotide or octreotide appear not to be associated with maternal or fetal adverse effects, though due to the very limited evidence their use should be considered only in selected cases (21,22). Cabergoline apparently can also be safely used in pregnancy, however it might not decrease tumor size efficiently and therefore is not indicated (21,23). Pegvisomant does not reduce tumor size and should not be used. No data on pasireotide are available in this situation. If there is no rapid or significant effect of medical therapy, surgery is indicated. Most experience with surgery is available for the second trimester; the first trimester should be avoided if possible (24). However, in emergency situations surgery should not be delayed, and in the third trimester, pre-term delivery should be considered. Not only due to its slow onset of action, radiotherapy obviously has no place in the therapy of acromegaly in pregnancy.

Two frequent complications of acromegaly – diabetes mellitus and hypertension – deserve special attention in pregnancy. Pregnancy and acromegaly both induce insulin resistance. Whereas many studies report the increased prevalence of diabetes in the nonpregnant women (25,26), data on gestational diabetes in acromegaly are scarce. A French multicenter and a single-center study reported increased risk of gestational diabetes in women with acromegaly, whereas a compilation of predominantly case reports published up to 2019 did not confirm this (17,27). This might be related to the lack of screening for gestational diabetes. Due to the possible deleterious effects of hyperglycemia during pregnancy, consequent screening for disturbed glucose homeostasis starting early in pregnancy appears advisable. In addition, GH excess induces sodium and fluid retention and thereby might further increase the risk for hypertension in pregnancy. There is no evidence that diabetes and hypertension should be treated differently in pregnant women with acromegaly than in women without acromegaly but it should be done strictly (17,27).

Disease activity frequently rebounds after delivery and therefore laboratory values, and in most cases MRI should be checked (14). Breastfeeding is usually possible, but women on somatostatin analogs should be informed that it is contraindicated according to the manufacturers (SPC).

The authors declare the following conflicts of interest:

M.H.S-R. has received honoraria for presentations from HRA Pharma; P. W. none; G. V. has received lecture and/or consulting fees from Ipsen, Pfizer, Novo Nordisk, Takeda, and HRA Pharma, and is Research Investigator in studies sponsored by Novartis, Recordati, Corcept, Chiasma, and Takeda; A. L. has received lecture and/or consulting fees from Ionis, Ipsen, Merck, Novartis Pfizer, and Sandoz.

References

1. Freemark M. Placental hormones and the control of fetal growth. *J Clin Endocrinol Metab*. 2010, 95:2054–2057.

2. Monaghan JM, Godber IM, Lawson N, et al. Longitudinal changes of insulin-like growth factors and their binding proteins throughout normal pregnancy. *Ann Clin Biochem*. 2004, 41:220–226.

3. Asvold BO, Eskild A, Jenum PA, et al. Maternal concentrations of insulin-like growth factor I and insulin-like growth factor binding protein 1 during pregnancy and birth weight of offspring. *Am J Epidemiol*. 2011, 174:129–135.

4. Dosouto C, Calaf J, Polo A, et al. Growth hormone and reproduction: Lessons learned from animal models and clinical trials. *Frontiers Endocrinol*. 10.404. https://doi.org/10.3389/fendo.2019.00404.

5. Li J, Chen Q, Wang J, et al. Does growth hormone supplementation improve oocyte competence and IVF

outcomes in patients with poor embryonic development? A randomized controlled trial. *BMC Pregnancy and Childbirth*. 2020, 20:310. https://doi.org/10.1186/s12884-020-03004-9.

6. Cozzolino M, Cecchino GN, Trojano DG, et al. Growth hormone cotreatment for poor responders undergoing in vitro fertilization cycles: A systematic review and meta-analysis. *Fertil Steril*. 2020, 114:97–107.

7. The ESHRE Guideline Group on Ovarian Stimulation, Bosch M, et al. ESHRE guideline: Ovarian stimulation for IVF/ICSI. Human Reproduction Open 2020; p. 1–3. https://doi.org/10.1093/hropen/hoaa009.

8. de Boer JA, Schoemaker J, and van der Veen EA. Impaired reproductive function in women treated for growth hormone deficiency during childhood. *Clin Endocrinol*. 1997, 46:681–689.

9. Giampetro A, Milardi D, Bianchi A, et al. The effect of treatment with growth hormone on fertility outcome in eugonadal women with growth hormone deficiency: Report of four cases and review of the literature. *Fertil Steril*. 2009, 91:930e7–930e11.

10. Tsilchorozidou T, and Conway GS. Uterus size and ovarian morphology in women with isolated growth hormone deficiency, hypogonadotrophic hypogonadism and hypopituitarism. *Clin Endocrinol*. 2004, 61:567–572.

11. Ipsa E, Cruzat VF, Kagize JN, et al. Growth hormone and insulin-like growth factor action in reproductive tissues.

Frontiers Endocrinol. 2019, 10:777. https://doi.org/10.3389/fendo.2019.00777.

12. Vila G, and Luger A. Growth hormone deficiency and pregnancy: Any role for substitution? *Minerva Endocrinol*. 2018, 43:451–457.

13. Vila G, Akerblad AC, Mattsson A, et al. Pregnancy outcomes in women with growth hormone deficiency. *Fertil Steril*. 2015, 104:1210–1217.

14. Luger A, Broersen LHA, Biermasz NR, et al. Functioning and nonfunctioning pituitary adenomas in pregnancy. An ESE clinical practice guideline. *Eur J Endocrinol*. 2021, 185:G1–G33

15. Casanueva FF, Barkan AL, Buchfelder M, et al. Criteria for the definition of Pituitary Tumor Centers of Excellence (PTCOE): A Pituitary Society statement. *Pituitary*. 2017, 20:489–498.

16. Grynberg M, Salenave S, Young J, et al. Female gonadal function before and after treatment of acromegaly. *J Clin Endocrinol Metab*. 2010, 95:4518–4525.

17. Caron P, Broussaud S, Bertherat J, et al. Acromegaly and pregnancy: A retrospective multicenter study of 59 pregnancies in 46 women. *J Clin Endocrinol Metab*. 2010, 95:4680–4687.

18. Katznelson L, Laws ER, Melmed S, et al. Acromegaly: An Endocrine Society Clinical Practice Guideline. *J Clin Endocrinol Metab*. 2014, 99:3933–3951.

19. van der Lely AJ, Gomez R, Heissler JF, et al. Pregnancy in acromegaly patients treated

with pegvisomant. *Endocrine*. 2015, 49:769–773.

20. ACOG Committee Opinion. Guidelines for diagnostic imaging during pregnancy and lactation. *Obstetrics Gynecol*. 1017, 130:e210–e216.

21. Chanson P, Vialon M, and Caron P. An update on clinical care for pregnant women with acromegaly. *Exp Rev Endocrinol Metab*. 2019, 14:85–96.

22. Abucham J, Bronstein MD, and Dias ML. Acromegaly and pregnancy: A contemporary review. *Eur J Endocrinol*. 2017, 177:R1–R12.

23. Abs R, Verhelst J, Maiter D, et al. Cabergoline in the treatment of acromegaly: A study in 64 patients. *J Clin Endocrinol Metab*. 1998, 83:374–378.

24. Graillon T, Cuny T, Castinetti F, et al. Surgical indications for pituitary tumors during pregnancy: A literature review. *Pituitary*. 2020, 23:189–199.

25. Alexopoulou O, Bex M, Kamenicky P, et al. Prevalence and risk factors of impaired glucose tolerance and diabetes mellitus at diagnosis of acromegaly: A study in 148 patients. *Pituitary*. 2014, 17:81–89.

26. Ciresi A, Amato MC, Pivonello R, et al. The metabolic profile in active acromegaly is gender-specific. *J Clin Endocrinol Meta*. 2013, 98: E51–E59.

27. Vialon M, Grunenwald S, Mouly C, et al. Gestational diabetes and acromegaly: Single-centre experience in 14 pregnancies. *Clin Endocrinol*. 2019, 91:805–809.

10

Gestational Diabetes

Serena Ottanelli, Federico Mecacci, and Moshe Hod

10.1 Introduction

Gestational Diabetes (GDM) is the most common metabolic disorder of pregnancy, and it is defined as a glucose intolerance resulting in hyperglycemia of variable severity with onset or first recognition during pregnancy. The International Diabetes Federation reports that 1 out of 6 (16.8 percent) pregnancies are affected by some sort of hyperglycemia, and among these, the majority (86.4 percent) are GDM. The prevalence of GDM is rapidly growing worldwide, because of the obesity epidemic, physical inactivity, and rising maternal age.

Hyperglycemia in pregnancy is associated with adverse outcomes for the fetus, with a higher incidence of perinatal morbidity but also with long term metabolic sequelae in offspring exposed in utero to maternal hyperglycemia. Maternal morbidity is also significantly increased, including short term complications (hypertensive disorders and cesarean deliveries) and long-term risk of type 2 diabetes and cardiovascular disease (1).

10.2 Metabolic Changes during Normal Pregnancy

In order to understand the pathophysiology of GDM, it is of utmost importance to recognize the metabolic alterations occurring in a normal pregnancy .

Pregnancy is characterized by complex endocrine-metabolic adaptations, including major changes in intermediate metabolism, that represent a necessary and indispensable adaptation to ensure a continuous supply of nutrients to the fetus in order to sustain its exponential growth. The mother's ability to regulate this metabolic balance is therefore essential for the health of both mother and fetus.

10.2.1 Carbohydrates Metabolism

Normal pregnancy has been identified as a "diabetogenic state" because of the progressive development of a state of insulin resistance (IR), that begins near mid-pregnancy and reaches its maximum value in the third trimester and returns to normal levels after delivery. This is a physiological condition in the second half of pregnancy to facilitate maternal catabolism in order to provide nutrients for fetal growth (2).

From a metabolic point of view, there are two different intervals during gestation. In the first half of pregnancy, maternal changes lead to the storage of energy and nutrients (anabolic phase). In contrast, late pregnancy is characterized by a decreased insulin sensitivity and increase in maternal glucose and free fatty acid concentrations, allowing greater substrate availability for fetal growth (catabolic phase).

During the first trimester of pregnancy, insulin sensitivity is higher than normal, resulting in an increase of peripheral glucose utilization and lower blood glucose levels, increased glycogen synthesis, and a reduction in hepatic gluconeogenesis. These changes will facilitate glucose and lipid uptake by adipose tissue, increasing the lipid stores. The second half of pregnancy is characterized by a state of insulin resistance, decreasing the uptake of glucose by maternal tissue sensible to insulin mainly the white adipose tissue and muscle. Catalano et al., by using the euglycemic-hyperinsulinemic clamp, estimated a 47 percent reduction in insulin sensitivity in obese women and a 56 percent reduction in normal weight women in the third trimester (2). The reduced insulin-mediated utilization of glucose switches the maternal energetic metabolism from carbohydrates to lipids, redirecting carbohydrates towards the growing fetal tissues (Figure 10.1).

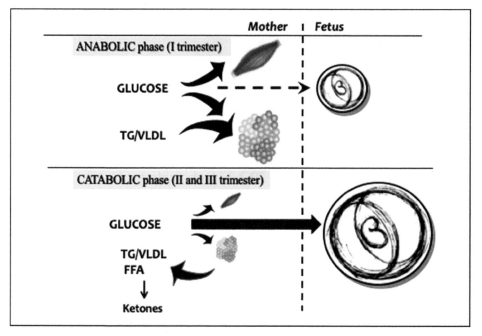

Figure 10.1 Metabolic adaptation to pregnancy. In early pregnancy, maternal metabolic changes are dominated by the storage of nutrients in body fat, while normal or possibly increased insulin sensitivity favors lipogenesis. Then increasing insulin resistance favors lipolysis to meet maternal energy needs with sparing of glucose for transfer to the fetus. *TG triglycerides, VLDL very low density lipoproteins, FFA free fatty acids.*

This reduction in insulin sensitivity is accompanied by a compensatory increase in insulin secretion and in β-cell mass and function, maintaining euglycemia (3).

Despite increased glucose production and insulin resistance, there is a trend towards lower plasma glucose concentrations during pregnancy, because of an increase in plasma volume in early pregnancy and given the high fetal glucose utilization in late gestation (4).

10.2.2 Lipids Metabolism

The metabolic changes occurring in the liver and adipose tissue have an impact on lipid metabolism. In early pregnancy, the increase in estrogen secretion and insulin levels inhibits lipolysis and promotes the creation of fat stores. Following an initial reduction during the first eight weeks of pregnancy, plasma levels of triglycerides and cholesterol tend to increase. The high plasma levels of triglycerides seem to be secondary to both an increased hepatic synthesis of very low density lipoproteins (VLDL) secondary to the elevation of estrogen levels, as well as a decreased lipoprotein lipase activity (LPL) in the adipose tissue determined by insulin resistance.

In the second half of pregnancy, the transition from an anabolic to a catabolic state determines an increase in circulating lipids and promotes their use as an energy source in the mother's tissues, preserving glucose and aminoacids which are transferred towards the fetus (5).

10.2.3 Placental and Maternal Hormones and Insulin Resistance

Though the specific mechanisms of the alteration of insulin secretion and action remain uncertain, they have been ascribed to the metabolic effects of several hormones of maternal and placental origin released in the maternal circulation.

10.2.3.1 Placental Hormones

Historically it was postulated that progesterone and human placental lactogen (hPL), produced by the placenta, were primarily responsible for insulin resistance of pregnancy. Results from animal models as well as human observational studies showed a parallel increase in these hormone levels during gestation and insulin resistance development. Furthermore, administration to nonpregnant patients decreased insulin sensitivity and determined a significantly higher plasma insulin responses after oral glucose administration (6).

Another placental product apparently playing a major role in this scenario is placental growth hormone (PGF); it seems to contribute to the insulin resistance in late pregnancy through up-regulation of the growth hormone/ insulin-like growth factor (IGF) axis with a possible inter-action with brown adipose tissue. In fact, its acti-vation has been demonstrated to improve insulin sensitivity and glucose homeostasis in adults. PGF levels were shown to be lower in women with GDM compared to normal pregnant women, and GDM pregnancies were found to have lower brown adipocyte activation (6,7).

Follistatin-like-3 is a circulating inhibitor of members of the transforming growth factor-beta family of proteins, highly expressed by the pla-centa. It enhances glucose tolerance and improves insulin sensitivity. Its levels were decreased in pregnancies complicated later by GDM (8). However, the lack of a standardized assay for FSTL-3 does not allow validating the use of this marker. Placental growth factor (PLGF) is a vas-cular endothelial growth factor-like protein usu-ally used, if low levels are detected, as predictor of intrauterine growth restriction and preeclampsia (PE) in the first trimester. On the contrary, high levels have been observed in those who will develop GDM later in gestation (9), but results needs to be fully elucidated.

10.2.3.2 Maternal Hormones

Several maternal hormones such as prolactin (PRL) and cortisol rise during pregnancy and have a well-known negative impact on insulin sensitivity. Another insulin metabolism marker is the sex hormone-binding globulin (SHBG), a protein negatively regulated by insulin, and inversely associated with insulin resistance. Low pre-pregnancy and first trimester levels of SHBG are predictive of GDM. It has been shown that women with pre-pregnancy SHBG in the lowest quartile had a four-fold increased risk of GDM (10).

10.2.3.3 Inflammation Molecules and Adipokines

More recently, new molecules linked to obesity and inflammation were considered as potential mediators of insulin resistance in pregnancy such as leptin, adiponectin, and Tumor necrosis factor alpha (TNF-α). These proinflammatory cell-signaling proteins are normally produced by maternal adipose tissue, but during pregnancy, the placenta also contributes to production of large amounts of these molecules.

In fact, the placenta seems to represent a major source of leptin, as shown by the fall in circulating leptin levels after delivery and by the lack of correlation between leptin levels and maternal adipose reserves. Serum leptin levels were significantly correlated with insulin sensitiv-ity index in the second and third trimester and are significantly in higher women who develop gesta-tional diabetes (11).

Adiponectin is produced in large quantities by adipose tissue, whereas the placenta seems not to be one of the sources. Levels of circulating adipo-nectin are inversely related to insulin resistance and are negatively correlated with adiposity. This molecule is considered as an anti-diabetes cyto-kine; in fact it enhances insulin signaling and fatty acid oxidation, inhibits gluconeogenesis, and stimulates insulin secretion, which farther down-regulates the production and release of other proinflammatory cytokines from adipocytes. It has been demonstrated that women that develop gestational diabetes had lower adiponectin levels at 16 weeks' gestation and in pre-conceptional period respect to controls with normal glucose tolerance in pregnancy (12).

TNF-α is a proinflammatory cytokine with numerous effects, including blocking insulin signal transduction; TNF-α levels correlated with insulin resistance in late pregnancy and were sig-nificantly higher in women with GDM than normal controls independent of obesity (11).

10.3 Pathophysiology of Gestational Diabetes

It is well known that the metabolic abnormalities in GDM include an increased insulin resistance, together with a reduced β-cell capacity; hypergly-cemia in pregnancy develops when the maternal insulin response is insufficient to maintain glu-cose tolerance (Figure 10.2).

Several studies by Catalano et al. demon-strated significantly decreased insulin sensitivity in GDM compared to normal pregnancy, and this feature was present prior to conception and per-sisted across pregnancy and postpartum. Therefore, in the majority of GDM cases, the metabolic and endocrine changes of pregnancy

93

Figure 10.2 Pathophysiology of insulin resistance in pregnancy and gestational diabetes. *HPL human placental lactogen, PGF placental growth hormone, PRL prolactin, TNF Tumor necrosis factor, PCOS polycystic ovarian syndrome, GKG glucokinase gene.*

seem to exacerbate an asymptomatic pre-existing state of chronic insulin resistance, unmasking previously unknown beta cell dysfunction, especially in high risk populations (overweight and obesity, polycystic ovarian syndrome [PCOS], advanced maternal age).

In a few cases inability to compensate for insulin resistance may reflect intrinsic alterations of the β-cell. In fact, only in a minority of cases (2–13 percent) antibodies against specific β-cell antigen are found, whereas only around 5–10 percent of women with GDM have some sort of monogenic diabetes (MODY) with mutations in GCK (glucokinase) gene – autosomal dominant genes influencing insulin production (13).

10.4 Risk Factors for Gestational Diabetes

GDM shares several nonmodifiable risk factors with T2DM, including advanced age, family history of diabetes, and ethnicity with a high prevalence of diabetes (including South Asian, Middle Eastern, and Black Caribbean).

After 35 years, the risk of GDM increases from 2 percent to 7 percent, and women older than 40 years have an OR 3.8 to develop GDM (14).

Belonging to an ethnic group such as South Asian or Middle Eastern nationalities, as well as having a low socioeconomic background, exposes one to a higher risk of GDM than the general population. However, immigrant women are at an increased risk of GDM across all ethnic groups. The reasons underlying the ethnic differences are likely to be multifactorial, including differences in body adiposity and insulin resistance, lifestyle, and genetic susceptibility (15).

Among modifiable risk factors, obesity and metabolic syndrome are crucial determinants of GDM. A meta-analysis of 20 cohort studies from America, Europe, and Australia estimated that the risk of GDM was approximately two-, four-, and eight-fold higher in overweight, obese, and severely obese women compared to normal weight women. It was estimated that the population attributable fraction of GDM relating to overweight and obesity was 46 percent. Obesity and metabolic syndrome before pregnancy are characterized by higher insulin resistance and chronic inflammation. In this group, pre-pregnancy counseling on diet change, physical exercise, and lifestyle changes are crucial in order to reduce the risk of GDM later in pregnancy. In PCOS, a hormonal and metabolic dysfunction,

Table 10.1. Risk assessment for gestational diabetes mellitus according to National Institute for Health and Care Excellence (NICE) and American Diabetes Association (ADA) guidelines

NICE	ADA

BMI above 30 kg/m^2
• Previous macrosomic baby weighing 4.5 kg or above
• Previous GDM
• Family history of diabetes (first-degree relative)
• Minority ethnic family origin with a high prevalence of diabetes:
   - South Asia: India, Pakistan, or Bangladesh
   - Black Caribbean
   - Middle Eastern (Saudi Arabia, United Arab Emirates, Iraq, Jordan, Syria, Oman, Qatar, Kuwait, Lebanon, or Egypt)
	Overweight or obese (BMI above 25 kg/m^2 or above 23 kg/m^2 in Asian Americans) adults who have one or more of the following risk factors
	• First-degree relative with diabetes
	• High-risk race/ethnicity (e.g., African American, Latino, Native American, Asian American, Pacific Islander)
	• History of CVD
	• Hypertension ($\geq$140/90 mmHg or on therapy for hypertension)
	• HDL cholesterol level <35 mg/dL (0.90 mmol/L) and/or a triglyceride level >250 mg/dL (2.82 mmol/L)
	• Women with polycystic ovary syndrome
	• Physical inactivity
	• Other clinical conditions associated with insulin resistance (e.g., severe obesity, acanthosis nigricans)

BMI, body mass index; CVD, cardiovascular disease; GDM, gestational diabetes mellitus; HDL, high-density lipoprotein.

the presence of associated obesity, insulin resistance, and hyperandrogenism contributes to the three-fold increased risk of GDM (16).

A summary of risk factors for GDM are outlined in Table 10.1.

10.5 Screening and Diagnosis

10.5.1 Diagnostic Thresholds

Though GDM is one of the most common medical conditions complicating pregnancy, considerable controversies remain regarding universal versus selective screening, the optimal time for screening, and appropriate diagnostic threshold.

The first diagnostic criteria for GDM were established more than 50 years ago, using a two-step approach, and they were designed to identify women at risk of developing diabetes after pregnancy.

The HAPO study, an international cohort study involving more than 25,000 women, provided for the first time the evidence of a strong, continuous relationship between maternal glucose levels and adverse perinatal outcomes and no cutoff was reported.

Following the HAPO study, after an extensive consensus process, the IADPSG in 2010 introduced new recommendations for overt diabetes early in pregnancy and for GDM universal screening with the 2 hour, 75 g oral glucose tolerance test (OGTT) from 24 to 28 weeks of gestation (17). Proposed diagnostic thresholds were based on an adjusted odds ratio threshold of 1.75 (compared with the odds at the HAPO cohort mean) for fetal complications (birth weight, cord C-peptide, and percent body fat above 90th percentile) (18).

The choice of these outcomes and thresholds produced debate and criticism, claiming that the selected outcomes were not the most clinically important to guide the diagnosis and that the value of 1.75 was arbitrary without lack of evidence to support treatment. One of the major concerns was the increase of GDM prevalence adopting IADPSG recommendations: The prevalence in the HAPO study population was 18 percent (10–25 percent), and several studies have reported a prevalence 3.5 higher using IADPSG criteria in different populations.

Since its publication, multiple organizations have endorsed the IADPSG criteria including the WHO (30), FIGO (1), ADA (31), and many local and national societies. Conversely, ACOG and SMFM still recommend the traditional approach of using the two-step screening strategy

Table 10.2. FIGO guidelines for the diagnosis of hyperglycemia in pregnancy, based on resource settings

Setting	Who to test and when	Diagnostic test	
Fully resourced settings	All women at booking/first trimester 24–28 weeks	Measure FPG, RBG, or HbA1c to detect diabetes in pregnancy If negative: perform 75-g 2-hour OGTT	**Interpretation as per IADPSG/WHO/IDF guidelines***
Fully resourced settings serving ethnic populations at high risk	All women at booking/first trimester 24–28 weeks	Perform 75-g 2-hour OGTT to detect diabetes in pregnancy If negative: perform 75-g 2-hour OGTT	
Any setting (basic); particularly medium to low-resource settings serving ethnic populations at risk	All women between 24 and 28 weeks	Perform 75-g 2-hour OGTT	

* **Diabetes in pregnancy** if Fasting Plasma Glucose ≥ 126 mg/dl (7.0 mmol/l) or Random Plasma Glucose ≥200 mg/dl (11.1 mmol/l) Or HbA1c ≥6.5 percent; **GDM** if at least one value at OGTT e ≥92-180-153 mg/dl.
FPG fasting plasma glucose; HbA1c glycate hemoglobin; RPG random plasma glucose; GDM gestational diabetes mellitus; OGTT oral glucose tolerance test.

with the 50 g glucose challenge test (GCT), and if abnormal, the 3 hour, 100 g OGTT is performed using the Carpenter and Coustan criteria or the National Diabetes Data Group (NDDG) criteria (32).

In original guidelines IADPSG recommended that a FPG in the range 5.1–6.9 mmol/L should be considered diagnostic for GDM if noted at any time during pregnancy, also in the first trimester; this threshold was arbitrary and was chosen as the same value as after 24 weeks. More recent data from Italy and China, where IADPSG diagnostic criteria were applied, demonstrated that early FPG ≥5.1 mmol/L is poorly predictive of later GDM at 24–28 weeks' gestation. Consequently, in 2016 IADPS members suggested that the use of the IADPSG fasting glucose threshold of ≥ 5.1 mmol/L for the identification of GDM in early pregnancy was not justified. So a first trimester FPG value of 92–126 mg/dl should be considered a risk factor for GDM, but not a diagnostic test (19).

10.5.2 Universal or Selective Screening

Apart from the different cut-off values, there is still no consensus about selective or universal screening. Selective testing based on clinical risk factors evolved from the view that in populations with low risk of GDM, subjecting all pregnant women to an OGTT was not considered cost-effective; however, most studies have found that if such a system were used, a significant proportion of GDM cases would be missed. Another problem of risk factor-based screening is the necessity of more complex protocols for testing, which results in lower compliance by both patients and healthcare providers. Given the high rates of hyperglycemia in pregnancy in most populations and considering that selective testing based on known risk factors has poor sensitivity for detection of GDM, universal testing is strongly recommended by FIGO, which adopts and supports the IADPSG/WHO/IDF position that all pregnant women should be tested for hyperglycemia during pregnancy (1) (Table 10.2).

10.6 Maternal and Fetal Complications

10.6.1 Short Term Complication for the Offspring

GDM is associated with several adverse fetal and neonatal outcomes that can be partly prevented by providing a tight maternal glycemic control (Figure 10.3).

Table 10.3. Perinatal outcomes in the HAPO cohort when IADPSG criteria for GDM are applied

Outcome	Frequency in GDM (%)	Frequency in non-GDM (%)	Frequency difference (%)
Preeclampsia	9.1	4.5	4.6
Delivery at <37 weeks	9.4	6.4	3.0
Primary cesarean delivery	24.4	16.8	7.6
Shoulder dystocia or birth injury	1.8	1.3	0.5
Intensive neonatal care	9.1	7.8	1.3
Clinical neonatal hypoglycaemia	2.7	1.9	0.8
Neonatal hyperbilirubinemia	10.0	8.0	2.0
Birthweight >90th percentile	16.2	8.3	7.9
Cord C-peptide >90th percentile	17.5	6.7	10.8
Percent body adipose tissue content >90th percentile	16.6	8.5	8.1

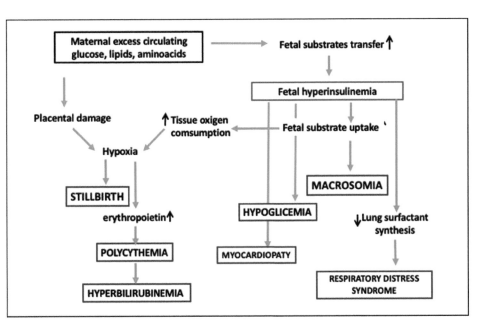

Figure 10.3 Intrauterine exposure to maternal hyperglycemia: fetal and neonatal complications.

The HAPO study provides useful data about the frequency of short term perinatal complications in pregnancy with relatively mild GDM in the absence of treatment (Table 10.3) and showed a clear linear association between maternal glucose levels and short term adverse pregnancy, including macrosomia, birth injury, shoulder dystocia, preterm delivery, PE, cesarean section, neonatal hypoglycemia, neonatal unit admission, and respiratory distress (17).

Physiopathology of fetal complications is explained by the well-known Pedersen's hypothesis: uncontrolled maternal hyperglycemia during pregnancy leads to significant higher glucose placental transfer because of the direct relationship between the maternal and fetal glucose concentrations, and consequently to a prolonged fetal hyperglycemia and hyperinsulinism that leads to accelerated fetal anabolism, increased fetal growth, and macrosomia. Moreover, the fetal hyperinsulinism once established might favor a high transplacental glucose transfer rate and an excessive growth of fetal fat mass, even under optimal later control of maternal glycemia. The

Pedersen hypothesis has been extended by Freinkel who introduced the concept of "fuel mediated teratogenesis," proposing that the placenta and the fetus develop in an ambient that is totally derived from maternal fuels (glucose, amino acids, lipids) which cross the placenta in a concentration dependent modality. Since all of these constituents are regulated by maternal insulin, alteration in its supply or action will influence the whole nutrient composition to which the fetus is exposed, leading to fetal hyperinsulinemia. Accelerated fetal growth in the fetus of a diabetic mother is asymmetric, with excessive growth of insulin sensitive tissue and consequently a normal head size but broader shoulders and increased thoracic and abdominal diameters compared with infants of mothers without diabetes. Macrosomia in GDM offspring is therefore associated not only with an increased risk of operative delivery (cesarean or instrumental vaginal), but also to adverse neonatal outcomes, such as shoulder dystocia and its associated complications: brachial plexus injury, fracture, and neonatal depression. Hyperinsulinemic neonates born from diabetic mothers have a higher risk of hypoglycemia in the immediate postpartum period and of respiratory distress, with a higher need of hospitalizations in neonatal intensive care units (20).

Early studies observed an increased incidence of stillbirth among women with GDM who were undiagnosed or suboptimally treated; in recent years, screening, diagnosis, and treatment of GDM have become more widespread and the association between GDM and intrauterine fetal death has become less clear. Due to the low prevalence of stillbirth, it is difficult to design and power a study to show a difference comparing women receiving an optimal treatment with those poorly controlled

Insulin stimulates fetal aerobic glucose metabolism and will hence increase oxygen demand of the fetus. If adequate supply is not available because of reduced oxygen delivery to the intervillous space as a result of thickening of the placental basement membrane (a common placental structural change in GDM), fetal hypoxemia will ensue and can lead to stillbirth. Therefore, we must consider that confounding factors associated with stillbirth such as obesity, metabolic syndrome, and advanced maternal age may play a role in women with GDM (21).

10.6.2 Short Term Complication for the Mother

Short term adverse obstetric outcome in GDM include operative delivery and birth trauma lacerations, cesarean section, and hypertensive disorders.

Even though GDM alone is not considered an indication for cesarean section, the increase in large for gestational age (LGA) or macrosomic infants among GDM women leads to an increase in cesarean delivery for various reasons, such as cephalopelvic disproportion or fetal distress. Since it is a major surgical procedure, it carries the risk of complications such as infection, bleeding, thrombosis, and wound dehiscence, especially in obese women.

Many studies reported an increase in cesarean delivery rate among GDM women compared to normal pregnant women, especially with nonelective indications; it is reported that a nonelective cesarean section rate for women with GDM is 19.5 percent, compared to 13.5 percent for nondiabetic women. The HAPO study found a direct correlation between maternal glycemia and cesarean section rate, with an overall frequency of 23.7 percent (17).

Several studies have reported increased risk for gestational hypertension and PE in pregnancies complicated by GDM, with a described risk of PE almost doubled in GDM compare to normoglycemic women. In the HAPO study, 5.9 percent of GDM women had gestational hypertension, and 4.8 percent had PE (17).

To understand this link between GDM and hypertensive disorders, it has been hypothesized that GDM and PE share a common etiologic pathway. It is well known that insulin resistance, together with a reduced beta cell capacity, is the most important feature in GDM pathogenesis. In addition, GDM and PE share many risk factors, all characterized by a reduced insulin sensitivity, including advanced maternal age, pre-pregnancy obesity, PCOS, and metabolic syndrome.

Recent studies also support an association between PE and increased insulin resistance, and a reduced insulin sensitivity has also been hypothesized to contribute to the pathophysiology of preeclampsia. Epidemiological studies have demonstrated an increased risk of PE in pregnancies complicated by insulin resistance, and compared to women who have normotensive pregnancies, women who develop PE are more insulin resistant prior to pregnancy in the first and second trimesters and years after pregnancy. Furthermore, insulin resistance in the third trimester of gestation was a significant independent predictor of PE after adjustment for these common risk factors, suggesting an independent effect. On these bases, some authors postulated that insulin resistance during pregnancy could be the common trigger leading to GDM and/or PE in predisposed women (22).

It is known that dysfunction of the vascular endothelium and dysregulation of angiogenesis are considered to play a central role in pathophysiology of the disease. Insulin resistance can affect maternal endothelial function, and there are some data that angiogenic and insulin-dependent pathways may influence each other.

It is well know that PCOS, which in more than half of the cases is associated with obesity and insulin resistance, has a close link with GDM. Some proteomic biomarkers of inflammation and oxidative stress (Transferrin, fibrinogen variants, kininogen-1, annexin 2, and peroxiredoxin) are hyperexpressed in women with PE and in women with PCOS, and are suggested to be the link between these diseases. Moreover, there is evidence of placental damage in women with PCOS as reduction trophoblast invasion, abnormal villus maturity, and absence of physiological change of the spiral vessels (23).

Several studies have demonstrated that diabetic insult also in later stage of gestation leads to alteration in placental function and structure; not only maternal insulin resistance and hyperglycemia, but also fetal hyperinsulinemia may have direct and indirect effects on the placenta. Ultrastructural morphology of feto-maternal surface in term placenta complicated by GDM show alteration in vasculosyncitial membranes, an important component of placental barrier, that have the role to maintain the exchange surface area between mother and fetal circulation; in particular a thickened placental barrier, decreased density of syncytiotrophoblast (ST) apical microvilli, and increased ST vacuoles were found. These alterations can be interpreted as a compensatory mechanism to maintain homeostasis at the maternal fetal interface, but cause placental damage that can lead to hypertensive disease; the same alterations have been reported in placenta from women with PE (24).

10.6.3 Maternal Long Term Complications

10.6.3.1 Type 2 Diabetes

Although maternal glucose tolerance often normalizes shortly after pregnancy, a large body of literature has shown that women with GDM have a substantially increased risk of developing type 2 diabetes (T2DM) later in life, supporting that the original diagnostic criteria for GDM by O'Sullivan and Mahan were based on the maternal risk of developing diabetes later in life, and not on perinatal risk.

The cumulative incidence of type 2 diabetes after GDM varied widely among studies. The differences were largely explained by various lengths of follow-up among studies, the heterogeneity of included ethnic groups, different criteria considered for diagnosis of GDM and overt diabetes, and the rapid increase of glucose metabolism disorders in the last years because of the increasing trend in overweight/obesity and advanced maternal age.

In the first systematic review on this topic Kim et al. reported that the incidence of T2DM ranged from 2.6 percent to over 70 percent in women with prior GDM, with a rapid increase in the first 5 years after GDM and maintaining a high level 10 year after GDM and onwards (25). More recently in a review including 20 studies, Bellamy et al. demonstrated that women with GDM had 7.43 times the likelihood of developing T2DM as pregnant women without GDM, the relative risk was 4.69 within 5 years of a pregnancy complicated by GDM, and more than doubled to 9·34 in those who were examined more than 5 years postpartum (26).

The most recent metanalysis of more than two million of women from 30 cohort studies confirmed that previous GDM was associated with a 7.76-fold risk of diabetes, and after adjusting for confounding factors the risk of diabetes in GDM versus non-GDM was markedly increased (OR 17.92). The relative increase in risk of developing diabetes was highest at 3–6 years after GDM (OR 16.6) and at <40 years of age (OR 14.7), although the increased risks remained markedly elevated thereafter (27).

Several antepartum and postpartum risk factors for T2DM in women with GDM have been identified.

Among anthropometric measures associated with development of T2DM, BMI is the strongest risk factor in women with GDM. Obesity parameters other than BMI were found to be associated with postpartum diabetes, such as waist circumference, skinfold thickness, and body fat weight, with waist circumference being the strongest predictor. Also, high visceral fat content, high homocysteine, high retinol binding protein-4 (RBP-4), and low adiponectin were associated with the severity of postpartum glucose intolerance. These findings highlight that increased adiposity or insulin resistance, with a reduced β-cells secretory capacity, may accelerate the progression to postpartum diabetes. Family history of diabetes, older age, and nonwhite ethnicity are significant risk factors for progression to diabetes after GDM regarding constitutional factors.

Major gestation-specific risk factors are the glycemic status in pregnancy, including high fasting blood glucose concentrations, higher fasting plasma glucose at diagnosis of GDM, and high glucose levels in oral glucose tolerance testing; other predictors during gestation are need for insulin therapy and early gestational age at diagnosis (less than 24 weeks of gestation). Additional risk factors are GDM in more than one pregnancy and multiparity; in fact, it has been hypothesized that more episodes of insulin resistance of pregnancy may contribute to the decline in beta-cell function that leads to type 2 diabetes in high-risk women. Breastfeeding has instead a protective role in relation to DM development in women with previous GDM. Although the etiology behind this long term beneficial effect has not been established yet, several hypotheses have been proposed, such as extra energy expenditure for milk production, visceral fat mobilization, and pancreatic beta-cell rescue by prolactin and/or oxytocin (28).

Therefore, a history of GDM provides a low-cost, natural screening test for future type 2 diabetes; the postpartum period provides a unique opportunity to identify and establish an early and appropriate treatment of women with T2DM in order to avoid long term disease complications. Furthermore, early postpartum screening is critically important to identify prediabetes and provide an opportunity to prevent or delay the onset of T2DM through diet, physical activity, weight management, and pharmacologic intervention.

10.6.3.2 Cardiovascular Disease

Women who develop GDM are also at higher risk of overt cardiovascular disease (CVD) later in life.

Several large population-based studies reported an increase risk of cardiovascular events for women with a history of GDM compared with women without GDM during and up to 26 years of postpartum follow-up (29,30). About the effect of GDM on the risk of CVD, it is still not clear whether GDM is associated with future CVD independent of future diabetes; some studies have demonstrated that a diagnosis of GDM alone contributes to this risk, with or without any subsequent type 2 diabetes. A Canadian study with 10 years of follow-up showed that women with GDM who did not subsequently develop T2DM still had 30 percent greater risk of CVD and 41 percent greater risk of CAD compared to women without GDM (31).

Mechanisms by which gestational diabetes results in an increased risk of cardiovascular disease several years after delivery have yet to be completely elucidated.

Women with a history of GDM have common risk factors of CVD, such as obesity, hypertension, atherogenic lipid profiles, lower insulin sensitivity, or higher age (the common soil hypothesis), but it has been suggested that the brief period of potentially intense glucose intolerance typical of GDM can lead to immediate and irreversible endothelial changes, having a significant impact on cardiovascular systems during women's reproductive years and maybe triggering the first step towards the development of atherosclerosis.

Finally, the higher CV risk in a mother with GDM later in life potentially can be due in part to a subclinical inflammation. It is well known that a low level of inflammation is another major risk factor for future CVD, and circulating levels of systemic inflammatory markers and some adipokines associated with endothelial dysfunction and atherosclerosis have been found higher in GDM mothers at various times postpartum compared to women with normal glucose tolerance (Figure 10.4).

10.6.4 Offspring Long Term Complications

It is now widely accepted that an adverse pre-conceptional and intrauterine environment is associated with epigenetic programming of the fetal metabolism and predisposition to chronic disorders later in life.

Diabetes in pregnancy has not only adverse implications for the fetus and the newborn but

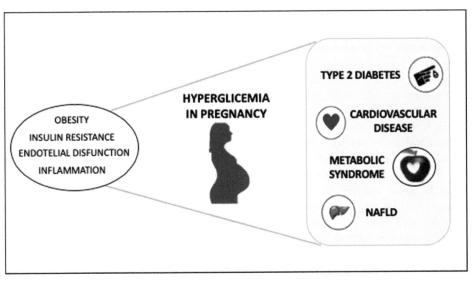

Figure 10.4 Maternal long term complications of gestational diabetes. *NAFLD nonalcoholic fatty liver disease.*

also determines long term effects on the offspring's health. Both animal and human studies have shown that fetal exposure to maternal diabetes during pregnancy is associated with later development of obesity, T2DM, and risk of CVD in the offspring.

The consequences of exposure to diabetes in utero on childhood overweight and obesity and the risk of T2D have been illustrated originally by studies in Pima Indians who have the highest rates of gestational diabetes.

More recently, a follow-up study in Denmark showed that 21 percent of the offspring of GDM women had pre-diabetes or diabetes at 18–27 years of age – an eight-fold increased risk compared with the general population; furthermore, the risk of overweight and metabolic syndrome was higher, and insulin sensitivity and secretion were reduced in this population (32).

The HAPO follow-up study that showed follow-up data in 4,832 children (683 of mothers with GDM and 4.149 controls) participating in the multiethnic multicenter HAPO study has recently been published; the authors confirmed the previous data and found a higher percentage of waist circumference, sum of skinfolds, and body fat percentage in offspring of mothers with GDM compared to controls at 11 years of age. Thus, GDM gives rise to a vicious cycle in which mothers with GDM have babies who are prone to develop metabolic disease later in life and GDM, that is a transgenerational transmission of the disease through epigenetic changes (33).

While it is well known that an optimal glycemic control during pregnancy can prevent short-term complications, the impact of the GDM treatment and of metabolic control on long term complications is less clear, and unfortunately current studies are not conclusive.

10.7 Management

The primary goal of GDM treatment is the normalization of maternal hyperglycemia, in order to prevent adverse effects on the mother and the fetus.

Two large randomized controlled trials have clearly shown that intervention with dietary advice, blood glucose monitoring, and insulin therapy if required is effective in reducing maternal and fetal short term complications (34,35). However, if the cornerstone of GDM management is to achieve an optimal glycemic control, the definition of optimal glycemic control in pregnancy is less clear. The current clinical guidelines recommend different targets, and the majority are higher respect to glycemic value founded in nondiabetic pregnancy. The use of lower glucose targets that better approximate normoglycemia can possibly permit optimal maternal and fetal outcomes (1,36,37).

10.7.1 Lifestyle Intervention and SBGM (Self Blood Glucose Monitoring)

Lifestyle interventions including nutritional therapy, physical activity, and weight management are an essential component of GDM management (38). The optimal diet must provide an adequate caloric intake, and a correct weight gain avoiding starvation ketosis.

The caloric intake is calculated based on pregestational BMI in accordance with IOM recommendations, with a minimum of 175 g carbohydrates per day, mainly with low glycemic index CHO. A low-glycemic-index diet has been shown in randomized trials to be associated with less frequent insulin use and lower birthweight than control diets. In obese women has been suggested a caloric restriction up to 30 percent of the required intake, and some evidence suggests that a modest weight reduction may be appropriate.

Lifestyle intervention also includes recommendations for daily physical activity (at least 150 minute per week), such as walking, cycling, and swimming. Diet and physical activity are sufficient to control the glycemic status in around 70 percent of GDM pregnancies.

Women with GDM are encouraged to self-monitor their fasting, pre-prandial and post-prandial blood glucose levels before and 1–2 hours after main meals. Continuous glucose monitoring has become more available in the last years and can replace finger tests in selected cases (38).

10.7.2 Pharmacological Therapy

When glycemic target are not obtained after 1–2 weeks of lifestyle interventions, daily glucose testing should be continued, and pharmacological treatment should be initiated. Ultrasonography evaluation of fetal growth and amniotic fluid can be used to guide the intensity of glucose control that is needed, and therefore the introduction or increase of pharmacological therapy.

10.7.2.1 Insulin Therapy

Insulin is one of the key strategies in managing diabetes in pregnancy, and is effective and safe for the fetus because it does not cross the placenta. In the last years short- and long-acting insulin analogues have replaced human-derived insulin, with a number of advantages for glycemic control. Short-acting analogues (Lispro and Aspart) have faster onset and shorter duration of action, determining a more overlapping peak to the one of the

endogenous insulin, and reducing the risk of post-meal hypoglycemia and improving glycemic control. The long-acting analogues (Glargine and Detemir) and their good pharmacokinetic characteristics allow to control basal glycemia providing a flat and protracted pharmacodynamic profile. Their use has increased in the last decade because of the rising attention to fasting glucose profile control rather than post meal glycemic values (39).

The insulin treatment can be a basal-bolus regimen using intermediate or long-acting insulin once or twice daily and a rapid-acting insulin before main meals, or a regimen using only one type of insulin (only rapid insulin before meals or only long acting insulin twice daily). Our study group has demonstrated that an optimal glycemic control can be achieved using only long-acting analogue twice daily in a large proportion of GDM women. In our study, women who required combined basal bolus therapy presented a specific phenotype: they were more often older, affected by GDM in previous pregnancy, and more insulin resistant (elevated fasting glucose values and more altered OGTT) compared to women who required only rapid analogues who were slimmer and had normal fasting glycemic values (40).

10.7.2.2 Metformin

Metformin is an insulin sensitizer and increases insulin-mediated peripheral glucose uptake, particularly in skeletal muscle. In randomized clinical trial, metformin and insulin have shown an equivalent effect on glycemic control; metformin seems to give better results for maternal weight gain and neonatal hypoglycemia despite a higher incidence of pre-term birth. No differences in birth weight, LGA, or small for gestational age were reported. However, at least one third of women with GDM who are treated with metformin also need additional treatment with insulin to reach a good glycemic control (41,42).

The main concern about metformin is that has been shown to freely cross the placental barrier reaching concentrations in fetal circulation up to 50 percent of that in the maternal serum; therefore, there is uncertainty about its long term effects on child health.

It has been demonstrated that children at 18 months of age exposed to metformin were heavier and taller than those exposed to insulin during pregnancy; however, motor, social, or linguistic development did not differ between the groups (43). At two years of age, children of the metformin group presented with a larger skinfold, although fat mass and body fat percentage, assessed by bioimpedance and DEXA, were not different (44). Moreover, in these children, no differences in blood pressure and neurodevelopmental tests were reported. Finally, a recent meta-analysis including studies with maximal follow-up duration of 9nineyears showed that children exposed in utero to metformin were heavier than controls, although the BMI z-score are comparable between groups (45).

The major international guidelines for treatment of GDM, including those from the ADA, FIGO, and NICE guidelines, all recommend lifestyle interventions and insulin as the cornerstones of GDM treatment but differ regarding the possible use of metformin in pregnancy. In conclusion, insulin remains the gold standard for pharmacotherapy of GDM, but metformin may be chosen in some women depending on the case and on patient compliance because it is easier to administer.

10.8 Prevention of Gestational Diabetes

Focusing on GDM prevention, a number of clinical trials of dietary and lifestyle changes, dietary supplements, and pharmacological medications have been conducted. Available trials on high-risk women for GDM undergoing mixed lifestyle interventions have showed either no effect or only a limited GDM reduction. The systematic reviews and meta-analysis that have been published on this topic recognized the wide variability in terms of diet and physical activity interventions (frequency, duration, advice only/more intensive support), patients' baseline characteristics (age, ethnicity), and heterogeneity of GDM (overt diabetes, "early" GDM, GDM). This may explain why most of them failed to show a benefit of those interventions in reducing GDM incidence, even though a reduced gestational weight gain was observed.

However, interventions may have been put in place simply too late, when the metabolic condition has already set in; in fact, there is some evidence that lifestyle intervention (diet, physical activity, or both) initiated before the 15th gestational week can reduce the risk of GDM (46).

Maternal pre-conception weight loss in obese women has shown to significantly reduce the risk of GDM: among those who lost more than 4.5 kg between two consecutive pregnancies, there was a 40 percent reduction in GMD rate (47).

Regarding pharmacological intervention during pregnancy, myo-inositol – an isomer of inositol with insulin sensitizing effects – has been shown in two small clinical trials to be effective in reducing the rate of GDM (66 percent decrease), macrosomia, and LGA babies, if a dose of 4 g daily was administered in early pregnancy in women at risk for GDM (both overweight and obese) (48).

The use of metformin in high-risk populations, such as overweight and obese women, showed no significant effect on GDM incidence or birth weight, even though it significantly reduced gestational weight gain and pre-eclampsia incidence (49,50). On the contrary, when metformin was used in pregnancy in women with PCOS, there was about a 10-fold reduction in the rate of GDM, together with a reduction in all PCOS related obstetric complications (51).

10.9 Conclusion

Pregnancy is a state of metabolic modifications, and maintaining glucose homeostasis is of upmost importance.

The rate of GDM is sharply increasing in association with the pandemic of obesity and of type 2 diabetes all over the world, although controversy remains over screening and diagnostic criteria.

Short term maternal and neonatal complications can be in large part prevented by providing a tight maternal glycemic control during pregnancy. However, GDM is not only a short term condition that confers increased risks of macrosomic babies, but a "window into future health" for the mother and the offspring. Therefore GDM represents an excellent opportunity to interrupt the vicious cycle that contributes to the growing burden of childhood obesity and cardiometabolic disorders in women and the future generation.

References

1. Hod M, Kapur A, Sacks DA, et al. The International Federation of Gynecology and Obstetrics (FIGO) initiative on gestational diabetes mellitus: A pragmatic guide for diagnosis, management, and care. *Int J Gynecol Obstet.* 2015, 131(S3):S173–211.

2. Catalano PM, Tyzbir ED, and Roman MN. Longitudinal changes in insulin release and insulin resistance in non obese pregnant women. *Am J Ob Gynecol.* 1991, 165: 1667–1672.

3. Di Cianni G, Miccoli R, Volpe L, et al. Intermediate metabolism in normal pregnancy and in gestational diabetes. *Diabetes Metabol Res Review.* 2003, 19:259–270.

4. Hernandez TL, Friedman JE, Van Pelt RE, et al. Patterns of glycemia in normal pregnancy: Should the current therapeutic targets be challenged? *Diabetes Care.* 2011, 34 (7):1660–1668.

5. Butte NF. Carbohydrate and lipid metabolism in pregnancy: Normal compared with gestational diabetes mellitus. *Am J Clin Nutr.* 2000, 71 (5):1256S–1261S.

6. Ryan EA, and Enns L. Role of gestational hormones in the induction of insulin resistance. *J Clin Endocrinol Metab.* 1988, 67:341–347.

7. Zhou J, Wu NN, Yin RL, et al. Activation of brown adipocytes by placentalgrowth factor. *Biochem Biophys Res Commun.* 2018, 504:470–477.

8. Powe CE. Early pregnancy biochemical predictors of gestational diabetes mellitus. *Curr Diab Rep.* 2017, 17(2):12.

9. Simpson S, Smith L, and Bowe J. Placental peptides regulating islet adaptation to pregnancy: Clinical potential in gestational diabetes mellitus. *Curr Opin Pharmacol.* 2018, 43:59–65.

10. Lorenzo-Almorós A, et al. Predictive and diagnostic biomarkers for gestational diabetes and its associated metabolic and cardiovascular diseases. *Cardiovasc Diabetol.* 2019, 30;18(1):140.

11. McIntyre HD, Chang AM, Callaway LK, et al. Hyperglycemia and Adverse Pregnancy Outcome (HAPO) study cooperative research group: Hormonal and metabolic factors associated with variations in insulin sensitivity in human pregnancy. *Diabetes Care.* 2010, 33:356–360.

12. Catalano PM, Hoegh M, Minium J, et al. Adiponectin in human pregnancy: Implications for regulation of glucose and lipid metabolism. *Diabetologia.* 2006, 49:1677–1685.

13. Buchanan, TA. Pancreatic B cell defects in gestational diabetes: Implications for the pathogenesis and prevention of type 2 diabetes. *J. Clin. Endocrinol. Metab.* 2001, 86:989–993.

14. Abouzeid M, Versace VL, Janus ED, et al. Socio-cultural disparities in GDM burden differ by maternal age at first delivery. *PLoS ONE.* 2015, 10 (2):e0117085.

15. Schwartz N, Nachum Z, and Green MS. The prevalence of gestational diabetes mellitus recurrence – Effect of ethnicity and parity: A metaanalysis. *Am J Obstet Gynecol.* 2015, 213 (3):310–317.

16. Palomba S, de Wilde MA, Falbo A, et al. Pregnancy complications in women with polycystic ovary syndrome. *Hum Reprod Update.* 2015, 21 (5):575–592.

17. HAPO Study Cooperative Research Group. Hyperglycemia and adverse pregnancy outcomes. *N Engl J Med.* 2008, 358:1991–2002.

18. International Association of Diabetes and Pregnancy Study Groups Consensus Panel. Metzger BE, Gabbe SG, Persson B, et al. International association of diabetes and pregnancy study groups recommendations on the diagnosis and classification of hyperglycemia in pregnancy. *Diabetes Care.* 2010, 33 (3):676–682.

19. McIntyre HD, Sacks DA, Barbour LA, et al. Issues with the diagnosis and classification of hyperglycemia in early pregnancy. *Diabetes Care.* 2016, 39(1):53–54.

20. Mitanchez D, Yzydorczyk C, Siddeek B, et al. The offspring of the diabetic mother – Short- and long-term implications. *Best Pract Res ClinObstet Gynaecol.* 2015, 29: 256–269.

21. Rosenstein MG, Cheng YW, Snowden JM, et al. The risk of stillbirth and infant death stratified by gestational age in women with gestational diabetes. *Am J Obstet Gynecol.* 2012, 206(4):309.e1–7.

22. Mastrogiannis DS, Spiliopoulos M, Mulla W, et al. Insulin resistance: The possible link between gestational diabetes mellitus and hypertensive disorders of pregnancy. *Curr Diab Rep.* 2009, 9(4):296–302.

23. Khan GH, Galazis N, Docheva N, et al. Overlap of proteomics biomarkers between women with pre-eclampsia and PCOS: A systematic review and biomarker database integration. *Hum Reprod.* 2015, 30:133–148.

24. Desoye G, and Hauguel-de MS. The human placenta in gestational diabetes mellitus: The insulin and cytokine network. *Diabetes Care.* 2007, 30(S2):S120–S126.

25. Kim C, Newton KM, and Knopp RH. Gestational diabetes and the incidence of

type 2 diabetes: A systematic review. *Diabetes Care*. 2002, 25:1862–1868.

26. Bellamy L, Casas JP, Hingorani AD, et al. Type 2 diabetes mellitus after gestational diabetes: A systematic review and meta-analysis. *Lancet*. 2009, 373(9677):1773–1779.

27. Guo J, Chen JL, Whittemore R, et al. Postpartum lifestyle interventions to prevent type 2 diabetes among women with history of gestational diabetes: A systematic review of randomized clinical trials. *J Women's Health*. 2016, 25 (1):38–49.

28. SH Golden, WL Bennett, K Baptist-Roberts, et al. Antepartum glucose tolerance test results as predictors of type 2 diabetes mellitus in women with a history of gestational diabetes mellitus: A systematic review. *Gend. Med*. 2009, 6 (S1):109–122.

29. Shah BR, Retnakaran R, and Booth GL. Increased risk of cardiovascular disease in young women following gestational diabetes mellitus. *Diabetes Care*. 2008, 31:1668–1669.

30. Tobias DK, Stuart JJ, Li S, et al. Association of history of gestational diabetes with long-term cardiovascular disease risk in a large prospective cohort of US women. *JAMA Intern Med*. 2017, 177 (12):1735–1742.

31. Retnakaran R, and Shah BR. Role of type 2 diabetes in determining retinal, renal, and cardiovascular outcomes in women with previous gestational diabetes mellitus. *Diabetes Care*. 2017, **40**:101–108.

32. Clausen, TD, et al. High prevalence of type 2 diabetes and pre-diabetes in adult offspring of women with gestational diabetes mellitus or type 1 diabetes: The role of intrauterine hyperglycemia.

Diabetes Care. 2008, 31:340–346.

33. Lowe, WL Jr., et al. Association of gestational diabetes with maternal disorders of glucose metabolism and childhood adiposity. *JAMA*. 2018, 320:1005–1016.

34. Crowther, CA, et al. Effect of treatment of gestational diabetes mellitus on pregnancy outcomes. *N Engl J Med*. 2005, 352:2477–2486.

35. Landon, MB, et al. A multicenter, randomized trial of treatment for mild gestational diabetes. *N Engl J Med*. 2009, 361:1339–1348.

36. American Diabetes Association. 13. Management of diabetes in pregnancy: sStandards of medical care in diabetes – 2020. *Diabetes Care*. 2020, 43(Suppl 1):S183–S192.

37. Italian National Guidelines (*Linee Guida Gravidanza Fisiologica*). Sistema nazionale per le linee guida dell'Istituto Superiore di Sanità. Available at: www.snlg-iss.it/cms/files/Lg .Gravidanza.pdf.

38. Martis R, Crowther CA, Shepherd E, et al. Treatments for women with gestational diabetes mellitus: An overview of Cochrane systematic reviews. *Cochrane Database Syst Rev*. 2018, 8:CD012327.

39 Brown J, Grzeskowiak L, Williamson K, et al. Insulin for the treatment of women with gestational diabetes. *Cochrane Database Syst Rev*. 2017, **11**: CD012037.

40. Mecacci F, Lisi F, Vannuccini S, et al. Different gestational diabetes phenotypes: Which insulin regimen fits better? *Front. Endocrinol*. 2021.

41. Rowan JA, Hague WM, Gao W, et al. MiG trial investigators: Metformin versus insulin for the treatment of gestational diabetes. *N Engl J Med*. 2008, 358: 2003–2015.

42. Balsells M, Garca-Patterson A, Sol. I, et al. Glibenclamide, metformin, and insulin for the treatment of gestational diabetes: A systematic review and meta-analysis. *BMJ*. 2015, 350:h102.

43. Ijas, H., Vaarasmaki, M., Saarela, et al. A follow-up of a randomised study of metformin and insulin in gestational diabetes: Growth and development of the children at the age of 18 months. *BJOG*. 2015, 122:994–1000.

44. Rowan JA, Rush EC, Plank LD, et al. Metformin in gestational diabetes: The offspring follow-up (MiG TOFU): Body composition and metabolic outcomes at 7–9 years of age. *BMJ Open Diabetes Res Care*. 2018, **6**:e000456.

45. van Weelden W, Wekker V, de Wit L, et al. Long-term effects of oral antidiabetic drugs during pregnancy on offspring: A systematic review and meta-analysis of follow-up studies of RCTs. *Diabetes Ther*. 2018, 9:1811–1829.

46. Shepherd E, Gomersall JC, Tieu J, et al. Combined diet and exercise interventions for preventing gestational diabetes mellitus. *Cochrane Database Syst Rev*. 2017, 11(11): CD010443.

47. Glazer NL, Hendrickson AF, Schellenbaum GD, et al. Weight change and the risk of gestational diabetes in obese women. *Epidemiology*. 2004, 15 (6):733–737.

48. Santamaria A, Alibrandi A, Di Benedetto A, et al. Clinical and metabolic outcomes in pregnant women at risk for gestational diabetes mellitus supplemented with myo-inositol: A secondary analysis from 3 RCTs. *Am J Obstet Gynecol*. 2018, 219(3):300. e1–300.

49. Dodd, JM et al. Effect of metformin in addition to

dietary and lifestyle advice for pregnant women who are overweight or obese: The GRoW randomised, double-blind, placebo-controlled trial. *Lancet Diabetes Endocrinol.* 2019, 7:15–24.

50. Chiswick, C, et al. Effect of metformin on maternal and fetal outcomes in obese pregnant women (EMPOWaR): A randomised, double-blind, placebo-controlled trial. *Lancet Diabetes Endocrinol.* 2015, 3:778–786.

51. Zeng XL, Zhang YF, Tian Q, et al. Effects of metformin on pregnancy outcomes in women with polycystic ovary syndrome: A meta-analysis. *Medicine (Baltimore).* 2016, 95 (36):e4526.

Obesity and Metabolic Syndrome in Pregnancy

Kent L. R. Thornburg, Amy M. Valent, Nicole E. Marshall, and Jonathan Q. Purnell

11.1 Obesity and the Global Chronic Disease Epidemic

While the death rate for all humans is 100 percent over a 150-year period, the causes of death and the age at which individuals die has changed dramatically over human history. In the past half century, there has been a dramatic global shift away from communicable (infectious) diseases (CD or ID) as the primary cause of death toward a larger portion of total mortality due to noncommunicable (NCD or chronic) diseases. In 1900 in the United States, the average life expectancy at birth was 50 years, and 4 out of the top 10 causes of mortality were communicable infectious diseases: diphtheria, gastrointestinal infections, tuberculosis, and pneumonia (1). A century later, life expectancy had increased to 80 years, and only one infectious disease remained in the top 10 causes of mortality – pneumonia – and it accounted for under 3 percent of all deaths; deaths were dominated by two chronic diseases – cardiovascular disease and cancer. Over the past two decades, the trend away from infectious diseases dominating population mortality has continued with the unexpected exception of pneumonia caused by SARS CoV-2.

The rise in global levels of chronic disease has become a pandemic in its own right. It is highly unlikely that history has seen such a massive increase in severe chronic disease heretofore. The impact is so severe that life expectancy at birth has been decreasing in the United States since 2016. The US Centers for Disease Control and Prevention (CDC) has determined that 60 percent of US residents have a chronic disease, and 40 percent suffer two or more chronic diseases (2).These are amazing numbers of affected people within a population of some 350 million. The causes underlying the current high prevalence of chronic disease are many and include genetic background and low levels of physical activity. One certain cause is the dramatic change in diet over the past three generations that now includes unprecedented increases in salt, fat, and sugar across the globe that may be associated with a changing gut microbiome (3).

11.2 The Prevalence of Obesity and Type 2 Diabetes Has Been Rising at Alarming Rates

Dramatic increases in the global prevalence of obesity and type 2 diabetes (T2DM) are prominent examples of the rise in incidence and prevalence of chronic diseases (4). The high prevalence of these diseases predict increases in the incidence of cardiovascular disease over the next two decades and a reduction in life expectancy. Obesity, defined as a body mass index (BMI) exceeding 30 kg/m^2, is now officially declared a disease in its own right and can no longer be considered a condition found in a small number of unfortunate people who seemed unable to control their appetites. Health economists and public health leaders in the United States and internationally have noted dramatic increases in obesity and T2DM beginning some 30 years ago. Obesity prevalence has more than doubled in some US states over that period of time, and the prevalence of T2DM has tripled. Figure 11.1 shows current prevalence of diabetes in global regions and projected increases in the following two decades. While some surveys show a decreasing incidence in recent years, the American Diabetes Association and the 2013–2016 National Health and Nutrition Examination Survey suggest rates are at an all-time high with a total of 13 percent (95 percent Confidence Interval, 12.0–14.1 percent) of the population affected. Obesity is the leading risk factor for type 2 diabetes. Barnes reported that "women with a body mass index of 30 kg/m^2 have a 28 times greater risk of developing T2DM than do women

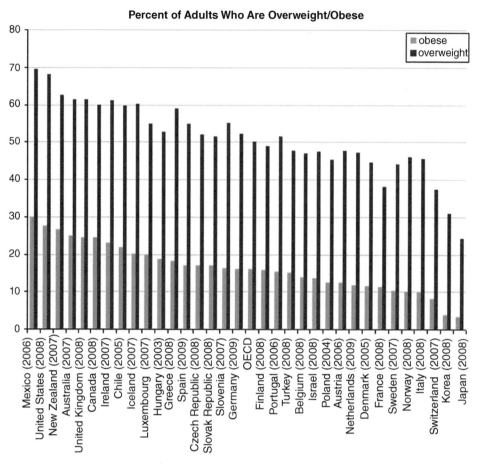

Percent of Adults Who Are Overweight/Obese

Figure 11.1 Estimated prevalence of diabetes in global regions (2019) and projected increases by 2045. From Statista free use license.

of normal weight"(5). Thus, obesity carries a high risk for T2DM, which leads to elevated risk for cardiovascular disease. Nearly 70 percent of adults with T2DM will develop cardiovascular disease.

11.3 Birthweight and Maternal BMI Predict Obesity in Offspring

Professor David Barker and colleagues were the first to show the inverse relationship between heart disease mortality and birthweight in an English population. Studies that followed have shown that babies born at the high end of the birthweight scale also have elevated risk for metabolic disorders and cardiac mortality. Thus, the mortality curve for cardiovascular disease is "U" shaped. Eriksson et al. (2001) showed a U shaped curve for prevalence of obesity among men and women in the Helsinki Birth Cohort (Figure 11.2) (7). However, birthweight was not the only significant factor predicting excessive weight gain. Both maternal

Figure 11.2 Showing a U-shaped trend for obesity in 1522 male adult offspring according to birthweight (7).

BMI at delivery and the BMI of male offspring at seven years were independently predictive. The take home message of these studies is that there are strong promoters of obesity that are passed to offspring during pregnancy that manifest during infancy, early childhood, and later in life. Both diabetes and obesity are associated with catch-up growth in babies born small, and an early adiposity rebound is characterized by a low birthweight followed by early childhood weight gain (8).

The number of women in the United States with obesity (BMI $\geq$30 kg/m^2) has been steadily rising for decades and now exceeds 40 percent (4,9), a disproportionate number of whom are Black and Hispanic (4). The number of pregnant women with overweight and obesity has been steadily rising for decades and now exceeds 50 percent (10). Since 2011, the incidence of class I obesity (BMI 30–34 kg/m^2) during pregnancy has increased by 6 percent, class II obesity (BMI 35–39 k/m^2) has increased by 10 percent, and class III (severe) obesity (BMI $\geq$40 kg/m^2) has increased by 14 percent (10). Women who carry exaggerated levels of fat have elevated risks for adverse pregnancy outcomes, as detailed below.

11.4 Obese Phenotypes and Metabolic Factors That Complicate Pregnancy

Although obesity is associated with adverse perinatal and long term outcomes for both the gestational carrier and offspring, not all obese pregnant women experience adverse outcomes. This highlights the remarkable heterogeneity of obesity-type among pregnant women with varying cardiovascular and metabolic manifestations, adipose distributions, degrees of fitness, nutritional health, and prior pregnancy complications differing among racial and ethnic groups (11). Obesity is a complex condition, and multiple factors including obesity-related comorbidities contribute to the increased risks for adverse pregnancy outcomes which include pregnancy loss (miscarriage and stillbirths), gestational diabetes (GDM), hypertensive spectrum disorder (HSD), and cesarean delivery in addition to adverse neonatal outcomes (Figure 11.3) (12). These risks increase as BMI increases (13).

Pregnant women with obesity have increased risks for adverse perinatal outcomes independent of diabetes status, suggesting other metabolic factors in addition to glucose contribute to the elevated risks during pregnancy. Even under controlled meal conditions, pregnant women with obesity have higher levels of fasting insulin, free fatty acids, triglycerides, and higher baseline glycemic profiles compared to normal weight pregnant individuals (14). Although a normal pregnancy is associated with changes in cytokine profiles across gestation to regulate the maternal immune system, obesity has been

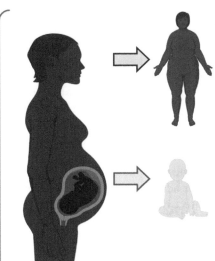

Obesity-related comorbidities:
Cardiovascular disease
Chronic inflammation
Dyslipidemia
Hypertension
Insulin resistance
Non-alcoholic fatty liver disease
Obstructive sleep apnea
Osteoarthritis
Secondary infertility
Type 2 diabetes mellitus

Potential contributory factors:
Chronic stress
Excessive gestational weight gain
Genetics
Insufficient physical activity
Mental health disorders
Poor nutrition quality
Trauma

Perinatal Outcomes:
Cesarean delivery
Endometritis & wound disruptor
Gestational diabetes
Hypertensive spectrum disorder
Postpartum weight retention
Pregnancy loss
Venous thromboembolism

Offspring outcomes:
Behavioral disorders
Childhood obesity
Congenital anomalies
Developmental delay
Increased adiposity
Large-for-gestational age
Metabolic dysfunction
Non-alcoholic fatty liver disease

Figure 11.3 Obesity related maternal co-morbidities, perinatal outcomes, and offspring outcomes.

associated with elevated plasma levels of pro-inflammatory markers including IL-6, TNF-α, and CSF-1 (15).

The pregnancy environment from early days and across gestation influences placental growth, development, and function. Pregnant women with obesity have heavier placentas, increased lipid accumulation in the placenta, and higher placental expression of cytokines, system A amino acid transporters 1 and 2, mTOR, and IGF-1, independent of diabetes status (16). The greater insulin resistance and pro-inflammatory environment observed in early pregnancy among women with obesity may well contribute to the differences in placental structure and function compared to lean individuals. However, the degree to which pro-inflammatory substances themselves cause adverse outcomes of pregnancy is not known.

11.5 Adverse Pregnancy Outcomes Associated with Obesity

According to the Centers for Disease Control and Prevention, the leading causes of pregnancy-related deaths are the following: cardiovascular conditions, hemorrhage, infection, venous thromboembolism, cardiomyopathy, mental health-related conditions, and HSD (17). Obesity is associated with all of these pregnancy complications in addition to several other pregnancy comorbidities, including pregnancy loss, cesarean delivery, and GDM and neonatal outcomes (large-for-gestational age [LGA], increased fat mass, birth injury, and behavioral and developmental disorders). Although obesity is not directly associated with postpartum hemorrhage, it confers risk for hemorrhage secondary to known factors associated with postpartum hemorrhage including prolonged labor, GDM, and HSD (18).

Several studies have demonstrated a dose effect predicting adverse outcomes with increasing BMI. Increased inter-pregnancy weight is associated with an elevated risk for adverse pregnancy outcomes, suggesting a direct role of pre-pregnancy weight leading to pregnancy complications. The pre-pregnancy metabolic milieu has an influence on follicular fluid composition and oocyte quality. This may explain poorer reproductive outcomes from normal weight maternal ova as BMI of the recipient mother increases. Pregnant women with obesity have higher rates

of elective pre-term birth secondary to pregnancy complications such as HSD. They also have increased rates of spontaneous pre-term deliveries and perinatal mortality, independent of other significant confounders at even modest increases in BMI (19,20).

Obesity complicates pregnancy care including therapeutic antibiotic drug-dosing, the need for specialized equipment and careful anesthesia management for operations performed during pregnancy or for delivery. Obesity is a risk factor for anesthetic complications that include intubation difficulties, hypoxemia during general anesthesia, respiratory impairment, epidural failure, hypotension, and prolonged fetal heart rate decelerations following regional anesthesia (16). Obesity is associated with an increased risk for congenital anomalies, but maternal anatomical characteristics, particularly with central obesity, pose a challenge to clearly identify prenatal structural abnormalities using ultrasound (21). Cesarean deliveries and failed trial of labor are higher in pregnant women with obesity which is further challenged by the limitations of performing an emergent delivery, increased risks for wound infection and endometritis, and higher rates of venous thromboembolism (12).

11.6 Physiology and Pathophysiology Leading to Obesity

Like other vital physiological systems (e.g., blood pressure and glucose levels), body weight is tightly regulated through feedback interactions between "sensing" organs and "response" systems. Broadly, three major organ systems comprise most of these interactions: the gastrointestinal tract and adipose tissue (the sensing organs) and the brain (the integrative and responding organ). On the sensing side, consumption and digestion of a meal triggers a release of gut hormones from the lining of the intestine and pancreas that act as afferent signals to the brain (hypothalamus and brainstem) conveying information about the types and amount (total calories) of food being consumed as well as an increasing sense of fullness as the meal progresses (22). At the same time, levels of the orexigenic (hunger) hormone, ghrelin, are immediately suppressed with meal initiation, typically nadir by 90 minutes and then start to rise again, conveying an increasing hunger signal to the brain until the next meal is initiated. In addition, leptin secretion occurs in proportion to fat mass and leptin levels convey a signal reflecting body weight to the same brain centers receiving input from meal-induced gut hormones (23). These brain centers are continually integrating these two sets of afferent signals to address two questions: Do we weigh what our brain thinks we should (leptin levels), and are we consuming sufficient calories to maintain that weight (gut hormone patterns and levels)? This process is commonly referred to as the body weight "set point," but is more accurately a set "range" since weight can often vary up or down by two to three kilograms at any time. If the brain senses that weight is changing, most commonly during weight loss (leptin levels are falling), or caloric intake is insufficient to maintain weight (gut hormone levels), or both are occurring simultaneously, these brain centers will set in motion physiologic responses that limit weight loss and bring the body weight back to baseline (Table 11.1).

For approximately 70 percent of our population up until the approximate age of 60 years, this body weight set point can rise and operate somewhere outside of what is considered a healthy weight range. As much as 70 percent of this weight gain is influenced by genetics, and several periods in women's lives represent vulnerable times when the set point can rise, including puberty, pregnancy, and menopause. Roughly half of women who become pregnant will return to their pre-pregnancy weight. The other half will retain some amount of their gestational weight gain with many crossing weight categories from normal to overweight or from overweight to obese (24). It is believed that underlying this unwanted weight gain and expression of overweight or obesity is development of leptin resistance requiring high leptin levels from increased fat mass before reestablishing homeostasis at a new, higher body weight set point, analogous to insulin resistance leading to higher insulin levels and, eventually, type 2 diabetes.

For people, once a set point is established at a higher body weight level, it does not return to the previous lower set point on its own, and the overweight or obese status becomes chronic. Lifestyle (diet and exercise) can influence the degree of expression of rise in the body weight set point as it is occurring but plays a limited role once a new set point is established, mainly influencing whether weight is maintained on the upper or lower limit of the set range. At this higher body weight set point, the brain regions involved with body weight regulation will respond to changes in sensing organ signaling during low-calorie states similarly to when the set point was in the normal weight range. This explains the phenomenon of weight "yo-yoing" experienced by patients with obesity during dieting. In this physiologic framework it is important to point out that the observed behaviors we exhibit when eating, including feeling satisfied with a meal and deciding when to stop eating or feeling like having a snack, are driven by internal biological signals (Table 11.1) that are not under our conscious control. In fact, they control us, and we cannot simply ignore them.

Table 11.1. Metabolic adaptations to weight loss in patients with obesity

Physiologic response or behavior	Proposed physiologic mediators	Clinical manifestation
↑ Hunger, ↓ meal-related fullness	↑ ghrelin, ↓ leptin, and ↓ postprandial satiety hormones	Increased food seeking, snacking, and binging behaviors
↓ Energy expenditure	Unknown	Partitioning of energy back into fat storage
↓ Fat oxidation	Unknown	Partitioning of energy back into fat storage
↓ T3, T4 levels	Reduced leptin signaling	Cold intolerance, hair loss, dry skin, weight retention
↓ Sympathetic nervous system	Reduced leptin signaling	Bradycardia during advanced fasting state

Therefore, most patients with obesity fail to sustain long term weight loss with calorie restriction alone not because of lack of willpower or inadequate effort, but because of activation of these counter-regulatory systems during weight loss and the promotion of a positive energy balance (Table 11.1), which remains active until body weight is fully restored. Therefore, advising patients with obesity to "eat less and move more" is well intentioned, but insufficient. To achieve meaningful and sustained weight loss, lifestyle improvements must be combined with interventions whose mechanisms of action involve those central brain centers responsible for weight regulation to allow establishment of a new, lower body weight set point, and then continued indefinitely, as described below.

11.7 Weight Management Approaches to Maternal Obesity

Several randomized trials have tested effects of lifestyle interventions to reduce gestational weight gain (GWG) among women with overweight and obesity as a means of reducing adverse maternal and neonatal outcomes (25). To date, this literature suggests that weight management during pregnancy for women with obesity results in only modest reduction in mean GWG with minimal impact on maternal or neonatal outcomes other than a possible reduction in LGA babies. Furthermore, studies that have followed maternal-child dyads for one year or longer after birth have not shown sustained long term benefit of weight management during pregnancy on childhood weight or obesity risk (26).

As a result of these findings, efforts to improve maternal-fetal health for women with obesity have shifted to the pre-conception period. Interventions for weight loss among nonpregnant adults include: (1) diet and lifestyle changes, which have consistently shown weight loss averaging close to 8 percent of baseline after one year that backtracks to 4 percent weight loss longer term (four years or longer) (27); (2) diet and lifestyle plus weight-loss medications, which may result in slightly more weight loss than lifestyle changes alone but are contra-indicated in women attempting pregnancy and would no longer be effective once stopped, risking a high rate of obesity recidivism as women begin trying to become pregnant and during gestation (28); and

Figure 11.4 Types of metabolic-bariatric surgery. Laparoscopic gastric band (A). Sleeve gastrectomy (B). Roux-en-Y gastric bypass (C). Biliopancreatic diversion with duodenal switch (D). The two most common current procedures are the sleeve gastrectomy (B) and gastric bypass (C). Both result in mild malabsorption of iron calcium and vitamin B12, but little or no impact on macronutrient absorption or uptake of water soluble vitamins, other minerals, and folate. Figures reproduced with permission from the American Society for Metabolic and Bariatric Surgery (https://asmbs.org/patients/bariatric-surgery-procedures).

(3) bariatric surgery (Figure 11.4), which is associated with a 20–25 percent weight loss after sleeve gastrectomy (SG) and 25–30 percent after Roux-en-Y gastric bypass (RYGB), with weight loss persisting for seven or more years (29).

11.8 Pregnancy and Prenatal Outcomes after Bariatric Surgery

Despite considerable heterogeneity in methodological approaches and surgical procedures studied, a recent meta-analysis of 20 cohort studies (involving ~2.8 million participants) including over 8,000 women who became pregnant after bariatric surgery showed several consistent findings regarding maternal health and fetal outcomes. As might be expected with large weight loss prior to conception, rates of GDM and maternal hypertensive disorders (including hypertension, preeclampsia, and eclampsia) were significantly reduced compared to women matched to their pre-surgery BMI and were not different than women matched to their pre-pregnancy BMI. Correspondingly, the likelihood of having a large baby (LGA or macrosomia) was significantly lower compared to both the pre-surgical and pre-pregnancy weight-matched control groups. However, these analyses have also consistently reported increased risk for premature birth and SGA babies in post-surgical women, regardless of whether they are compared to women matched to their pre-surgery or pre-pregnancy weight. Fortunately, uncertainty whether birth defect rates might be higher in women who underwent bariatric surgery (30) was recently addressed when a study of over 2,900 women who conceived and delivered after RYGB found a significant reduction in any major birth defect and no neural tube defects (RR 0.67; 95 percent CI 0.52–0.87) compared to nonsurgical women matched for pre-surgery BMI and diabetes status (31).

11.9 Postnatal Outcomes for Children Born to Mothers after Bariatric Surgery

Only a handful of studies to date have explored the effect of surgically-induced preconception weight loss on longer-term health of the baby, including growth, propensity for obesity, and expression of weight-related comorbidities. One of the earliest such studies compared weights of children born to 113 mothers after they underwent the now rarely used biliopancreatic diversion (BPD), which induces significant malabsorption (32), to weights of their siblings born prior to surgery (total number of children was 172, aged 6–18 years old) (33). It was shown that compared to their pre-surgical siblings, rates of overweight were reduced in both sexes of the children born after bariatric surgery, and obesity rates were ~50 percent lower in boys but not girls (33). In a follow-up study of a smaller number of women (n = 49) from the same group that included more extensive metabolic phenotyping, offspring born after bariatric surgery not only had

lower rates of obesity than their pre-surgical siblings (again only in boys, not girls), but they also exhibited less insulin resistance and better lipid profiles (34). Birthweight and macrosomia were reduced in the children born after bariatric surgery, but in contrast to the larger cohort studies (above), low-birth weight rates were not different. However, other studies report inconsistent benefits on childhood growth for children born to mothers after bariatric surgery compared to their pre-surgery siblings depending on the weight metric used (overweight versus obesity), length of follow-up, and offspring's sex (35,36), while still others failed to demonstrate benefit on offspring body weights (37).

While these reports provide foundational support for the potential benefits of preconception weight loss from bariatric surgery on future fetal risk for chronic diseases of adulthood (33,34), significant limitations and mixed results in this literature prevent confidence in their findings. These limitations include small numbers of participants with poor generalizability to the general population due to lack of inclusion of mothers from minority groups; limited datasets that do not include possible confounding maternal-fetal pregnancy outcomes such as parity, gestational weight gain, birth order, GDM, weight for gestational age, and SGA prevalence; and reporting outcomes after bariatric procedures that are either currently rarely used (biliopancreatic diversion or BPD) (33,34,38), or no longer recommended due to poor weight loss efficacy (vertical and horizontal bandied gastroplasties, laparoscopic gastric banding) or unacceptable side effects (jejunoileal bypass) (35,37,39). These procedural differences alone could account for the lack of consistency in childhood outcomes between studies. Finally, low birthweight typically reflects maternal undernutrition or placental dysfunction but can also be influenced by anemia and micronutrient deficiencies. In patients who undergo RYGB or SG, macronutrient malabsorption is considered physiologically inconsequential (40), but levels of vitamin B12 and ferritin are lower and anemia may be exacerbated.

11.10 Neonatal Issues Associated with Maternal Obesity

While the majority of offspring of women with obesity will not experience perinatal or neonatal complications, maternal obesity is associated with increased risk for congenital anomalies, stillbirth/neonatal death, extremes of fetal growth including fetal growth restriction and macrosomia/large for gestational age, childhood obesity/increased adiposity, metabolic dysfunction, non-alcoholic fatty liver disease, behavioral disorders, and developmental delay. Some of these complications may be related in part to suboptimal nutrition without exclusive human milk feeding, as lactation difficulties are more common among women with obesity.

In additional to perinatal morbidity, maternal obesity is associated with increased offspring mortality. The relative risk for fetal death (spontaneous death of a fetus during pregnancy or labor), stillbirth (death of a fetus in the second half of pregnancy), and infant death (death of a live-born infant before age one) demonstrate moderate to strong increase per each five-unit increase in maternal BMI in a dose-response fashion (20). This has been ascribed to not only an increase in obstetric complications among women with obesity, but also a significant increase in placental dysfunction among women with obesity (41). In addition, macrosomia is a risk factor for stillbirth which is more common among women with obesity, the combination of maternal obesity and fetal macrosomia is associated with a six-fold increase in rate of stillbirth compared to women with normal weight and macrosomic infants (42).

Abnormal fetal growth patterns are more common among women with obesity, including increased risk for fetal growth restriction and fetal macrosomia (43). Fetal growth restriction is associated with increased risk of perinatal death, cognitive delay, and adult-onset diseases including obesity, type 2 diabetes, and cardiovascular disease. In addition to those risks, fetal macrosomia, defined as birth weight above 4 or 4.5 kg, and LGA (birth weight >90 percent for gestational age) are also associated with many of the same risks as found among growth restricted infants but also increased risk of shoulder dystocia and subsequent sequela including neonatal fractures and brachial plexus injury (44). Abnormal fetal growth patterns have lifelong metabolic and developmental implications for the offspring including increased risk for later adiposity (45) and metabolic dysfunction.

Maternal obesity is implicated in increased risk for offspring cardiometabolic morbidity including obesity, increased adiposity, metabolic syndrome (insulin resistance/hyperglycemia, hypertension, hyperlipidemia, increased adiposity), and nonalcoholic fatty liver disease (NAFLD) in numerous clinical, epidemiologic, and animal studies, with evidence of sex differences (46). Maternal overweight and obesity during pregnancy is associated with a significantly increased risk for childhood obesity, with up to a 264 percent increased odds for childhood obesity among offspring of mothers with pre-pregnancy obesity (47). Childhood adiposity is more difficult to assess due to the variation in techniques used to quantify fat mass; however, there is consistent evidence that maternal obesity is associated with increased offspring adiposity, regardless of maternal glycemia (46). While it remains unclear whether metabolic syndrome as defined can be diagnosed during childhood per adult criteria, a longitudinal study of children born to mothers with and without obesity and/or gestational diabetes found a doubling of the risk for development of metabolic syndrome by age 11 among offspring of mothers with obesity, independent of diabetes status. A significant rise in NAFLD has been noted in the pediatric population, and there is evidence for a 68 percent increase in liver fat among newborns born to mothers with obesity and GDM compared to the offspring of women with normal weight and normal glycemia (48). These findings strongly support a relationship between maternal obesity during pregnancy and childhood cardiometabolic health, which provides additional evidence supporting the developmental origins of health and disease and the importance of optimizing maternal preconception weight status to decrease offspring metabolic dysfunction.

There is increasing evidence that maternal obesity during pregnancy is associated with altered offspring mental and behavioral health, including increased risk for development of attention deficit hyperactive disorder (ADHD), autism spectrum disorders (ASDs), anxiety, depression, schizophrenia, and eating disorders. In addition to metabolic changes, maternal perinatal obesity is thought to impact neuroendocrine and immunologic function that may result in disruption of fetal neural pathway development essential for behavior regulation and cognition (49). This may be driven by alterations in gut microbiota composition among women with obesity compared to their normal weight peers which could result in altered gut microbiota in the developing fetus (50). Maternal obesity has been associated with early childhood reduced cognitive development compared to normal weight peers after adjustment for socioeconomic variables and paternal BMI, suggesting a potential intrauterine effect.

11.11 Lactation Issues Associated with Maternal Obesity

Exclusive breastfeeding, defined as providing only human milk through direct feeding or expressed milk for the first six months of life, is recommended by the World Health Organization and the American Academy of Pediatrics for optimal infant nutrition (51). Length of lactation and exclusive breastfeeding are associated with numerous health outcomes, including lower rates of infection and obesity and normal intelligence. Maternal benefits of breastfeeding include lower rates of diabetes, obesity, heart disease, and breast cancer.

Women with obesity face several challenges in meeting lactation targets, starting with lower rates of intention to breastfeed and initiation efforts. The breastfeeding disparities between women with normal weight and women with obesity start prior to delivery, as women with obesity are less likely to report intention to breastfeed and report a shorter intended duration of breastfeeding compared to their normal weight peers. Breastfeeding initiation is decreased among women with obesity compared to women with normal weight in the majority of studies, with an odds ratio ranging from 1.19 to 3.65. Women with obesity have a shorter duration of providing any human milk to their infants, even after adjusting for confounding factors, which was statistically significant in 11 of 18 included studies. Cessation of exclusive breastfeeding occurred earlier in women with obesity compared to women with normal weight in the majority of studies (52), but demonstrated variation by race/ethnicity with differences more pronounced among Hispanic women (53).

Maternal obesity-related metabolic differences may serve as a potential etiology for the weight-related disparities in lactation outcomes. Women with obesity have been demonstrated to have an increased risk for low milk transfer, defined as less than 9.2 g per feeding, at 60 hours postpartum compared to women of normal weight (54). There

is also evidence that obesity may interfere with prolactin release in response to infant suckling in the first postpartum week, which may help explain the increase incidence of delayed lactogenesis – the onset of copious milk production – among women with obesity. Low milk supply perception is more commonly reported among women with obesity compared to women of normal weight, and hence it is no surprise that insufficient milk as the indication for breastfeeding cessation is more commonly reported among women with higher BMI.

Other studies have suggested that anatomic, psychosocial, and cultural factors including larger breast size, greater discomfort with breastfeeding around others, and decreased familial/peer support may be to blame for weight-related lactation disparities (55). However, despite concerted efforts targeted at these factors, there has not been a corresponding increase in exclusive breastfeeding or breastfeeding duration among women with obesity, suggesting that additional studies are needed to address lactation disparities.

11.12 Management Considerations in Pregnancies Complicated by Obesity

Clinical management of pregnant women with obesity ideally begins prior to pregnancy, but regardless of the reproductive stage of the patient, lifestyle modifications and interventions are the mainstay (Figure 11.5). The US Preventative Services Taskforce (USPSTF) and the US Department of Health and Human Services recommend for pregnant women to achieve at least 150 minutes of moderate-level aerobic activity per week and 2–3 days per week of resistance activity, with no more than 2 consecutive days of inactivity (56).

The recent US Department of Agriculture dietary guidelines report advising all pregnant women to consume and adhere to a diet enriched with vegetables, fruits, whole grains, nuts, legumes, fish, and vegetable oils and with limited amounts of meat, added sugars, and refined grains to reduce the risk for adverse perinatal outcomes (57). Because of the short and long term risks associated with excessive gestational weight gain in pregnancy, the National Academy of Medicine (formerly Institute of Medicine)

Figure 11.5 Important clinical management strategies to optimize the health of pregnant people with obesity.

updated the gestational weight gain guidelines to serve providers with a platform for practice, suggesting a total pregnancy weight gain of 5–9.1 kg (25–42 pounds) for women with obesity (58,59).

Many of the interventions focusing on pregnant women with obesity are designed to reduce excessive weight gain. Lifestyle interventions initiated during pregnancy have not reduced adverse perinatal outcomes such as gestational diabetes or preeclampsia. However, regardless of the lifestyle modification strategy (trainer led sessions, meal replacements, the Mediterranean Diet, the Dietary Approaches to Stop Hypertension [DASH] diet, modified Diabetes Prevention Program [DPP], parent–educator intervention, or telehealth approach), studies have consistently demonstrated reductions in excessive gestational weight gain without increasing small-for-gestation age infants (25,60). The long term benefit of improving pre- or inter-pregnancy lifestyle habits or limiting excessive gestational weight gain is unknown.

Obesity is associated with an increased risk for higher insulin resistance, GDM, and HSD in addition to other obesity-related comorbidities. Addressing these risks and optimizing health prior to pregnancy is preferred but once an individual is pregnant, recognition of these elevated

risk factors and developing strategies and goals to help reduce the risks of adverse outcomes is key. Pregnant women with obesity and with additional risk factors for insulin resistance require ruling out T2DM early in pregnancy with an oral glucose tolerance test and repeat screening during the standard 24–28 week gestation period even if early testing is within normal laboratory limits. The increased risk for congenital anomalies among women with obesity and GDM suggest that a first trimester examination, including a nuchal translucency evaluation, should be investigated, as well as a comprehensive anatomic ultrasound performed to identify potential structural abnormalities. Obesity increases the risk for anesthetic complications, and women with class III obesity should consider an anesthesia consultation and investigate whether institutional equipment and protocols are available to safely care for high BMI persons in labor and delivery. Prior studies have demonstrated a reciprocal link between obesity and depression, and both are associated with adverse pregnancy outcomes (61). Pregnant women should be screened for depression and anxiety during pregnancy and postpartum with appropriate referral for those at increased risk of perinatal depression to counseling interventions. The medical, physical, mental, and physiologic complexities of obesity suggest that individualized care with a multidisciplinary approach is the best way to manage such cases.

Acknowledgments

The authors thank Kim Rogers and Lisa Rhuman for outstanding editorial assistance.

References

1. Jones DS, Podolsky SH, and Greene JA. The burden of disease and the changing task of medicine. *The New England Journal of Medicine*. 2012, 366:2333–2338.

2. (NCCDPHP) CsNCfCDPaHP. Chronic Diseases in America. In: (NCCDPHP) NCfCDPaHP, ed.: Center for Disease Control and Prevention, 2021.

3. Turnbaugh PJ, Ley RE, Mahowald MA, et al. An obesity-associated gut microbiome with increased capacity for energy harvest. *Nature*. 2006, 444:1027–1031.

4. Hales CM, Carroll MD, Fryar CD, et al. Prevalence of Obesity and Severe Obesity Among Adults: United States, 2017-2018. NCHS data brief 2020:1-8.

5. Barnes AS. The epidemic of obesity and diabetes: Trends and treatments. *Texas Heart Institute Journal*. 2011, 38:142–144.

6. Percent of Adults Who Are Overweight/Obese. In: Global Sherpa, 2011.

7. Eriksson J, Forsén T, Tuomilehto J, et al. Size at birth, childhood growth and obesity in adult life. *International Journal of Obesity and Related Metabolic Disorders: Journal of the International Association for the Study of Obesity* 2001, 25:735–740.

8. Rolland-Cachera MF, Deheeger M, Maillot M, et al. Early adiposity rebound: Causes and consequences for obesity in children and adults. *International Journal of Obesity*. 2005, 30 Suppl (4): S11–S17.

9. Hales CM, Fryar CD, Carroll MD, et al. Trends in obesity and severe obesity prevalence in US youth and adults by sex and age, 2007–2008 to 2015–2016. *JAMA*. 2018, 319:1723–1725.

10. Deputy NP, Dub B, and Sharma AJ. Prevalence and trends in prepregnancy normal weight - 48 states, New York City, and District of Columbia, 2011–2015. *MMWR Morbidity and Mortality Weekly Report*. 2018, 66:1402–1407.

11. Neeland IJ, Poirier P, and Després JP. Cardiovascular and metabolic heterogeneity of obesity: Clinical challenges and implications for management. *Circulation*. 2018, 137:1391–1406.

12. ACOG Practice Bulletin No 156: Obesity in pregnancy. *Obstetrics and Gynecology*. 2015, 126:e112–e126.

13. Villamor E, and Cnattingius S. Interpregnancy weight change and risk of adverse pregnancy outcomes: A population-based study. *Lancet*. 2006, 368:1164–1170.

14. Harmon KA, Gerard L, Jensen DR, et al. Continuous glucose profiles in obese and normal-weight pregnant women on a controlled diet: Metabolic determinants of fetal growth. *Diabetes Care*. 2011, 34: 2198–2204.

15. Hedman AM, Lundholm C, Andolf E, et al. Longitudinal plasma inflammatory proteome profiling during pregnancy in the Born into Life study. *Scientific Reports*. 2020, 10:17819.

16. Catalano PM, and Shankar K. Obesity and pregnancy: mechanisms of short term and long term adverse consequences for mother and child. *BMJ (Clinical Research Ed.)*. 2017, 356:j1.

17. Davis NL SA, and Goodman, DA. Pregnancy-Related Deaths: Data from 14 U.S. Maternal Mortality Review Committees, 2008-2017. Centers for Disease Control and Prevention, US Department of Health and Human Services, 2019.

18. Ende HB, Lozada MJ, Chestnut DH, et al. Risk factors for atonic postpartum hemorrhage: A systematic review and meta-analysis. *Obstetrics and Gynecology*. 2021, 137:305–323.

19. Cnattingius S, Villamor E, Johansson S, et al. Maternal obesity and risk of preterm delivery. *JAMA*. 2013, 309:2362–2370.

20. Aune D, Saugstad OD, Henriksen T, et al. Maternal body mass index and the risk of fetal death, stillbirth, and infant death: A systematic review and meta-analysis. *JAMA*. 2014, 311:1536–1546.

21. Best KE, Tennant PW, Bell R, et al. Impact of maternal body mass index on the antenatal detection of congenital anomalies. *BJOG: An International Journal of Obstetrics and Gynaecology*. 2012, 119:1503–1511.

22. Pucci A, and Batterham RL. Endocrinology of the gut and the regulation of body weight and metabolism. In: Feingold KR, Anawalt B, Boyce A, Chrousos G, de Herder WW, Dungan K, et al., eds. *Endotext*. South Dartmouth, MA: MDText.com, Inc. 2000.

23. Barsh GS, and Schwartz MW. Genetic approaches to studying energy balance: Perception and integration. *Nature Reviews Genetics*. 2002, 3:589–600.

24. Wallace JM, Bhattacharya S, and Horgan GW. Weight change across the start of three consecutive pregnancies and the risk of maternal morbidity and SGA birth at the second and third pregnancy. *PLoS ONE*. 2017, 12:e0179589.

25. Peaceman AM, Clifton RG, Phelan S, et al. Lifestyle interventions limit gestational weight gain in women with overweight or obesity: LIFE-Moms prospective meta-analysis. *Obesity*. 2018, 26:1396–1404.

26. Phelan S, Clifton RG, Haire-Joshu D, et al. One-year postpartum anthropometric outcomes in mothers and children in the LIFE-Moms lifestyle intervention clinical trials. *International Journal of Obesity*. 2005, 2020(44):57–68.

27. Knowler WC, Barrett-Connor E, Fowler SE, et al. Reduction in the incidence of type 2 diabetes with lifestyle intervention or metformin. *New England Journal of Medicine*. 2002, 346:393–403.

28. Tchang BG, Kumar RB, and Aronne LJ. Pharmacologic treatment of overweight and obesity in adults. In: Feingold KR, Anawalt B, Boyce A, Chrousos G, de Herder WW, Dungan K. et al., eds. *Endotext*. South Dartmouth, MA: MDText.com, Inc. 2000.

29. Courcoulas AP, King WC, Belle SH, et al. Seven-year weight trajectories and health outcomes in the Longitudinal Assessment of Bariatric Surgery (LABS) Study. *JAMA Surgery*. 2018, 153:427–434.

30. Benjamin RH, Littlejohn S, and Mitchell LE. Bariatric surgery and birth defects: A systematic literature review. *Paediatric*

and Perinatal Epidemiology. 2018, 32:533–544.

31. Neovius M, Pasternak B, Näslund I, et al. Association of maternal gastric bypass surgery with offspring birth defects. *JAMA*. 2019, 322:1515–1517.

32. Elder KA, and Wolfe BM. Bariatric surgery: A review of procedures and outcomes. *Gastroenterology*. 2007, 132:2253–2271.

33. Kral JG, Biron S, Simard S, et al. Large maternal weight loss from obesity surgery prevents transmission of obesity to children who were followed for 2 to 18 years. *Pediatrics*. 2006, 118: e1644–1649.

34. Smith J, Cianflone K, Biron S, et al. Effects of maternal surgical weight loss in mothers on intergenerational transmission of obesity. *The Journal of Clinical Endocrinology and Metabolism*. 2009, 94:4275–4283.

35. Willmer M, Berglind D, Tynelius P, et al. Children's weight status, body esteem, and self-concept after maternal gastric bypass surgery. *Surgery for Obesity and Related Eiseases: Official Journal of the American Society for Bariatric Surgery*. 2015, 11:927–932.

36. Barisione M, Carlini F, Gradaschi R, et al. Body weight at developmental age in siblings born to mothers before and after surgically induced weight loss. *Surgery for Obesity and Related Diseases: Official Journal of the American Society for Bariatric Surgery*. 2012, 8:387–391.

37. Willmer M, Berglind D, Sørensen TI, et al. Surgically induced interpregnancy weight loss and prevalence of overweight and obesity in offspring. *PLoS ONE*. 2013, 8: e82247.

38. Guénard F, Deshaies Y, Cianflone K, et al. Differential

methylation in glucoregulatory genes of offspring born before vs. after maternal gastrointestinal bypass surgery. *Proceedings of the National Academy of Sciences of the United States of America*. 2013, 110:11439–11444.

39. Berglind D, Müller P, Willmer M, et al. Differential methylation in inflammation and type 2 diabetes genes in siblings born before and after maternal bariatric surgery. *Obesity*. 2016, 24:250–261.

40. Svane MS, Bojsen-Møller KN, Martinussen C, et al. Postprandial nutrient handling and gastrointestinal hormone secretion after Roux-en-Y gastric bypass vs sleeve gastrectomy. *Gastroenterology*. 2019, 156:1627–1641.e1.

41. Nohr EA, Bech BH, Davies MJ, et al. Prepregnancy obesity and fetal death: A study within the Danish National Birth Cohort. *Obstetrics and Gynecology*. 2005, 106:250–259.

42. Ikedionwu CA, Dongarwar D, Yusuf KK, et al. Pre-pregnancy maternal obesity, macrosomia, and risk of stillbirth: A population-based study. *European Journal of Obstetrics, Gynecology, and Reproductive Biology*. 2020, 252:1–6.

43. Marshall NE, Guild C, Cheng YW, et al. Maternal superobesity and perinatal outcomes. *American Journal of Obstetrics and Gynecology*. 2012, 206(417):e1–6.

44. Beta J, Khan N, Khalil A, et al. Maternal and neonatal complications of fetal macrosomia: Systematic review and meta-analysis. *Ultrasound in Obstetrics & Gynecology: The Official Journal of the International Society of Ultrasound in Obstetrics and Gynecology*. 2019, 54:308–318.

45. Desai M, and Ross MG. Fetal programming of adipose tissue: Effects of intrauterine growth

restriction and maternal obesity/high-fat diet. *Seminars in Reproductive Medicine*. 2011, 29:237–245.

46. Kislal S, Shook LL, and Edlow AG. Perinatal exposure to maternal obesity: Lasting cardiometabolic impact on offspring. *Prenatal Diagnosis*. 2020, 40:1109–11025.

47. Heslehurst N, Vieira R, Akhter Z, et al. The association between maternal body mass index and child obesity: A systematic review and meta-analysis. *PLoS Medicine*. 2019, 16:e1002817.

48. Brumbaugh DE, Tearse P, Cree-Green M, et al. Intrahepatic fat is increased in the neonatal offspring of obese women with gestational diabetes. *The Journal of Pediatrics*. 2013, 162:930–936. e1.

49. Cirulli F, Musillo C, and Berry A. Maternal obesity as a risk factor for brain development and mental health in the offspring. *Neuroscience*. 2020, 447:122–135.

50. Basu S, Haghiac M, Surace P, et al. Pregravid obesity associates with increased maternal endotoxemia and metabolic inflammation. *Obesity*. 2011, 19:476–482.

51. Breastfeeding and the use of human milk. *Pediatrics*. 2012;129:e827–841.

52. Marshall NE, Lau B, Purnell JQ, et al. Impact of maternal obesity and breastfeeding intention on lactation intensity and duration. *Maternal & Child Nutrition*. 2019, 15: e12732.

53. Kugyelka JG, Rasmussen KM, and Frongillo EA. Maternal obesity is negatively associated with breastfeeding success among Hispanic but not Black women. *The Journal of Nutrition*. 2004, 134:1746–1753.

54. Chapman DJ, and Pérez-Escamilla R. Maternal perception of the onset of lactation is a valid, public health indicator of lactogenesis stage II. *The Journal of Nutrition*. 2000, 130:2972–2980.

55. Amir LH, and Donath S. A systematic review of maternal obesity and breastfeeding intention, initiation and duration. *BMC Pregnancy and Childbirth*. 2007, 7:9.

56. Piercy KL, and Troiano RP. Physical activity guidelines for Americans from the US Department of Health and Human Services. *Circulation Cardiovascular Quality and Outcomes*. 2018, 11:e005263.

57. Agriculture USDo SU. Dietary Guidelines for Americans, 2020–2025. In: USDoHaH, ed. Vol. 9th Edition. 2020.

58. ACOG Committee opinion no. 548: Weight gain during pregnancy. *Obstetrics and Gynecology*. 2013, 121:210–212.

59. Voerman E, Santos S, Inskip H, et al. Association of gestational weight gain with adverse maternal and infant outcomes. *JAMA*. 2019, 321:1702–1715.

60. Poston L, Bell R, Croker H, et al. Effect of a behavioural intervention in obese pregnant women (the UPBEAT study): A multicentre, randomised controlled trial. *The Lancet Diabetes & Endocrinology*. 2015, 3:767–77.

61. Luppino FS, de Wit LM, Bouvy PF, et al. Overweight, obesity, and depression: A systematic review and meta-analysis of longitudinal studies. *Archives of General Psychiatry*. 2010, 67:220–229.

Chapter 12

Hormones and Pre-term Birth

Emily M. Frier, Sarah J. Stock, Stephen Lye, and Oksana Shynlova

12.1 The Problem of Pre-term Birth

12.1.1 Epidemiology and Demographics

Pre-term birth (PTB), or delivery before 37 weeks' gestation, is a substantial and complex global burden. In 2014, approximately 14.8 million babies were born pre-term (1). Despite advances in neonatal care, complications of PTB remain the leading global cause of death in children under five years of age (1), and in 2018, were responsible for 35 percent of 2.5 million neonatal deaths (2). Survivors of PTB are exposed to both short- and long-term complications, with potentially lifelong effects on physical and neurodevelopmental health (1).

Pre-term birth is a major health inequality: rates of PTB, and the degree of resultant morbidity and mortality, are strongly associated with a country's level of income and geographical location (2). PTB rates range from 5 to 18 percent; in 2014, the global rate of PTB, based on data analysis and regression modelling from 107 countries, was estimated as 10.6 percent (1). The majority of pre-term babies are born in low- and middle-income countries (3); over 80 percent of all PTB in 2014 occurred in Asia and sub-Saharan Africa (1). However, high-income countries do contribute to the global burden of PTB, particularly the USA, which in 2012 had a PTB rate of 12 percent, comparable with 13 percent in India, and contrasting with 7.8 percent in the UK. In 2010 the USA was ranked sixth of the ten countries in the world with the highest numbers of PTB (3).

Blencowe et al. reviewed trends in PTB rates in 65 countries within the Millennium Development Goal regions "Developed countries" and "Latin America and the Caribbean," where birth data from 1990 to 2010 was reliable and sufficient (over 10,000 livebirths per year): Only three countries recorded a reduction in PTB rate over this time (3). Most other countries had stable or increasing rates of PTB; the highest average annual increase in PTB rate was found in Caribbean regions, at 1.5 percent (3). Increasing PTB rates partly represent improved registration of cases of extremely PTB, rather than genuine increased rates (3), which is further affected by changes in classification of births around the threshold of viability (1). Nevertheless, plausible theories for increasing PTB rates are advancing maternal age and increasing use of assisted reproductive technology (both associated with increased rate of multiple pregnancy, which is strongly associated with PTB) and the global obesity epidemic (3). The rising rate of provider-initiated PTB is most responsible for the increase in PTB (4).

The disparity in survival from PTB between regions is stark. In the UK, the current survival rate for babies born alive at 25 weeks, who receive active management, is 70–78 percent (5). However, in low- and middle-income countries, lack of basic neonatal support, such as antibiotics or maintenance of warmth, means that only half of all babies born before 34 weeks' gestation survive (3).

12.1.2 Definitions, Clinical Presentation, and Risk Factors for PTB

12.1.2.1 Definitions and Clinical Presentation

Pre-term birth is defined by the World Health Organization as delivery before 37 completed weeks of gestation, or fewer than 259 days since the start of a woman's last normal menstrual period (1, 2). The standard definition of PTB rate, endorsed by the WHO, is "number of liveborn preterm births (before 37 completed weeks, whether singleton or multiple) divided by the number of livebirths" (1). However, methods of determining gestational age (GA) are highly variable between higher- and lower-resource countries (3), and inclusion of viability assessment in the definition causes further variation in reporting practice across different settings (1). The International Classification of Diseases (ICD-10) system recommends that all babies with any signs of life at birth should be considered a "livebirth", rather than using a GA threshold to define fetal viability (1). However, in practice, definitions of viability, and thresholds used for stillbirth registration, are variable and often include birthweight or GA (1). This affects data capture of livebirths, as extremely PTB can be underrepresented or misclassified as stillbirths (3).

Gestational age, which correlates inversely with neonatal mortality and morbidity, can be used to categorise PTB as extremely pre-term (<28 weeks), very pre-term (28 to <32 weeks) and moderately pre-term (32 to <37 weeks) (3). "Moderately pre-term" births, which account for over 80 percent of PTB, can be further divided into "moderate" (32 to <34 weeks) and "late" pre-term / "near term" (34 to <37 weeks) (4).

As perinatal care advances, the GA at which babies can be considered "viable" is reducing (5). The British Association of Perinatal Medicine (BAPM) recently published guidance recommending that management decisions for babies born between 22 to 27 weeks' gestation should not be based on GA alone, but on an individualized risk assessment for each baby, accounting for multiple prognostic factors, and the wishes of the parents (5).

Pre-term labor (PTL) is defined as the onset of labor before 37 completed weeks, in the form of regular contractions, accompanied by cervical change (4); when contractions occur without cervical change, a diagnosis of "threatened pre-term labor" is made (6). Fewer than 20 percent of women presenting with threatened PTL deliver pre-term (7). Over two thirds of cases of PTB are "spontaneous" (sPTB), when delivery is preceded by spontaneous onset of either uterine contractions and/or cervical dilatation, or by pre-term pre-labor rupture of membranes (PPROM). The remaining 30 percent of cases are provider-initiated PTB, for maternal or fetal concerns (4).

Pre-term birth is increasingly recognized as a multifactorial syndrome, initiated by the complex, dynamic interplay of several mechanisms, with a range of phenotypic characteristics (8). The exact biological mechanisms involved in the PTB

Figure 12.1 Pre-term Birth Syndrome classification proposed by Villar et al, modified from (10). "Caregiver (provider)-initiated" PTB is subdivided based on whether the delivery can be deemed clinically necessary or "discretionary", or whether a clinical indication is absent ("iatrogenic"), or unknown (10).

syndrome are poorly understood, although pathways include activation of maternal and fetal hypothalamic pituitary-adrenal axis, functional withdrawal of progesterone (9), and inflammatory decidual activation, typically by intrauterine infection or haemorrhage (4). Villar et al. proposed a new conceptual framework to subclassify PTB based on five phenotypic components (Figure 12.1) (10). This system recognizes PTB is the product of multiple overlapping factors, and that in the majority of cases, it is not possible to identify a specific discernible cause.

12.1.2.2 Risk Factors

Many clear risk factors associated with PTB have been identified, which can be classified as per Table 12.1 (4,11).

Demographic, Social & Environmental

Such risk factors frequently coexist. It is difficult to elucidate relative contributions of individual risks, and residual bias is likely in most observational studies.

Maternal Age – Maternal age below 20 years is associated with increased risk of PTB (12), as is advanced maternal age, even after attempted adjustment for potential confounding factors such as an increased likelihood of pre-existing maternal disease or pregnancy complications. The adjusted odds ratio (aOR) for PTB in mothers over 40 is 1.20 (95 percent CI 1.06–1.36) (12).

Table 12.1. Risk factors for pre-term birth

Demographic, social and environmental	Obstetric and gynecological factors	Risks of current pregnancy

• Maternal age
• Race and Ethnicity
• Pre-pregnancy BMI & Nutrition
• Family history
• Social deprivation & Poverty
• Smoking
• Illicit drug use
• Domestic violence
• Maternal education
• Psychological stress & Depression
• Pollution
	• Previous PTB
	• Previous late miscarriage
	• Previous second stage Caesarean section
	• Short interpregnancy interval (<6 months)
	• Previous uterine curettage
	• Previous cervical surgery
	• Congenital uterine anomalies
		• Assisted Reproductive Technology
		• Multiple pregnancy
		• Maternal medical comorbidities
		• Fetal anomaly
		• Polyhydramnios or Oligohydramnios
		• Antepartum hemorrhage
		• Infection:
		  - Vaginal and Intra-uterine
		  - Non-genital
		• Abdominal surgery (second & third trimesters)
		• Male fetus

Race & Ethnicity – In the UK and USA, rates of PTB in Black, African-American and Afro-Caribbean women are 16–18 percent, contrasting with 5–9 percent in white women, when attempts to adjust for potential confounders, including socioeconomic status, are made (4). Race impacts upon GA at delivery and initiation of parturition: Compared with white women, Black women are three times more likely have an extremely PTB, which is typically preceded by PPROM rather than uterine contractions and/or cervical dilatation (4). Furthermore, recurrence of PTB is commoner in Black women (9).

Racial differences in PTB are complex and likely to be multifactorial. In Black women only, associations have been found between sPTB and the Tumor Necrosis Factor-α-308 (TNF-α-308) A allele, which may serve as a genetic marker for PTB susceptibility (9). Racial disparities in PTB rates are increasingly recognized to be a product of significant inequalities surrounding access and provision of healthcare, further compounded by cultural differences in health-seeking behaviors, and potential low-grade but long-term psychological stressors resulting from racial discrimination.

Body Mass Index (BMI) – Women who are clinically underweight pre-pregnancy, defined as BMI $\leq 18.5 kg/m^2$, have an aOR of 1.3 (95 percent CI 1.2–1.3) for sPTB (11). Low BMI frequently indicates chronic malnutrition, associated with deficient intake of essential nutrients including vitamin D, zinc, iron, folate, and selenium (4), and increased rates of maternal anemia, all of which are established risk factors for PTB (12). Causal mechanisms may include hypo-perfusion of the uterus secondary to a relatively lower plasma volume in thinner women, and increased risk of maternal infection from a lack of essential vitamins and minerals (4).

The association between raised BMI and PTB is more controversial (4). Few studies can adjust for all confounders, as obesity itself involves a complex interaction of biological, behavioral, and socioeconomic factors. Furthermore, obesity is associated with increased rates of obstetric complications, such as congenital anomalies or preeclampsia (PE), which increase the risk of both spontaneous and provider-initiated PTB (4). A meta-analysis of 1.5 million women found mild obesity (BMI 30–34.9) may actually protect against sPTB (aOR 0.83, 95 percent CI 0.75–0.92) (13). However, after stratification of results by gestation, the risk of PTB under 32 weeks consistently increased with rising BMI (BMI > 40 – aOR 2.27 [95 percent CI 1.76–2.94]) (13).

Family History – Epidemiological studies provide evidence of strong familial clustering of PTB, and most support a primary maternal origin of genetic heritability, with limited impact of paternal or fetal genes (9). The risk of PTB is significantly higher in mothers born pre-term themselves (OR 1.49, 95 percent CI 1.12–1.99) (9).

Social Deprivation & Poverty – Social deprivation increases risk of PTB, and typically occurs alongside other risks, including lack of social support, low rates of maternal education, unemployment (aOR 1.32, 95 percent CI 1.21–1.9), malnutrition, domestic violence (OR 1.91, 95 percent CI 1.6–2.3), and increased rates of smoking and illicit drug use (12). Coexistence of these risks underpins the health inequalities surrounding PTB.

Smoking – Tobacco use confers an OR of 1.4 for sPTB (95 percent CI 1.3–1.4) (11), potentially by activating a systemic inflammatory response (4).

Psychological Stress – Women experiencing significant psychological stress, depression, or anxiety are at increased risk of PTB after adjustment for confounding factors such as increased smoking (4). Postulated mechanisms include activation of neuroendocrine pathways via raised maternal serum corticotrophin-releasing hormone (CRH) and cortisol levels, causing either premature or excessive activation of placental-fetal endocrine pathways, and/or proinflammatory modulation of the immune response, where stress alters Th1–Th2 ratio, thereby increasing susceptibility to maternal infection (14).

Obstetric & Gynecological Factors

Previous PTB – The most significant risk factor for PTB is a history of previous PTB (11). Recurrence risk ranges from 15 to 50 percent, increases with number of previous PTBs (12), and is inversely related to GA of previous PTB.

Previous Second Stage Cesarean Section – A cohort study reported that a history of previous emergency full dilatation cesarean birth confers an aOR of 3.29 (95 percent CI 2.02–5.13) for sPTB (15). Cervical trauma is commoner at second stage cesarean section and may impair the ability of the cervix to retain a subsequent pregnancy to term (15).

Previous Uterine Curettage or Cervical Surgery – Uterine curettage in the context of previous surgical termination of pregnancy or surgical management of miscarriage may cause cervical trauma (OR 1.7 [CI 95 percent 1.5–1.9] for sPTB <28 weeks) (11). Previous conization, trachelectomy, or large loop excision of the transformation zone has an OR of 2.0 (95 percent CI 1.4–3.0) for sPTB (11), which may result from cervical weakness, increased risk of ascending infection (11), or directly from dysplasia (6).

Risks of Current Pregnancy

Multiple Pregnancy – Twin or higher order pregnancies account for only 3 percent of all live births, but result in 15–20 percent of all PTB (4). One third of PTB in twin pregnancies is provider-initiated, resulting from increased rates of obstetric complications and intervention (16) and postulated causative mechanisms for increased risk of sPTB and PPROM include uterine overdistention, and increased secretion of CRH from a larger placental mass (4,16).

Infection
-Intra-uterine or vaginal
Intra-uterine infection is responsible for at least 25–40 percent of PTB, although given the limitations of conventional culture techniques, this is likely to be an underestimate (4). Infection is present in the majority of PTB before 30 weeks but is rarely implicated in late PTB (17). Bacteria either ascend from the vagina and cervix, spread through the placenta (hematogenous dissemination), enter through the fallopian tubes via the abdominal cavity, or can be introduced during an invasive procedure (17). When bacteria invade the choriodecidual space, the decidua and fetal membranes are activated to release a cascade of proinflammatory cytokines, which trigger the innate immune response. This provokes synthesis of prostaglandins, which initiate uterine contractions, and metalloproteases, which degrade fetal membranes, resulting in PPROM, and cervical softening (17).

Bacterial vaginosis (BV) is an imbalance of the vaginal microbiota, whereby naturally-occurring lactobacilli are reduced, and mixed anaerobes are increased. Although BV is associated with PTB, the responsible mechanisms remain unclear, and there is insufficient evidence to support universal screening of low-risk women for BV (11). Its presence may serve instead as a marker of intrauterine colonization by similar micro-organisms, such as *U. urealyticum* and *M. hominis*, commonly associated with PTB.

- Nongenital
A range of nongenital infections including appendicitis, pyelonephritis, malaria, and periodontal disease are associated with PTB (4). There is insufficient evidence to support antibiotic treatment of asymptomatic bacteriuria (12).

123

Neuro-developmental
- Cerebral palsy, most commonly spastic dysplegia
- Cognitive impairment
- Sensory impairment (visual / auditory)
- Disorders of executive functioning
- Specific learning difficulties (such as dyslexia)

Behavioral & Psychiatric
- Attention defecit hyperactivity disorder
- Social maladaptation
- Anxiety
- Depression

Other
- Chronic lung disease of prematurity
- Higher rates of hospital readmission, especially LRTI
- Increased use of outpatient care
- Chronic medical disorders (such as hypertension), into adulthood

Figure 12.2 Long-term sequelae of PTB; data derived from Saigal et al. (20). Recognized behavioral and psychiatric complications from PTB frequently persist into adolescence and adulthood (20). *LRTI = Lower Respiratory Tract Infection.*

Male fetus – Over 55 percent of PTB occurs in male babies, in which rates of neonatal mortality are higher compared to females born at a similar gestation (3).

12.1.3 Impact of PTB

12.1.3.1 Neonatal Morbidity and Mortality

Complications of PTB are responsible for 16 percent of global deaths in children under five, and the relative contribution of PTB to child mortality is increasing: Neonatal deaths (NNDs) contributed 47 percent of all under-5 deaths worldwide in 2018, compared with 40 percent in 1990 (2). In almost all middle- and high-income countries, PTB is the commonest cause of child mortality (3). PTB also increases a baby's risk of dying from neonatal infection (3).

Morbidity and mortality from PTB are directly related to GA at delivery (3). In high-income countries, over 90 percent of babies born before 28 weeks survive (3), providing stark contrast with low-income countries, where only 10 percent survive (3). Survival rates from PTB have improved over the last 20 years, particularly at the lower limit of viability (18). However, the lower the GA at birth, the higher the risk of "severe impairment," as defined by British Association Perinatal Medicine (BAPM): severe cognitive impairment, severe cerebral palsy, and/or blindness or profound hearing impairment (5). In the UK, the risk of

severe impairment in survivors of extreme PTB increases from 1 in 7 at 24–24+6 weeks' gestation to 1 in 4 at 23–23+6 weeks (5).

Morbidity from PTB is significant: major complications include respiratory distress syndrome (19), necrotizing enterocolitis (NEC), sepsis, retinopathy of prematurity, intraventricular hemorrhage (IVH), seizures, and hypoxic ischaemic encephalopathy (1). Longer term sequelae of PTB are shown in Figure 12.2.

The pre-term brain is vulnerable to injury in several areas by multiple mechanisms, including IVH, or via the fetal inflammatory response, characterized by raised fetal plasma interleukin-6 secondary to maternal intra-amniotic infection. This is strongly associated with periventricular leukomalacia, which is the commonest cause of white matter injury in pre-term neonates (18).

Pre-term birth can have a profound psychological, social, and financial impact on individuals and their families. The costs associated with PTB have a significant economic impact on society, long after a baby is discharged from the Neonatal Intensive Care Unit (20).

12.1.3.2 Maternal Morbidity and Mortality

Physical maternal morbidity from PTB usually originates from the pathology which led to the delivery, whether this was sPTB or provider-initiated – for example, significant obstetric hemorrhage (6). Emergency cesarean sections for extremely pre-term infants often require a vertical uterotomy (classical incision), as the lower uterine segment is frequently poorly formed (6). The associated operative risks can be serious, with increased risk of uterine rupture and abnormally invasive placenta in future pregnancies.

A cohort study found that women who delivered pre-term had a 1.7-fold mortality risk within the 10 years after delivery, compared with women who delivered at term (21). Median length of follow up was 23 years, and co-sibling analyses were used to control for unmeasured shared genetic or early-life environmental factors. Most deaths were cancer-related; 14.0 percent were cardiovascular.

Pre-term birth and threatened PTL can cause major psychological distress to mothers and their partners (20). Parents endure prolonged uncertainty regarding their baby's prognosis, and extremely pre-term babies typically require a protracted stay in a neonatal intensive or high dependency care unit, which can be emotionally disturbing for parents, and potentially impede maternal-infant bonding (6).

12.2 Hormonal Regulation of Parturition

12.2.1 Role of Hormones in Pregnancy and Labor

12.2.1.1 Progesterone

The role of steroid hormones throughout pregnancy is well established, especially for progestogens, estrogens, and glucocorticoids. Progesterone (P4) is the primary sex hormone with essential roles in establishment and maintenance of pregnancy, and initiation of labor; it supports fetal growth and development by ensuring quiescence of uterine muscle (myometrium) throughout pregnancy, preventing decidual activation, and promoting a tolerant maternal immune environment (22,23). P4 mediates its actions via two nuclear progesterone receptor isoforms – PRA and PRB – which are ligand-activated transcription factors encoded by a single gene. Upon binding P4, cytoplasmic PRA and PRB homo- or hetero-dimerize, translocate to the nucleus, and bind P4 response elements (24) on the promoters of P4-responsive genes to regulate gene transcription. PRs are expressed equally in all human P4

target tissues (including myometrium), and while PRB often has greater transcriptional activity, PRA has repressor activity over PRB. P4 also mediates rapid nongenomic effects through binding progesterone membrane components (PGRMC) or membrane-coupled progestin receptors (mPR) (Figure 12.3).

The fundamental question remains as to how the pregnant uterus can swiftly transform from a quiescent state into a contracting state required for parturition. In virtually all species other than humans and nonhuman primates, a fall in tissue/plasma P4 levels is a critical initiating event prior to the onset of labor (25). In humans, women do not experience systemic withdrawal of P4; instead, the plasma levels of both P4 and E2 rise progressively with advancing gestation, peaking at parturition. P4 ensures uterine quiescence by suppressing the expression of contraction-associated proteins (CAPs), such as gap junction protein (Cx43), oxytocin receptor (OXTR), prostaglandin receptor (PGFR), prostaglandin endoperoxide synthase 2 (PTGS2), and ion channels within the myometrium. In addition, P4 exerts an anti-inflammatory action by inhibiting the production of cytokines/chemokines and immune cell migration to the uterus, and acts on the decidua to prevent the induction of the pro-inflammatory prostaglandin (PG) PGF2a.

It was reported that PR isoforms play a central role in regulating myometrial function during labor. Novel research studied the molecular mechanisms leading to "functional" P4 withdrawal in the uterine tissue that trigger the onset of term labor (TL) (22). Prior to and during labor, an increase in the ratio of PRA to PRB isoforms occurs that reduces myometrial responsiveness to P4 and the concentration of receptor coregulators that are essential for PR function. Importantly, cellular metabolism of P4 results in reduced P4 levels and P4/PRB function in myometrium (22). Associated with this localized P4 withdrawal, we discovered that nuclear PRs become unliganded (in association with both TL and PTL) (22). We demonstrated that unliganding of PRA switches this receptor from a transcriptional repressor to a transcriptional activator of CAP genes and hence contributes to myometrial activation. The mechanism by which P4 could be locally withdrawn during labor is currently unknown. We speculate that altered P4 metabolism in the term human myometrium could result in local removal of the

Emily M. Frier et al.

Figure 12.3 Mechanisms of genomic and nongenomic actions of steroid hormones on myometrial cells
Estrogen (E2) mediates its genomic actions on target genes by binding to its specific nuclear estrogen receptors, ERα and ERβ, ligand-activated transcription factors that require homo-dimerization before binding to estrogen response elements (EREs) on the promoter of target genes. E2/ER regulates myometrial contractility through MAPK/ERK pathway by induction of pro-labor CAPs (Cx43, PTGS2, OXTR, PGFR), endothelin, thromboxane A2, contractile machinery proteins and membrane ion channels (Na+, Ca2+, K+). E2 also exerts its effects through binding to the ligand-activated receptor in the plasma membrane (GPER /GPR30) and through the activation of intracellular signaling pathways (MAPK/PLC/PI3K/PKA) (nongenomic regulation) which in turn cause the phosphorylation of substrate proteins and transcription factors (e.g., AP-1) that positively or negatively regulate gene transcription. Progesterone (P4) that plays a major role in myometrial quiescence during pregnancy, mediates its actions via two nuclear progesterone receptor isoforms, PRA and PRB, which are ligand-activated transcription factors. Upon binding P4, cytoplasmic PRA and PRB homo- or hetero-dimerize, translocate to the nucleus, and bind to specific DNA sequences called P4 response elements (24) on the promoters of P4-responsive genes to regulate gene transcription (genomic action). P4 also mediates rapid nongenomic effects through binding progesterone receptor membrane components (PGRMC1/2) or membrane-coupled progestin receptors (mPR). Androgen (A) signaling primarily occurs through the nuclear androgen receptor (AR), a steroid receptor and ligand-activated transcription factors. Within the nucleus, dimerization of ligand-bound AR units at promoter elements results in the transcriptional regulation of AR target genes (genomic action). Androgens play a major role in myometrial relaxation during pregnancy via non-genomic, AR-independent pathways, by penetration into the lipid bilayer and affecting Cs2+ transients (VOCCs, ROCCs, gap junctions). During term parturition they regulate cervical remodeling. *This Figure is made using BioRender software.*

hormone by the increased expression of the P4-methabolizing enzyme 20α-hydroxysteroid dehydrogenase (20a-HSD) (22). Moreover, we suggest that functional withdrawal of P4 down-regulates the transcription of genes that promote uterine quiescence, reducing the inhibitory effect of P4 on inflammation and increasing sensitivity of the myometrium to uterotonic agents.

12.2.1.2 Estrogens

The term "estrogens" refers to a group of primary female sex hormones, namely estrone (E1),

estradiol (E2), estriol (E3), and estretrol (E4). During pregnancy, levels of E2 and E3 are increased in the circulation, creating an estrogenic milieu towards term (23). The most common and potent form of estrogen during female reproductive years is E2. At the cellular level, E2 mediates its genomic actions on target genes by binding to its specific nuclear receptors, ERα and ERβ (Figure 12.3). In addition to the full-length ERα isoform, several shorter isoforms have been identified (for example, ERΔ7, a dominant negative isoform of ERα). Estrogen receptors (ERs) act as ligand-activated transcription factors and require homo-dimerization before binding to their ligand or to specific DNA sequences called estrogen response elements (EREs). The myometrial expression of both ER isoforms remains low through most of gestation due to inhibitory action of P4 as well as ERΔ7, which binds with and blocks ERα actions, thereby making the myometrium insensitive to the high-circulating E2. Cells often coexpress both ER and PR, with E2 being an important regulator of PR expression as the PR gene promoter contains several EREs.

Estrogens, particularly E2, have pro-labor actions in the uterus inducing biochemical and physical changes needed for labor and delivery. Although both hormones, E2 and P4, are equally abundant in the maternal system during gestation, P4 inhibits the actions of E2, reducing responsiveness to this hormone until term. A substantial body of evidence indicates that E2 plays a significant role in human parturition, since both uterine E2 and ERα are upregulated and activated at term. In addition, the combination of two factors (the local/functional withdrawal of P4 and the down-regulation of ERΔ7) activates E2 signaling, increasing myometrial sensitivity and responsiveness to E2. It is largely accepted that E2 and ERα promote myometrial activation at term through stimulation of biochemical changes in myocytes: induction of pro-labor CAPs (Cx43, PTGS2, OXTR, PGFR), endothelin, thromboxane A2, and contractile machinery proteins (myosin light chain kinase and calmodulin), and modify membrane ion channels (Na+, Ca2+, K+). Changes in ion channel results in a relative depolarization of myocytes, increasing excitability. Increases in uteronin receptor expression increases sensitivity to these agonists, while increases in the formation of gap junctions increases the capacity for synchronous labor contractions (22). E2 also stimulates the production of PGs by maternal decidua and fetal membranes and cervical expression of proteolytic enzymes, Matrix Metalloproteases (MMPs). MMPs and PGs promote cervical ripening and enhance spontaneous rupture of the fetal membranes. Moreover, at term, E2 induces migration of immune cells to the uterus and antagonises anti-inflammatory actions of P4/PRs by induction of pro-inflammatory cytokines and chemokines (such as TNFa) (26).

Studies in various species (rodents, sheep, human) have shown that the ERa gene is relatively low throughout gestation expression but rises at parturition, with the MAPK/ERK cascade being the principal pathway through which E2/ER regulates myometrial contractility in labor (27). Multiple studies have reported lower P4:E2 ratios in laboring women at term and pre-term, mostly due to a marked decrease in P4 levels and increase in circulating E2 levels. E2 levels were shown to be increased in women experiencing infectious PTB; Hepatitis E virus (HEV) infection caused increased secretion of E2 and expression of ERs, which was associated with PRB, low birthweight babies, and increased fetal mortality due to placental dysfunction (24).

12.2.1.3 Androgens

Androgens are male sex steroids fundamental for the defeminization and masculinization of male fetuses during development, and for the maintenance of male secondary sexual characteristics in adulthood (28). In women, the major androgens – dehydroepiandrosterone (DHEA), dehydroepiandrosterone sulphate (DHEAS), an drostenedione (A4), testosterone, and dihydrotestosterone (DHT) – are synthesized within the ovaries, the adrenal glands, and in fat cells (28). They act in an endocrine, paracrine, or intracrine manner, as pro-hormones for biosynthesis of estrogens.

Androgen signalling primarily occurs through the androgen receptor (AR), a steroid receptor belonging to the nuclear receptor 3-ketosteroid group C (NR3C) subfamily of ligand-activated transcription factors (Figure 12.3). Within the nucleus, dimerization of ligand-bound AR units at promoter elements results in the transcriptional regulation of AR target genes, leading to either activated or suppressed gene expression, depending on the coregulatory proteins with which this AR-dimer is interacting (genomic action) (29). Multiple studies suggest that increased androgens might regulate key molecular processes during pregnancy and term parturition, in particular cervical remodelling. Additionally, androgens play a major role in myometrial relaxation during pregnancy via nongenomic, AR-independent pathways, which is critical for the maintenance of pregnancy (28).

It appears androgens and their receptor are also fundamental for appropriate fetal growth and development *in utero*. In nonpregnant women, excess androgen production is associated with polycystic ovarian syndrome (PCOS) and can result in subfertility. During normal pregnancy, there is a physiologic systemic increase in androgen levels due to additional production by the fetus and placenta; androgens act as substrates for estrogen formation in the placenta (28). Abnormal androgen levels at the beginning of pregnancy have been associated with midtrimester loss or recurrent miscarriages. It is known that specific mechanisms are activated to protect both the mother and fetus from pregnancy-induced androgen excess; however, in some cases, high androgen levels are recorded during gestation and are associated with comorbidities such as PCOS and gestational diabetes mellitus (GDM), which could lead to PTB and present risks for fetus(es) and mother (29). Women with PCOS have a 6 percent higher risk of PTB, as PCOS is also associated with an increase in many inflammatory mediators.

Pathological pregnancy-induced hyperandrogenic conditions also include *hyperreactio luteinalis*, which is caused by high β-human chorionic gonadotrophin (β-hCG) levels and is highly associated with adverse pregnancy outcomes, such as PE and PTB (28). Increased testosterone levels in the maternal circulation in the third trimester have been associated with PE, suggesting testosterone as a predictive marker for PE. In addition, increasing maternal age (which is negatively associated with maternal androgen levels in pregnancy) is known to be a risk factor for PTB. Even though there is no association between fetal sex and maternal serum concentrations of any androgen (28), the dynamic state of androgen biosynthesis and bioavailability is fundamental for the appropriate development of fetuses, and any perturbations to these processes (for example, elevated testosterone) can have adverse developmental outcomes such as intrauterine growth restriction (30).

12.2.1.4 Thyroid Hormones

Pregnancy is a stress test of maternal thyroid function. Maternal subclinical hypothyroidism and hyperthyroidism occur in 10 percent of all pregnancies and are risk factors for PTB. Multiple epidemiological studies have also investigated the links between mild thyroid function abnormality (such as presence of thyroid antibodies) and risk of PTB (31). The prevalence of thyroid autoantibodies in women of reproductive age is common (6–20 percent), but it is higher in women with a

history of miscarriage and subfertility (31–33 percent). The rate of PTB is doubled in women with thyroid autoantibodies. Until recently, it remained unclear whether thyroid antibodies were risk factors for, or only markers of PTB, as the thyroid autoimmunity could be the main cause of hypothyroidism or an indicator of an activated autoimmune state (32). There is evidence that in nonpregnant women positive for thyroid antibodies, there is an alteration of cytokine expression by peripheral T lymphocytes. In pregnant women, the presence of thyroid autoantibodies can reflect a generalized activation of the immune system and its dysregulation at the fetal-maternal interface. Earlier meta-analysis (32) reported a statistically significant association between the presence of thyroid autoantibodies (including both thyroid peroxidase antibody, TPO-Ab, and thyroglobulin antibody, TG-Ab) and PTB (32). Later meta-analysis of prospective cohort studies specified that only presence of TPO-Ab in pregnant women increased the risk of PTB, whereas pregnant women with positive TG-Ab had no obvious increased risk of PTB (31). The most recent meta-analysis confirmed that in addition to TPO-Ab positivity, pregnant women without overt thyroid disease, but with subclinical hypothyroidism or isolated hypothyroxinemia, were at a significantly higher risk of PTB (33), anemia, and PE, as well as a higher rate of cesarean and neonatal morbidities. According to another meta-analysis, supplementation with levothyroxine to correct a deficiency of thyroid hormones showed beneficial effect in pregnant women with subclinical hypothyroidism and thyroid autoimmunity, namely a reduced risk of PTB (34).

12.2.2 Corticotropin-Releasing Hormone, Stress and PTB

Towards the end of pregnancy, the myometrium gradually increases its sensitivity towards uterotonins (oxytocin [OX] and PGs). This activation of the myometrium and the associated changes in hormonal milieu described above may be linked to increasing levels of the hypothalamic neuropeptide CRH, known as "the placental clock." Normally, maternal plasma CRH levels rise exponentially with advancing gestation, and peak during TL (35). CRH is produced by the combined action of fetal adrenals and the placenta, contributing to fetal lung maturation by the synthesis of surfactant protein A (SP)-A in fetal lungs and synthesis of E2 in placenta. In the myometrium, CRH directly stimulates the Nuclear Factor kB (NFkB) pathway, promoting inflammatory gene expression and leukocyte recruitment (36), and activates the AP-1 pathway, increasing the expression of CAPs, such as Cx43.

It is reported that increased psychological stress is associated with higher incidence of PTB. Physiological changes induced by stress include the production of glucocorticoids and uterotonic PGs, which may trigger the initiation of sPTB. Importantly, stress causes a premature increase in CRH plasma levels (comparable to those found during TL) and may stimulate sPTB (36). CRH may induce the synthesis and production of uterotonics PGF2α and PGE2, leading to activation of the uterine myometrium and the initiation of contractions. Thus, CRH is considered as a mediator of stress-induced PTB.

12.2.3 Physiologic Inflammation and Labor Onset

Pregnancy is a unique condition that modulates the maternal immune system in order to prevent rejection of the fetal allograft, as well as protect the mother and the baby from adverse consequences of the maternal immune response to pathogens. A successful pregnancy is associated with marked changes in the maternal immune system. At early gestation, uterine changes during implantation, placentation, and decidualization are associated with a strong pro-inflammatory response. During mid-pregnancy, when rapid fetal growth and development occurs, the predominant immunological feature is an anti-inflammatory state. Finally, at term, the successful delivery of the fetus requires reactivation of inflammatory process for parturition.

Numerous studies indicate that physiologic uterine inflammation at term is induced by mechanical and endocrine factors that cause the release of numerous pro-inflammatory cytokines and chemokines (including Inter Leukin-1β (IL-1β), IL-6, TNFα, C-C Motif Chemokine Ligand 2 (CCL2), and chemokine (C-X-C motif) ligand 8 (CXCL8)) by different uterine tissues, and is associated with the infiltration of inflammatory cells into the cervix, myometrium, fetal membranes, and amniotic cavity, even in the absence of infection (37). Thus, spontaneous TL is thought to be a physiological inflammatory process (37). The common pathway of parturition involves cervical ripening (dilatation and effacement), myometrial and membrane/decidual activation, and is associated with further induction of an inflammatory cascade within uterine tissues leading to massive infiltration of leukocytes, predominantly neutrophils and monocytes/macrophages (37). These immune cells are a rich source of pro-inflammatory cytokines and PGs, contributing to their tissue-specific expression. Cytokines mediate activation of the pro-inflammatory transcription factors, such as NF-κB and AP-1, which subsequently induce biochemical and molecular changes within the uterus (37). This pro-inflammatory environment promotes the contraction of the uterus, expulsion of the baby, and detachment of the placenta.

Disorder of immune function during pregnancy may cause pregnancy complications, including PTB and PE. It has been proposed that cellular stress can trigger both fetal membrane weakening and labor onset (38) through the production of molecules known as Danger Associated Molecular Patters (DAMPs) or Alarmins, including heat shock proteins, extracellular matrix breakdown products, circulating histones, and nucleic acid fragments – such as cell free DNA, mitochondrial DNA, and extracellular RNA, HMGB1, and various interleukins (IL-1a) (39). Alarmins can trigger myometrial inflammation through their interaction with Pattern Recognition Receptors (PRRs), including Toll-like receptors (TLRs), which can induce uterine activation by upregulating pro-inflammatory cytokines such as TNFa, IL-6, and PGs expression (38).

12.2.4 Infection and PTB

Depending upon the population, about half of PTB cases are attributed to infection, particularly intra-uterine infection with the presence of microbial invasion of the amniotic cavity and characterized by a positive amniotic fluid culture for microorganisms. Infection is the only pathological process for which a firm causal link with PTB has been established and for which a defined molecular pathophysiology is known (40). The evidence in support of this link includes: (1) sub-clinical intra-uterine infection (absence of clinical signs and symptoms) is associated with PTB; (2) intrauterine infection or systemic administration of microbial products to pregnant animals can result in PTB, whilst antibiotic treatment of ascending intrauterine infections in experimental models of chorioamnionitis can prevent sPTB; and (3) patients with elevated concentrations of pro-inflammatory cytokines (for example, IL-6, TNFα) and MMPs in amniotic fluid at the time of mid-trimester amniocentesis are at risk for subsequent PTB (40). Unfortunately, prevention and treatment of infection-associated PTB remains an unsolved problem. Importantly, accumulating evidence suggests that intra-amniotic infection may be a chronic condition. Chronic intra-uterine infection may persist between pregnancies and cause repeat sPTB (17). Regardless of the underlying cause, a common element in both infectious and noninfectious PTB is the presence of an inflammatory state.

12.3 Prediction and Management of Pre-term Birth

12.3.1 Prediction, Prevention, and Management of PTB in Humans

12.3.1.1 Prediction of PTB

Accurate prediction of women most likely to experience PTB enables appropriate and timely interventions to be offered, to prevent or delay the onset of PTL and to reduce adverse neonatal outcomes associated with PTB. However, approximately two thirds of PTB occurs in women without recognized risk factors for PTB (12). Furthermore, women presenting with signs and symptoms of threatened PTL generate significant diagnostic uncertainty: Almost 80 percent remain pregnant after 7 days (7).

Targeting therapies to women who are most likely to benefit avoids a "treat-all" approach for women presenting with symptoms of PTB, thereby preventing unnecessary intervention (7).

In the context of PTB, screening and surveillance targets high-risk populations, specifically women with previous sPTB or mid-trimester loss, in which there is robust evidence confirming benefit from different preventive interventions (6).

Cervical Length

Cervical length (CL) and effacement can be assessed on ultrasound which is transvaginal

(TVU), transabdominal, and transperineal (41). CL is inversely related to risk of PTB (42), and CL <10th centile may represent reduced or insufficient cervical function(42). TVU-measured CL is most predictive of PTB between 14 to 34 weeks' gestation (41).

Symptomatic women: The National Institute for Health and Care Excellence recommends that assessment of threatened PTL ≥30 weeks should include TVU-measured CL, using a cut-off ≤15mm to diagnose and treat PTB (43). Meanwhile, detection of a long cervix on TVU is protective, may help avoid overtreatment: Negative predictive values (NPV) for CL thresholds 15–25 mm approach 95 percent (6).

Asymptomatic women:

- "Low risk": Although a universal cervical screening approach is attractive, there is insufficient evidence to support this. The UK National Screening Committee highlighted uncertainty over which CL threshold should trigger intervention, and its low sensitivity of 35–40 percent (12 42).
- "High risk": Identification of a short cervix in this population enables early prophylactic intervention to reduce risk of PTB. In women with previous sPTB, CL <25 mm is deemed the optimal cut-off to predict increased PTB risk (44).

Fetal Fibronectin and Other Biomarkers

Fetal Fibronectin (fFN) is an adhesive glycoprotein located at the maternal-fetal interface of the amniotic membranes, between the chorion and decidua, which functions a biochemical marker of PTB if detectable in cervicovaginal secretions after 22 weeks (45). Disruption to the choriodecidual interface – typically inflammatory (42), infective, or mechanical (6) – causes release of fFN into cervicovaginal fluid, which can be sampled at speculum examination. Primary clinical use of fFN is as a qualitative test, using 50ng/mL as a cut-off to confirm or refute diagnosis of PTB, and its high NPV (7) can prevent unnecessary intervention, including hospital admission.

Where TVU is unavailable or unacceptable, the National Institute for Health and Care Excellence (NICE) recommends use of qualitative fFN to predict PTB and to inform management decisions, including discharge from hospital (43).

In the UK, measurement of qualitative fFN utilizes a bedside test called the Rapid fFN 10Q System

(Hologic), which rapidly yields fFN concentration from a vaginal swab sample (7). Studies report increasing specificity as fFN threshold increases (46), with improved stratification of individual patient PTB risk by use of specific incremental thresholds (10, 50, 200, 500 ng/mL). This improves PPV, both in high-risk asymptomatic women, and in women symptomatic of PTB (6).

Screening for fFN is not currently recommended in multiple pregnancies (16), nor in asymptomatic, "low-risk" women (42).

In the context of intact membranes, the European Association of Perinatal Medicine recommends assessment of additional biomarkers in cervicovaginal secretions (43,46), including placental alpha macroglobulin-1 ("PartoSure"), and phosphorylated insulin-like growth factor binding protein-1 ("Actim Partus") (46), which have sensitivities of 69 percent and 74 percent for delivery within 7 days, respectively (46).

Recent studies have identified gene expression signatures in maternal blood that are predictive of imminent delivery in women in threatened PTL as well as subsequent PTB in asymptomatic women (47,48). These findings support the role of maternal immune cells in the initiation of labor.

12.3.1.2 Management: Prevent and Delay PTB

Interventions aimed at reducing morbidity and mortality associated with PTB can be categorized as *primary* (directed at all women, before or during pregnancy), *secondary* (to eliminate or reduce risk in women with known risk factors) or *tertiary* (to prevent delivery or improve outcomes from PTB, after parturition has started) (42). The majority of interventions are tertiary, and aim to reduce the burden associated with PTB, rather than the rate of PTB per se (42).

Goodfellow et al. highlighted the paucity of evidence to support individual risk-reducing measures in the "low-risk" population (12), with the exception of smoking cessation (42), screening and treatment for *Chlamydia trachomatis* under 20 weeks (12), midwife-led continuity of care models (12), and zinc supplementation (12). This reflects the multifactorial etiology of PTB, which may be better addressed in the low-risk population through "bundles" of prevention care.

Effective secondary preconceptual interventions are limited to specific cases, such as surgical correction of uterine malformations (42), and insertion of

Figure 12.4 Preventive treatments for PTB (based on NICE guidelines (43). NICE advises on indications for preventive interventions based on past obstetric history and/or CL on mid-trimester TVU. Few trials have compared prophylactic progesterone with prophylactic elective cervical cerclage in the population of women with previous mid-trimester loss/previous sPTB, and finding of a short cervix; these women can be offered either intervention. *sPTB = spontaneous PTB. CL = Cervical length.*

transabdominal cerclage (typically limited to women with grossly disrupted or absent vaginal cervix, or in whom previous elective transvaginal cerclage has been unsuccessful) (49).

Detection and treatment of vaginal infection in "at-risk" women has yielded conflicting results; treatment of BV does not prevent PTB in all women with previous PTB, although detection and treatment of infection before 20 weeks may be more effective (11,42). Increased rates of PTB have been reported in high-risk women receiving metronidazole and clindamycin (6,42).

The main preventative treatments for PTB are cervical cerclage and progesterone therapy; indications are shown in Figure 12.4 (43).

Progesterone

Feasible mechanisms by which P4 supplementation reduces PTB include antagonism of oxytocin, maintenance of cervical integrity, and anti-inflammatory effects (42).

A systematic review concluded that prenatal administration of P4 versus placebo significantly reduced rate of delivery <34 weeks, when given to women with a previous sPTB (RR 0.31, 95 percent CI 0.14–0.69) and to women with short cervix on TVU (RR 0.64, 95 percent CI 0.45–0.90) (50). For women with prior sPTB, this review was sufficiently powered to detect the association between P4 supplementation and improved neonatal outcomes, confirming reduced rates of NND

(RR 0.45, 95 percent CI 0.27–0.76) and NEC (RR 0.30, 95 percent CI 0.10–0.89) (50). The OPPTIMUM trial of vaginal P4 for women at high-risk of PTB included childhood follow up to two years of age, and found no significant differences in cognitive scores or neurodevelopmental impairment in babies exposed to P4 compared to placebo (51).

There is insufficient evidence to support use of P4 supplementation in multiple pregnancies (16,50). Iams et al. postulates this shows P4 acts primarily through modulation of inflammation or cervical ripening, rather than prevention of uterine contractility (42).

Cervical Cerclage

Several potential mechanisms lead to cervical shortening or effacement, including congenital factors, biochemical effects secondary to hormones or inflammation, and biophysical influences such as uterine distention or contractile activity (42). Cervical cerclage (cervical stitch or suture), involves placing a suture around the cervix to prevent pregnancy loss or PTB secondary to cervical weakness (49). The efficacy of cerclage depends upon the pathophysiology underlying PTB; as such, its use is limited to specific subgroups of women (42). Elective cerclage may be history-indicated or ultrasound-indicated, while emergency ("rescue") cerclage is examination-indicated. A meta-analysis of RCTs confirmed prophylactic cerclage reduces PTB in women with CL <25 mm on TVU, but only in singleton pregnancies where there is a history of previous sPTB (RR 0.63, 95 percent CI 0.48–0.85) (52). Prophylactic cerclage was ineffective in women with short cervices alone, and in twin pregnancies it was disconcertingly associated with significantly increased rates of PTB <35 weeks (RR 2.15, 95 percent CI 1.15–4.01) (16).

In clinical practice, women with previous PTB or mid-trimester loss are offered ultrasound surveillance of CL, and subsequently offered cerclage if CL <25 mm (6). History-indicated cerclage in the absence of cervical shortening has a weaker evidence base; typically women with ≥3 previous sPTBs or mid-trimester losses are offered cerclage, between 12–15 weeks (6,49).

NICE recommends consideration of rescue cerclage for women from 16 to 27+6 weeks' gestation who present with cervical dilatation and exposed but unruptured fetal membranes, in the absence of bleeding, infection, or uterine contractions (43). A systematic review and meta-analysis concluded that rescue cerclage for women with cervical dilatation between 14 to 27 weeks significantly improved neonatal survival compared with expectant management (53).

Cervical Pessary

Arabin pessaries are flexible, silicone devices designed to be inserted round the cervix, to support it and thereby prevent PTB (54). Their benefits are uncertain and may be limited to asymptomatic women with short cervix on TVU (6,54).

Tocolysis

Tocolysis is the act of slowing or suppressing uterine contractions, designed to defer PTB in women in established PTL. Tocolytic agents do not appear to reduce the rate of PTB, nor do they sufficiently prolong pregnancy to enable significant intrauterine growth and development, but they do enable sufficient time for critical interventions to be implemented, which can improve neonatal outcomes (42,55), such as optimizing site of delivery via in-utero transfer to an appropriate higher-care neonatal unit, and administration of Antenatal Corticosteroid Therapy (ACT) (5). Tocolytics are contraindicated in the presence of bleeding or infection, where the harms of prolonging a pregnancy may outweigh the benefits (43).

Several classes of tocolytic drugs exist, which suppress contractions either by targeting contractile proteins in the myometrium by blockage of myosin phosphorylation, or by inhibition of myometrial stimulants (such as prostaglandins or oxytocin) (56). Side effects typically occur when nonmyometrial tissue is responsive to the cellular effects of that particular agent (56). Due to the adverse side effect profile, NICE advise against using betamimetics for tocolysis, and instead recommend calcium channel blockers as first-line (43). Insufficient evidence exists to support the use of tocolysis in multiple pregnancies (16).

12.3.1.3 Management: Reduce Morbidity and Mortality of PTB
Antenatal Corticosteroid Therapy (5)

Respiratory distress syndrome affects approximately half of babies born before 28 weeks' gestation (57). The use of ACT in humans to prevent Respiratory Distress Syndrome (RDS) in pre-term infants was first demonstrated in 1970s and ACT has since become the mainstay of care for women at risk of imminent PTB (57). Administration of ACT promotes fetal lung maturity by increasing synthesis of surfactant, lung compliance, and reducing vascular permeability (42). A Cochrane systematic review reported that a single course of ACT given to women before PTB reduced the most significant complications of PTB, namely, perinatal mortality (RR 0.85, 95 percent CI 0.77–0.93), neonatal mortality (RR 0.78, 05 percent CI 0.70–0.87) and RDS (RR 0.71, 95 percent CI 0.65–0.78) (57). ACT is also neuroprotective: The Cochrane review also reported that ACT reduced risk of IVH (RR 0.58, 95 percent CI 0.45–0.75), likely due to its vasoconstrictive effects in the fetal brain, and several studies have shown ACT is associated with a reduction in periventricular leukomalacia (18). Ten of the 21 studies included in the review took place in low- and middle-income countries, suggesting that the benefits of ACT are applicable to a range of settings (57).

National guidance from the UK recommends that women at high risk of imminent PTB, from 24 to 34+6 weeks, should be offered a course of ACT (79). Guidance from the UK and the USA recommends that ACT may be considered at 23+0 to 23+6 weeks, based on individual patient decisions surrounding neonatal resuscitation (43,58). BAPM recommends active, survival-focused management, including ACT, for babies deemed to be "moderate risk" (<50 percent chance mortality, or survival with severe impairment, in the context of active care), but emphasizes the paucity of evidence on ACT use below 24 weeks (5,57).

The optimal window for administration of ACT is 2–7 days before delivery. However, over 60 percent of women receiving ACT deliver outside of this timeframe (58), reinforcing the importance of accurate PTB prediction, to target therapies to women at highest risk of imminent PTB while avoiding overtreatment (7). Current guidance advises against regularly scheduled repeat courses of ACT (58,79).

Animal studies and studies of multiple courses of ACT have raised concerns regarding potential adverse long term effects of in utero ACT exposure, including impaired fetal growth, increased risk of cardiovascular disease and type 2 diabetes, and decreased brain growth (57,58).

Magnesium Sulphate

As neonatal care advances, survival rates of preterm infants, particularly those born at the extremes of viability, are improving, but this occurs in parallel with an increase in the incidence of neurological disability, including cerebral palsy (CP). A wide spectrum of neurological sequelae from PTB exists, from insult to the developing central nervous system. Perinatal neuroprotection aims to reduce these: The main agents currently in clinical use are ACT and magnesium sulphate. Alternative treatments, including N-acetylcysteine and melatonin, are under investigation (18).

A Cochrane review confirmed that administration of magnesium sulphate to women at risk of PTB substantially reduced risks of CP in the infant (RR 0.68, 95 percent CI 0.54–0.87; number needed to treat = 63) (59). The review also found that magnesium sulphate reduced significant gross motor dysfunction in early childhood (RR 0.61, 95 percent CI 0.44–0.85), without affecting paediatric mortality (RR 1.04, 95 percent 0.92–1.17) or maternal morbidity. The optimal regimen of administrating magnesium sulphate remains unclear (43,59) and the smallest possible therapeutic dose is recommended (18): As a peripheral vasodilator, dose-related side effects include flushing and sweating. Magnesium toxicity risks respiratory depression, respiratory arrest, and cardiac arrest (59). The review highlighted the need to investigate potential long-term consequences of magnesium sulphate therapy (59).

Postulated mechanisms for the neuroprotective effect of magnesium sulphate focus on its antagonism of The N-methyl-D-aspartate (NMDA) receptors on oligodendroglial progenitor cells, which prevents glutamate-mediated excitotoxicity, which would otherwise cause oligodendroglial progenitor cell death (18).

National guidelines from O&G committees in Australia, Canada, and the UK endorse the use of intravenous magnesium sulphate for neuroprotection in women up to 29+6 weeks' gestation, in whom PTB is expected to occur within 24 hours (18).

Antibiotics

Asymptomatic intrauterine infection is commonly a precursor of PPROM (4), management of which involves surveillance for and protection against infection. Antibiotic prophylaxis in PPROM prolongs pregnancy, and reduces maternal chorioamnionitis and neonatal morbidity (42): First-line antibiotic recommended is erythromycin, either for 10 days, or until the woman is in established labor (whichever occurs first) (43). Co-amoxiclav is contra-indicated in PPROM as it has been associated with increased rates of neonatal NEC (42,43).

Antibiotics to treat asymptomatic *Mycoplasma hominis*, *Streptococcus agalactiae*, *Ureaplasma urealyticum*, or *Trichomonas vaginalis* have been ineffective at preventing sPTB (12,17). Furthermore, antibiotics do not prolong pregnancy in women with threatened PTL and intact membranes (17). Intrapartum antibiotics, however, are recommended for all women in active PTL to prevent neonatal infection with group B streptococcus (GBS), given its increased prevalence in PTB (12), and significantly higher associated neonatal morbidity and mortality in pre-term infants (6,42).

12.3.2 Animal Models and Interventions of the Future

Most information about the pathophysiological mechanisms of PTB has been obtained using animal models. Ethical considerations do not allow *in vivo* human experiments, which are limited to observations and necessary medical interventions. Animal models of PTB have allowed detailed investigation of the earliest cellular/molecular events that initiate premature uterine contractions or cervical changes. Different animal models of PTB have used pregnant mice (60,61), rabbits, guinea pigs, sheep, and nonhuman primates (rhesus monkeys and macaque (62,63). Mouse models of PTB are popular and have several advantages to examine detailed factors involved in the PTB process: mice have a short gestational length (18–22 days), are easy to breed, and allow tight control of experimental variables, while minimizing costs. Also, the mouse immune system is well characterized, their genome is completely sequenced (which simplifies genetic manipulation), providing an array of knockout and transgenic mice suitable for studying the role of specific genes in the process of PTB (64). Moreover, molecular and biochemical changes associated with murine labor are similar to humans, including transient increases in myometrial CAPs (OTR, CX43, and PTGS2) (60,64).

12.3.2.1 Noninfectious (Sterile) Models

As described in Section 12.2, progesterone is the major pregnancy hormone that promotes relaxation and represses myometrial contractions. In rodents, P4 is produced in the ovary by corpora lutea. In virtually all species including rodents, a fall in tissue/plasma P4 levels due to luteolysis is a critical initiating event prior to the onset of labor. Experimental removal of the ovaries during early pregnancy causes termination of pregnancy in the mouse (65). Since there is no model of sPTB in mice, PR blockade by RU486 (mifepristone) provides a model of hormonal withdrawal or noninfectious "sterile" PTB (60). Pregnant mice and rats treated with RU486 experienced PTB, the premature increase of Cx43 gene expression, an increase in multiple cytokines (66), and leukocyte infiltration into the myometrium, decidua, and cervix (63). In contrast, administration of P4 or medroxyprogesterone acetate (MPA) in late pregnancy in rodents (to maintain elevated plasma progestin concentrations) blocks the onset of labor, and prevents increased expression of CAPs and ECM genes (60).

Growing evidence suggests that alarmin molecules found in amniotic fluid, such as IL-1α, are central initiators of sterile intra-amniotic inflammation (IAI) (67). Intra-amniotic administration of IL-1α causes PTB and neonatal mortality by inducing activation of the NOD-like receptor family, pyrin domain containing 3 (NLRP3) inflammasome.

12.3.2.2 Infectious Models

There is abundant evidence that infection-induced inflammation can cause PTB in humans, and animal models have been developed to investigate this relationship using bacteria, bacterial products, or inflammatory molecules (68). PTB can be induced in the mouse by exposure to (1) heat-killed *Escherichia coli*, (2) lipopolysaccharide (LPS, the major component of the outer membrane of Gram-negative bacterial cell walls), or (3) peptidoglycan, a component of Gram-positive bacterial cell walls. In mice and nonhuman primates, Group B Streptococcus caused IAI and PTB (62). The mechanism by which intrauterine infection initiates PTB is through TLRs; their stimulation results in the induction of transcription factor NF-κB, and initiates the inflammatory cascade as manifested by cytokines and production of PGs by uterine tissues, causing myometrial contractions and PTB (69). Different routes of administration of infectious or inflammatory agents were used to induce premature parturition. Most mouse models of infectious PTB utilize either intraperitoneal injection of LPS (a systemic inflammation model) or intrauterine or intravaginal infusion of LPS (localized inflammation model) during the last third of gestation (usually, gestational day 15 or 17).

Systemic mouse models represent human PTB associated with conditions that promote bacteraemia or sepsis (such as pyelonephritis) or viral infection (such as influenza). Systemic inflammation activates tissue macrophages to generate "early response" cytokines IL-1 and TNF-α, pointing to pathophysiology of infection-induced labor (70). Inflammatory activation can induce PTB, even in the absence of intrauterine infection. Systemic administration of IL-1 and TNF-α in mouse, rabbit, and intra-amniotic injection in nonhuman primate models, as well as intraperitoneal injections of PGF$_{2\alpha}$ in mice were capable of inducing PTB (63). Models of systemic inflammation, however, are limited, as most women in PTB have no features of systemic illness.

In contrast, models of local inflammation mimic clinical conditions of PTB more accurately. Intrauterine inoculation of pregnant mice with heat-killed *E.coli* can induce PTB, indicating the role of systemic inflammatory response to bacterial pathogens (68). This mouse model was refined using intrauterine administration of high dose LPS, resulting in the activation of the NF-kB pathway in the maternal uterus and the fetal brain, up-regulation of PGs, cytokine synthesis, and induction of PTB (60). Vaginal administration of high dose of LPS in mice or PGE2 in Guinea pigs produced subclinical cervical inflammation and caused PTB (63). Exposure to a prenatal inflammation is a known risk factor for neurobehavioral disorders including cerebral palsy and autism. To study the impact of inflammation on the fetal brain, a low dose of intrauterine LPS, insufficient to induce PTB in mice but capable of stimulating expression of multiple cytokines in maternal plasma and amniotic fluid was administered to pregnant mice. The study found that intrauterine inflammation, even in the absence of pre-term parturition, was sufficient to induce fetal brain injury (71).

Genetic ablation or "knockout" (KO) of single or multiple genes has been used to analyze molecular pathways regulating parturition in the mouse. Targeted disruption of PGHS-1 prolonged gestation in mice resulted in NND, whereas double KO of oxytocin and PGHS-1 genes restored the normal onset of labor by allowing luteolysis in the absence of elevated PGF$_{2\alpha}$ production (72). In addition, genetic inactivation of the CB1 receptor resulted in aberrant secretions of CRH and corticosterone during late gestation, altered P4 and E2 levels, and PTB induction (73). In mice with an IL-1 type 1 receptor KO, exposure to bacterial infection caused PTB, suggesting that IL-1 is sufficient but not necessary for the onset of labor. However, TNF-α/IL-1β double KO mice were protected from PTB under these circumstances (74). Mice with an anaphylotoxin C5a receptor KO had normal pregnancies and were protected from RU486-induced or vaginal LPS-induced PTB, indicating the role of the complement cascade in labor initiation (75). A few studies have examined genes regulating myometrial contractile function: A conditional Cx43 KO resulted in the prolongation of pregnancy, suggesting an important role for intercellular communication through gap junctions in normal uterine contraction during parturition, while overexpressed calcium-activated K$^+$ channel isoform 3 (KCNN3) caused blockage of uterine contractility, an absence of TL, and LPS-induced PTB in mice (63). These genetic manipulations in mice provide important information regarding the physiological pathways that may be relevant to human parturition.

12.3.2.3 Prevention of PTB: Animal Models

The importance of finding new therapeutic targets for PTB prevention cannot be overstated. Unfortunately, the development of drugs to inhibit uterine contractile activity has not reduced the incidence of PTB, likely because they target a late stage event in the labor cascade, when irreversible changes in uterine tissues have already occurred. Different therapeutic approaches to delay PTB (42) have targeted the control of inflammation and the regulation of P4 in uterine tissues. As discussed in Section 12.3.1.2, P4 treatment can prevent PTB and improve neonatal outcome in specific patient populations (50), possibly by repression of myometrial contractility including down-regulation of CAPs, increase in cAMP, or inhibition of myosin phosphorylation (76). In a mouse model of infection-induced PTB, pre-treatment with MPA inhibited cervical ripening; down-regulated expression of cytokines, Ptgs2, and Cx43; and delayed PTB (60). These data indicate that, in the context

135

of intrauterine infection, P4 has anti-inflammatory actions and acts to decrease myometrial contractility. Progestins can also prevent RU486-induced PTB by inhibiting cervical ripening (66). We assessed the prophylactic potential of a nonmetabolizable selective progesterone receptor modulator (SPRM), Promegestone/R5020, using LPS-induced and RU486-induced PTB mouse models and found that Promegestone prevents pre-term parturition by limiting inflammation of uterine/fetal tissues and inhibiting the expression of pro-contractile genes/proteins in the myometrium (77).

A therapeutic approach to prevent PTB by targeting the inflammatory cascade at an earlier stage – either by blocking pro-inflammatory mediators, up-regulating endogenous, or administrating exogenous anti-inflammatory mediators – is under investigation. A protective effect of indomethacin, lactoferrin, prostaglandin synthesis inhibitors, betamethasone, anti-TNF-α, MMP inhibitor GM6001, and anti-inflammatory prostaglandin 15d-PGJ$_2$ (a metabolite of PGD$_2$) on the incidence of systemic LPS-induced PTB in mice has been reported (63). Infection-induced PTB was prevented through selective inhibition of phosphodiesterase type-4 by rolipram and small guanosine triphosphatase RhoA/Rho-kinase inhibitor Y-27632. Recent study using an *in vivo* animal model of LPS-induced IAI reported that a specific inhibitor of NLRP3, MCC950, reduced

IAI-induced PTB and neonatal mortality (61). Unfortunately, few have progressed to pre-clinical trials because of side effects.

Pharmacological blockade of chemokine action without overall immune suppression has been proposed as a novel means of reducing uncontrolled inflammation. Broad Spectrum Chemokine Inhibitors (BSCIs) have been developed to block concurrently multiple chemokine signalling pathways; we explored whether BSCIs may reduce uterine inflammation and decrease the rates of PTB in two animal models (78). We found that administration of BSCI (FX125L) to pregnant macaques powerfully suppressed uterine contractility, the cytokine response, and PTB induced by Group B Streptococcus (62). In mice, BSCI blocked LPS-induced PTB by inhibiting the influx of neutrophils, reducing inflammation, and decreasing cytokine levels in maternal blood and in the myometrium and decidua (78).

Knowledge gained using animal models of PTB suggests that novel anti-inflammatory drugs (such as BSCI), and synthetic progestins effectively delay pre-term parturition. Based on our current understanding of the importance of infection/inflammation in the aetiology of PTB, it can be anticipated that both may be future therapeutic candidates for prevention of PTB.

References

1. Chawanpaiboon S, Vogel JP, Moller A-B, et al. Global, regional, and national estimates of levels of preterm birth in 2014: A systematic review and modelling analysis. *The Lancet Global Health.* 2019, 7(1):e37–e46.

2. UNICEF, WHO, World Bank Group and United Nations. United Nations Inter-agency Group for Child Mortality Estimation (UN IGME). Levels & Trends in Child Mortality: Report 2019, Estimates Developed by the United Nations Inter-Agency Group for Child Mortality Estimation. New York: 2019.

3. Blencowe H, Cousens S, Oestergaard MZ, et al. National, regional, and worldwide estimates of preterm birth rates in the year 2010 with time trends since 1990 for selected countries: A systematic analysis and implications. *The Lancet.* 2012, 379(9832):2162–2172.

4. Goldenberg RL, Culhane JF, Iams JD, et al. Epidemiology and causes of preterm birth. *The Lancet.* 2008, 371 (9606):75–84.

5. Mactier H, Bates SE, Johnston T, et al. Perinatal management of extreme preterm birth before 27 weeks of gestation: A framework for practice. *Archives of Disease in Childhood: Fetal and Neonatal Edition.* 2020, 105(3):232.

6. Hezelgrave N, and Shennan A. Threatened and actual preterm labor. In: James D, Steer P, Weiner C, B G, SC R, (Eds.), *High-Risk Pregnancy Management Options.* 2. Fifth Ed, 2017; 1624–1647. Cambridge: Cambridge University Press.

7. Stock SJ, Wotherspoon LM, Boyd KA, et al. Quantitative fibronectin to help decision-making in women with symptoms of preterm labour (QUIDS) part 1: Individual participant data meta-analysis and health economic analysis. *BMJ Open.* 2018, 8(4): e020796.

8. Barros FC, Papageorghiou AT, Victora CG, et al. The distribution of clinical phenotypes of preterm birth syndrome: Implications for prevention. *JAMA Pediatrics.* 2015, 169(3):220–229.

9. Rood KM, and Buhimschi CS. Genetics, hormonal influences, and preterm birth. *Seminars in Perinatology.* 2017, 41 (7):401–408.

10. Villar J, Papageorghiou AT, Knight HE, et al. The preterm birth syndrome: A prototype phenotypic classification. *Am Journal of Obstetrics and Gynecology.* 2012, 206 (2):119–123.

11. Cobo T, Kacerovsky M, and Jacobsson B. Risk factors for spontaneous preterm delivery. *International Journal of Gynecology & Obstetrics.* 2020, 150(1):17–23.

12. Goodfellow L, Care A, and Alfirevic Z. Controversies in the prevention of spontaneous preterm birth in asymptomatic women: an evidence summary and expert opinion. *BJOG: An International Journal of Obstetrics & Gynecology.* 2020.

13. Torloni MR, Betrán AP, Daher S, et al. Maternal BMI and preterm birth: A systematic review of the literature with meta-analysis. *The Journal of Maternal-Fetal & Neonatal Medicine.* 2009. 22(11):957–970.

14. Hobel C, and Culhane J. Role of psychosocial and nutritional stress on poor pregnancy outcome. *Journal of Nutrition.* 2003, 133(5 Suppl 2):1709s–1717s.

15. Williams C, Fong R, Murray S, et al. Caesarean birth and risk of subsequent preterm birth: A retrospective cohort study. *BJOG: An International Journal of Obstetrics & Gynecology.* 2020.

16. Murray SR, Stock SJ, Cowan S, et al. Spontaneous preterm birth prevention in multiple pregnancy. *The Obstetrician & Gynaecologist.* 2018, 20(1):57–63.

17. Goldenberg RL, Hauth JC, and Andrews WW. Intrauterine infection and preterm delivery. *New England Journal of Medicine.* 2000, 342 (20):1500–1507.

18. Chang E. Preterm birth and the role of neuroprotection. *BMJ: British Medical Journal.* 2015, 350:g6661.

19. Gravett MG, Witkin SS, Haluska GJ, et al. An experimental model for intraamniotic infection and preterm labor in rhesus monkeys. *American Journal of Obstetrics and Gynecology.* 1994, 171 (6):1660–1667.

20. Saigal S, and Doyle LW. An overview of mortality and sequelae of preterm birth from infancy to adulthood. *The Lancet.* 2008, 371 (9608):261–269.

21. Crump C, Sundquist J, and Sundquist K. Preterm delivery and long term mortality in women: National cohort and co-sibling study. *BMJ.* 2020, 370:m2533.

22. Shynlova O, Nadeem L, Zhang J, et al. Myometrial activation: Novel concepts underlying labor. *Placenta.* 2020, 92: 28–36.

23. Smith R, Smith JI, Shen X, et al. Patterns of plasma corticotropin-releasing hormone, progesterone, estradiol, and estriol change and the onset of human labor. *The Journal of Clinical Endocrinology and Metabolism.* 2009, 94(6):2066–2074.

24. Singh S, Daga MK, Kumar A, et al. Role of oestrogen and its receptors in HEV-associated feto-maternal outcomes. *Liver International.* 2019, 39 (4):633–639.

25. Menon R, Bonney EA, Condon J, et al. Novel concepts on pregnancy clocks and alarms: Redundancy and synergy in human parturition. *Human Reproduction Update.* 2016, 22 (5):535–560.

26. Mendelson CR, Gao L, and Montalbano AP. Multifactorial regulation of myometrial contractility during pregnancy and parturition. *Frontiers in Endocrinology.* 2019, 10(714): 1–17.

27. Welsh T, Johnson M, Yi L, et al. Estrogen receptor (ER) expression and function in the pregnant human myometrium: estradiol via ERα activates ERK1/2 signaling in term myometrium. *Journal of Endocrinology.* 2012, 212 (2):227–238.

28. Makieva S, Saunders PTK, and Norman JE. Androgens in pregnancy: Roles in parturition. *Human Reproduction Update.* 2014, 20(4):542–559.

29. Meakin AS, and Clifton VL. Review: Understanding the role of androgens and placental AR variants: Insight into steroid-dependent fetal-placental growth and development. *Placenta.* 2019, 84:63–68.

30. Carlsen SM, Jacobsen G, and Romundstad P. Maternal testosterone levels during pregnancy are associated with offspring size at birth. *European Journal of Endocrinology.* 2006, 155 (2):365–370.

31. He X, Wang P, Wang Z, et al. Thyroid antibodies and risk of preterm delivery: A meta-analysis of prospective cohort studies. *European Journal of Endocrinology.* 2012, 167 (4):455–464.

32. Thangaratinam S, Tan A, Knox E, et al. Association between thyroid autoantibodies and miscarriage and preterm birth: Meta-analysis of evidence. *BMJ.* 2011, 342:d2616.

33. Korevaar TIM, Derakhshan A, Taylor PN, et al. Association of thyroid function test abnormalities and thyroid autoimmunity with preterm birth: A systematic review and meta-analysis. *JAMA: The Journal of the American Medical Association.* 2019, 322 (7):632–641.

34. Rao M, Zeng Z, Zhou F, et al. Effect of levothyroxine supplementation on pregnancy

137

loss and preterm birth in women with subclinical hypothyroidism and thyroid autoimmunity: A systematic review and meta-analysis. *Human Reproduction Update.* 2019, 25(3): 344–361.

35. Chen Y, Holzman C, Chung H, et al. Levels of maternal serum corticotropin-releasing hormone (CRH) at midpregnancy in relation to maternal characteristics. *Psychoneuroendocrinology.* 2010, 35(6):820–832.

36. You X, Liu J, Xu C, et al. Corticotropin-Releasing Hormone (CRH) promotes inflammation in human pregnant myometrium: The evidence of CRH initiating parturition? *The Journal of Clinical Endocrinology and Metabolism.* 2014, 99(2): E199–E208.

37. Shynlova O, Lee Y-H, Srikhajon K, et al. Physiologic uterine inflammation and labor onset: Integration of endocrine and mechanical signals. *Reproductive Sciences.* 2013, 20 (2):154–167.

38. Menon R, Behnia F, Polettini J, et al. Placental membrane aging and HMGB1 signaling associated with human parturition. *Aging.* 2016, 8 (2):216–230.

39. Padron JG, Saito Reis CA, and Kendal-Wright CE. The role of danger associated molecular patterns in human fetal membrane weakening. *Frontiers in Physiology.* 2020, 11(602): 1–18.

40. Romero R, Espinoza J, Gonçalves LF, et al. Inflammation in preterm and term labour and delivery. *Seminars in Fetal and Neonatal Medicine.* 2006, 11(5):317–326.

41. Berghella V, and Saccone G. Cervical assessment by ultrasound for preventing preterm delivery. *Cochrane*

Library: Cochrane Reviews. 2019, 9(9):Cd007235.

42. Iams JD, Romero R, Culhane JF, et al. Primary, secondary, and tertiary interventions to reduce the morbidity and mortality of preterm birth. *The Lancet.* 2008, 371 (9607):164–175.

43. National Collaborating Centre for Ws, Children's H. *National Institute for Health and Care Excellence: Clinical Guidelines. Preterm Labour and Birth.* London: National Institute for Health and Care Excellence (UK) National Collaborating Centre for Women's and Children's Health; 2015.

44. Owen J, Yost N, Berghella V, et al. Mid-trimester endovaginal sonography in women at high risk for spontaneous preterm birth. *JAMA.* 2001, 286 (11):1340–1348.

45. Berghella V, and Saccone G. Fetal fibronectin testing for reducing the risk of preterm birth. *Cochrane Database of Systematic Reviews.* 2019, 7.

46. Excellence NIfHaC. *Biomarker Tests to Help Diagnose Preterm Labour in Women with Intact Membranes.* London: NICE; 2018.

47. Heng Y, Pennell C, Chua HN, et al. Whole blood gene expression profile associated with spontaneous preterm birth in women with threatened preterm labor. *PLoS ONE.* 2014, 9:e96901.

48. Heng YJ, Pennell CE, McDonald SW, et al. Maternal whole blood gene expression at 18 and 28 weeks of gestation associated with spontaneous preterm birth in asymptomatic women. *PLoS ONE.* 2016, 11 (6):e0155191.

49. Gibb D, and Saridogan E. The role of transabdominal cervical cerclage techniques in maternity care. *The*

Obstetrician & Gynaecologist. 2016, 18(2):117–125.

50. Dodd JM, Jones L, Flenady V, et al. Prenatal administration of progesterone for preventing preterm birth in women considered to be at risk of preterm birth. *Cochrane Database of Systematic Reviews.* 2013, (7):CD004947.

51. Norman JE, Marlow N, Messow C-M, et al. Vaginal progesterone prophylaxis for preterm birth (the OPPTIMUM study): A multicentre, randomised, double-blind trial. *The Lancet.* 2016, 387(10033):2106–2116.

52. Berghella V, Odibo AO, To MS, et al. Cerclage for short cervix on ultrasonography: Meta-Analysis of trials using individual patient-level data. *Obstetrics & Gynecology.* 2005, 106(1).

53. Ehsanipoor RM, Seligman NS, Saccone G, et al. Physical examination-indicated cerclage: A systematic review and meta-analysis. *Obstet Gynecol.* 2015, 126(1):125–135.

54. Hermans FJR, Schuit E, Bekker MN, et al. Cervical pessary after arrested preterm labor: A randomized controlled trial. *Obstetrics & Gynecology.* 2018, 132(3).

55. Haas DM, Caldwell DM, Kirkpatrick P, et al. Tocolytic therapy for preterm delivery: Systematic review and network meta-analysis. *BMJ: British Medical Journal.* 2012, 345: e6226.

56. Caritis S. Adverse effects of tocolytic therapy. *BJOG: An International Journal of Obstetrics & Gynaecology.* 2005, 112(s1):74–78.

57. McGoldrick E, Stewart F, Parker R, et al. Antenatal corticosteroids for accelerating fetal lung maturation for women at risk of preterm birth. *Cochrane Database of Systematic*

Reviews. 2020, 12(12): CD004454.

58. ACOG. Committee Opinion No. 713: Antenatal Corticosteroid Therapy for Fetal Maturation. *Obstetrics and Gynecology*. 2017, 130 (5):1159.

59. Doyle LW, Crowther CA, Middleton P, et al. Magnesium sulphate for women at risk of preterm birth for neuroprotection of the fetus. *Cochrane Database of Systematic Reviews*. 2009, (1): CD004661.

60. Elovitz MA, and Mrinalini C. Animal models of preterm birth. *Trends in Endocrinology and Metabolism*. 2004, 15 (10):479–487.

61. Faro J, Romero R, Schwenkel G, et al. Intra-amniotic inflammation induces preterm birth by activating the NLRP3 inflammasome. *Biology of Reproduction*. 2019, 100 (5):1290–1305.

62. Coleman M, Orvis A, Wu T-Y, et al. A broad spectrum chemokine inhibitor prevents preterm labor but not microbial invasion of the amniotic cavity or neonatal morbidity in a non-human primate model. *Frontiers in Immunology*. 2020, 11(770).

63. Shynlova O, and Lye SJ. Regulation of parturition. In: Croy BA, Yamada AT, DeMayo FJ, Adamson SL (Eds), *The Guide to Investigation of Mouse Pregnancy*. 2014; 373–389. Boston: Academic Press.

64. Bryan FM, and Michael JT. Are animal models relevant to key aspects of human parturition? *American Journal of Physiology-Regulatory, Integrative and Comparative Physiology*. 2009, 297 (3):525–545.

65. Dinny Graham J, and Clarke CL. Physiological action of

progesterone in target tissues. *Endocrine Reviews*. 1997, 18 (4):502–519.

66. Holt R, Timmons BC, Akgul Y, et al. The molecular mechanisms of cervical ripening differ between term and preterm birth. *Endocrinology*. 2011, 152 (3):1036–1046.

67. Motomura K, Romero R, Garcia-Flores V, et al. The alarmin interleukin-1α causes preterm birth through the NLRP3 inflammasome. *Molecular Human Reproduction*. 2020, 26 (9):712–726.

68. Hirsch E, and Wang H. The molecular pathophysiology of bacterially induced preterm labor: Insights from the murine model. *The Journal of the Society for Gynecologic Investigation: JSGI*. 2005, 12 (3):145–155.

69. MacIntyre DA, Sykes L, Teoh TG, et al. Prevention of preterm labour via the modulation of inflammatory pathways. *The Journal of Maternal-Fetal & Neonatal Medicine*. 2012, 25 (Suppl 1):17–20.

70. Mulligan MS, and Ward PA. Immune complex-induced lung and dermal vascular injury. Differing requirements for tumor necrosis factor-alpha and IL-1. *The Journal of Immunology*. 1992, 149 (1):331–339.

71. Elovitz MA, Brown AG, Breen K, et al. Intrauterine inflammation, insufficient to induce parturition, still evokes fetal and neonatal brain injury. *International Journal of Developmental Neuroscience*. 2011, 29(6):663–671.

72. Gross GA, Imamura T, Luedke C, et al. Opposing actions of prostaglandins and oxytocin determine the onset of murine labor. *Proceedings of the National Academy of Sciences*

(PNAS). 1998, 95 (20):11875–11879.

73. Wang H, Xie H, and Dey SK. Loss of cannabinoid receptor CB1 induces preterm birth. *PLoS ONE*. 2008, 3 (10):1–8.

74. Hirsch E, Filipovich Y, and Mahendroo M. Signaling via the type I IL-1 and TNF receptors is necessary for bacterially induced preterm labor in a murine model. *American Journal of Obstetrics and Gynecology*. 2006, 194 (5):1334–1340.

75. Gonzalez JM, Romero R, and Girardi G. Comparison of the mechanisms responsible for cervical remodeling in preterm and term labor. *Journal of Reproductive Immunology*. 2012, 97(1):112–119.

76. Soloff MS, Jeng Y-J, Izban MG, et al. Effects of progesterone treatment on expression of genes involved in uterine quiescence. *Reproductive Sciences*. 2011, 18(8):781–797.

77. Shynlova O, Nadeem L, Dorogin A, et al. The selective progesterone receptor modulator, Promegestone, delays term parturition and prevents infection-mediated preterm birth in mice. *AJOG*. 2022, 226(2):249. e1–249.e21.

78. Shynlova O, Dorogin A, Li Y, et al. Inhibition of infection-mediated preterm birth by administration of broad spectrum chemokine inhibitor in mice. *Journal of Cellular and Molecular Medicine*. 2014, 18 (9):1816–1829.

79. Stock SJ, Thomson AJ, Papworth S; the Royal College of Obstetricians, Gynaecologists. Antenatal corticosteroids to reduce neonatal morbidity and mortality. *BJOG: An International Journal of Obstetrics & Gynecology*. 2022.

Chapter 13

Thyroid Dysfunction in Pregnancy and Postpartum

Luigi Bartalena, Eliana Piantanida, Adriana Lai, and Maria Laura Tanda

13.1 Thyroid Physiology in Pregnancy

Pregnancy is characterized by relevant, physiological changes in thyroid economy underpinned by the following situations: (1) the mother has to provide thyroid hormones to the fetus, whose thyroid gland is not fully functioning until 16–18 weeks' gestation; (2) an increase in synthesis and secretion of the major thyroid hormone binding protein (thyroxine-binding globulin, TBG) occurs, triggered by maternal estrogens; (3) enhanced renal iodine clearance and, consequently, increased iodine loss take place, which, together with fetal iodine requirements, account for the increase in daily iodine demand during pregnancy; and (4) thyroid hormones undergo increased peripheral degradation, mainly related to the activity of placental deiodinase type 3, which reduces monodeiodination of the prohormone, thyroxine (T4), to the metabolically active hormone, triiodothyronine (T3), and inactivates T3 to nonmetabolically active metabolites (1). All of the above events concur to cause an increased requirement for thyroid hormone synthesis from the mother's thyroid gland, which is satisfied – in the first trimester of pregnancy – through thyroid stimulation by human Chorionic Gonadotropin (hCG); this hormone, produced by the trophoblasts, binds to the thyrotropin (TSH) receptor on thyroid follicular cells (1). Although hCG is a weaker thyroid stimulator than the physiological ligand – TSH – its high concentrations in the first trimester of pregnancy suffice to satisfy the increased thyroid hormone demand. Further to the above changes, in the first trimester of pregnancy, serum total T4 and T3 concentrations are increased (due to increased TBG-related thyroid hormone binding capacity), serum free T4 (FT4) and free T3 (FT3) concentrations are transiently increased, and serum TSH concentration is transiently decreased to suppressed (1). To adapt to the above changes, thyroid size tends to increase during pregnancy, especially in iodine-deficient areas.

13.2 Hyperthyroidism in Pregnancy

13.2.1 Definition, Epidemiology, and Etiology

Thyrotoxicosis and hyperthyroidism are not synonyms: While hyperthyroidism is a condition related to an excessive thyroid hormone production, thyrotoxicosis indicates a state of increased serum thyroid hormone circulating levels, which do not necessarily reflect thyroid hyperfunction, but may also be due to an excessive thyroid hormone intake (iatrogenic or factitious thyrotoxicosis) or to a thyroid-destructive process (subacute thyroiditis, painless thyroiditis, amiodarone-induced thyroiditis). Hyperthyroidism may be overt (presence of symptoms and signs associated with increased serum FT4 and FT3 concentrations and decreased/suppressed serum TSH levels) or subclinical (absent/limited clinical manifestations, normal serum FT4 and FT3 concentrations, but decreased/suppressed serum TSH).

In the general population outside pregnancy, the prevalence of overt hyperthyroidism varies between 0.2 percent and 1.3 percent in iodine-replete geographical areas (2), and a recent European meta-analysis reported a mean prevalence of 0.75 percent, considering women and men together (3). Overt hyperthyroidism is however far more prevalent in women than in men (2.7 percent versus 0.23 percent) (2). Sublinical hyperthyroidism is even more frequent and may affect 1 to 5 percent of the general population (4).

In iodine-sufficient geographical areas, hyperthyroidism is most frequently due to Graves' disease, which usually peaks in the third to fifth decade of life, thus coinciding with childbearing age (5). Conversely, in iodine-deficient

Table 13.1. Causes of thyrotoxicosis/hyperthyroidism and hypothyroidism in pregnancy

Thyrotoxicosis/Hyperthyroidism

Graves' disease

Gestational Transient Thyrotoxicosis

Toxic Adenoma or Toxic Multinodular Goiter

Trophoblastic disease

Familial gestational hyperthyroidism

Constitutive activation of the TSH receptor

Subacute or painless thyroiditis

Factitious or iatrogenic thyrotoxicosis

Struma ovarii

Hypothyroidism

Chronic Autoimmune Thyroiditis

Iodine deficiency

Inadequate levothyroxine replacement therapy for hypothyroidism

Previous thyroidectomy

Previous radioactive iodine treatment for hyperthyroidism

Bold: most common causes

geographical areas, thyroid hyperfunction is more frequently caused by autonomous nodules (either a single toxic adenoma or multinodular toxic goiter), but the latter usually have their peak of incidence at an older age and are uncommon in women <40 years of age (6,7). Thus, in pregnancy hyperthyroidism is most commonly caused by Graves' disease, an autoimmune disorder in which the ultimate cause of hyperthyroidism is the uncontrolled thyroid stimulation by autoantibodies interacting with the TSH receptor on the surface of thyroid follicular cells (TSH receptor antibody, TSHR-Ab) (8) (Table 13.1). The incidence of Graves' disease is 55–80 cases/100,000/year in women >30 years of age, 35–50 cases/100,000/year in women <30 years of age (7,9). An incidence of 5.9 cases of Graves' hyperthyroidism per 1000 pregnant women/year women has been reported in USA (10), but Graves' hyperthyroidism is less likely to occur *de novo* during pregnancy, with an estimated risk of 0.05 percent, as thyroid autoimmune phenomena usually improve during gestation (7,11).

The other major cause of hyperthyroidism in pregnancy is gestational transient thyrotoxicosis (GTT). This condition is caused by extremely high serum hCG concentrations which may cause either subclinical or overt hyperthyroidism. The underpinning mechanism is binding of hCG to the TSH receptor. When hyperthyroidism is overt, the pregnant woman also has hyperemesis gravidarum. Hyperthyroidism is transient, remits after peaking around the tenth week of gestation, and is observed in 0.3–1 percent of pregnant women (11) (Table 13.1). Very rarely, hyperthyroidism may be due to trophoblastic disease (hydatidiform mole or choriocarcinoma) associated with very high serum hCG concentrations (7). Another very rare cause of hyperthyroidism in pregnancy is familial gestational hyperthyroidism due to a mutation in the TSH receptor, making it hyperresponsive to hCG (12). Other conditions enlisted in Table 13.1 should be considered as extremely rare causes of hyperthyroidism in pregnancy.

13.2.2 Clinical Features and Diagnosis

Clinical manifestations of hyperthyroidism may to some extent overlap with symptoms and signs commonly observed during pregnancy, including palpitations, heat intolerance, tremors, and warm skin. Diagnosis of hyperthyroidism relies on the finding of increased serum free thyroid hormone concentrations associated with suppressed serum TSH levels. Caution should be used in the interpretation of results, as free thyroid hormone assays may be flawed in pregnancy by the increase in circulating TBG and other thyroid hormone-binding proteins (13). Differentiation between Graves' disease and GTT may not be easy on clinical grounds (Table 13.2). Patients may lose weight or fail to gain weight in spite of polyphagia. The presence of emesis favors the diagnosis of GTT. Family history of thyroid autoimmune diseases, personal history of a previous diagnosis of Graves' disease or antithyroid drug (ATD) treatment, the presence of Graves' orbitopathy, the main extrathyroidal manifestation of Graves' disease (14), or the presence of a diffuse goiter support the diagnosis of hyperthyroidism due to Graves' disease. Although serum hCG concentration is usually higher in patients with GTT than in patients with Graves' hyperthyroidism, the diagnostic value of serum hCG measurement is limited, due to considerable overlap between the two conditions (15). Thyroid ultrasonography is useful if nodular thyroid disease is suspected, but there is no sound evidence that it helps to differentiate Graves' disease from GTT. Serum TSHR-Ab measurement is the clue test for the differential diagnosis, because positive TSHR-Ab tests establish the diagnosis of Graves' disease (Table 13.2) (8). Thyroid scan cannot be performed in pregnancy (16).

13.2.3 Maternal-Fetal Consequences of Hyperthyroidism

Information on the possible consequences of subclinical hyperthyroidism is limited (11). However, some data indicate that high serum FT4 levels within the normal range may be associated with a decrease in birth weight and an increased risk of small-for-gestational age newborns (17), as well as with lower child IQ and low grey matter and cortex volume (18).

Overt and uncontrolled hyperthyroidism can cause complications both to the mother and the fetus and can negatively impact on pregnancy outcome (Table 13.3). Thyroid storm – a life-threatening manifestation of very severe hyperthyroidism – as well as congestive heart failure have been reported, although infrequently, in pregnant women with uncontrolled Graves' hyperthyroidism (7). In a large cohort from the USA, hyperthyroidism was associated with an increased risk of preeclampsia (odds ratio [OR] 1.8), pre-term birth (OR 1.8), induction of labor (OR 1.4), and maternal admission to the intensive care unit (OR 3.7) (19). Nationwide studies from Denmark have reported a higher risk of

Table 13.2. Clinical and diagnostic features of Graves' disease (GD) and gestational transient thyrotoxicosis (GTT)

	GD	GTT
Family history of thyroid autoimmune disease	+	−
Symptoms of hyperthyroidism	+	+
Emesis	−	+
Previous diagnosis of or treatment for Graves' disease	+	−
Graves' orbitopathy	+	−
High serum free thyroid hormone levels	+	+
Decreased/suppressed serum TSH levels	+	+
High serum human Chorionic Gonadotropin levels	+	++
Positive serum TSH-receptor antibody tests	+	−

Table 13.3. Maternal, fetal/neonatal, and pregnancy possible risks from uncontrolled hyperthyroidism and hypothyroidism during pregnancy

	Hyperthyroidism	Hypothyroidism
Maternal	• thyroid storm • congestive heart failure • preeclampsia • admission to intensive care unit	• preeclampsia • postpartum hemorrhage • gestational hypertension
Fetal/Neonatal	• low birth weight • small for gestational age • stillbirth • lower IQ • low grey matter and cortex volume • intrauterine growth restriction • attention deficit hyperactivity disorder • epilepsy • neonatal hyperthyroidism	• low birth weight • small for gestational age • stillbirth • neonatal respiratory distress • lower IQ • delay in language development • decrease in motor skill • attention deficit hyperactivity disorder • autism spectrum disorder • epilepsy
Pregnancy	• miscarriage • pre-term delivery • induction of labor	• miscarriage • pre-term delivery • placental abruption

spontaneous abortion, stillbirth, intrauterine growth restriction, and attention deficit hyperactivity disorder in the offspring of hyperthyroid mothers compared to euthyroid mothers (20,21) (Table 13.3). Because maternal TSHR-Abs cross the placenta, fetal hyperthyroidism may occur, potentially associated with fetal loss or stillbirth (7). This condition may also develop when the mother has been previously treated with either radioactive iodine (RAI) or thyroidectomy, but still has circulating TSHR-Abs. Exposure of the fetus to increased thyroid hormone concentration might be associated with the subsequent occurrence of seizures (22). Finally, maternal TSHR-Abs may be responsible for neonatal hyperthyroidism, which occurs a few days after birth and remits when maternal TSHR-Abs are cleared from the newborn, but, nevertheless, requires prompt treatment (7). Taken together, the high rate of detrimental effects of uncontrolled hyperthyroidism in pregnancy underscore the need for a rapid restoration and stable maintenance of euthyroidism, because this is associated with a good prognosis for both the mother, the fetus, and the outcome of pregnancy (7).

13.2.4 Treatment of Hyperthyroidism in Pregnancy

GTT usually does not need any treatment. However, in more severe cases associated with emesis, supportive measures – including control of vomiting and dehydration – may be required, and hospitalization may be needed (16). Current guidelines do not recommend using ATDs, but in selected cases consider the possible use of small doses of β-blockers for a limited period of time (16).

In the general population, Graves' hyperthyroidism can be treated either conservatively (ATDs) or with a definitive therapy (RAI treatment or thyroidectomy) causing thyroid ablation and hypothyroidism (23). Each treatment modality has advantages and disadvantages, indications and contraindications, as recently reviewed (24), but ATDs represent the first-line treatment worldwide in most cases (24). During pregnancy (and breastfeeding) RAI is absolutely contraindicated, while thyroidectomy should be limited to the very rare cases of pregnant women who have intolerance to or major adverse events from ATD

treatment, and should be performed in the second trimester of pregnancy (23). Therefore, thionamide ATDs (carbimazole, methimazole, and propylthiouracil) represent the treatment of choice for Graves' hyperthyroidism during pregnancy (23). Carbimazole is rapidly metabolized to methimazole. Both methimazole and propylthiouracil are effective in controlling hyperthyroidism, mainly by reducing thyroid hormone synthesis; in addition, propylthiouracil exerts an inhibitory effect on peripheral monodeiodination of the prohormone, T4, to the metabolically active hormone, T3. Thionamides may be associated with adverse events, usually mild; however, adverse events may rarely be severe, including agranulocytosis, hepatoxicity, and, very rarely, pancreatitis (24). The major concern regarding thionamide ATDs relates to the (low) risk of possible teratogenic effects associated with their use in early pregnancy, which are reported in Table 13.4. These effects have in the past been associated mostly with exposure to methimazole/carbimazole during the first 6–10 weeks of gestation (so called carbimazole/methimazole embriopathy), and include aplasia cutis, dysmorphic facies, choanal or esophageal atresia, abdominal wall defects, and ventricular septal defects (25). However, it is now established that also propylthiouracil may have a similar prevalence of teratogenic effects, but the latter are usually less severe (26) (Table 13.4). In a study from

Table 13.4. Possible birth defects in newborns born to mothers exposed to thionamide antithyroid drugs during early pregnancy

Thionamide	Defect
Carbimazole/ Methimazole	• aplasia cutis • choanal atresia • esophageal atresia • omphalocele • omphalomesenteric duct anomalies • ventricular sept defects • urinary defects • athelia • eye anomalies
Propylthiouracil	• face and neck defects • urinary defects • circulatory defects • digestive defects • situs inversus

143

Denmark, birth defects (all degree) were found in 9 percent of children exposed to methimazole, 8 percent of children exposed to propylthiouracil, and about 6 percent of those not exposed to either drug (26). It should be noted that, on the other hand, several studies failed to find any association between ATD use and birth defects (27), and hyperthyroidism *per se* may be associated with a risk of fetal malformations (27). Current guidelines recommend that, if ATD treatment needs to be continued during pregnancy, propylthiouracil should be used until the sixteenth week of pregnancy (16). While the American Thyroid Association guidelines stated that, afterwards, there is insufficient evidence to recommend continuing propylthiouracil or switching back to methimazole, the European guidelines (23) and a recent position paper by experts of Italian Endocrine and Gynecologic Scientific Societies (27) suggested to replace propylthiouracil with methimazole after the sixteenth week of pregnancy, as propylthiouracil seems to be associated with an increased risk of maternal hepatotoxicity. During pregnancy, thyroid function should be tightly controlled, and serum free thyroid hormone concentrations should be maintained in the upper third of normal reference range using the lowest dose of thionamides to maintain euthyroidism and to prevent fetal hypothyroidism and goiter (23). In women whose hyperthyroidism is stably controlled with low ATD doses (e.g., ≤5–10 mg of methimazole daily), an attempt to discontinue ATD treatment can be made, particularly in the second to third trimester of pregnancy (23). As indicated above, low doses of β-blockers can be used for a short period of time, if really necessary to control tachycardia, while long term treatment with these drugs should be avoided, as it has been associated with intrauterine growth restriction, fetal bradycardia, and neonatal hypoglycemia (23). Breastfeeding is allowed if low doses of ATDs (e.g., ≤5–10 mg of methimazole daily) are used; the tablet should be taken after breastfeeding (23). The postpartum period is a risk factor for the relapse of previously in remission Graves' hyperthyroidism (28).

If hyperthyroidism is due to hyperfunctioning nodules, management does not differ from that of Graves' disease and is based on the use of ATDs, postponing definitive therapy by RAI treatment or surgery.

13.2.5 Counseling for Women with Graves' Disease Planning Pregnancy

Hyperthyroid women in childbearing age should be informed that pregnancy has to be avoided until hyperthyroidism is kept under stable control (at least two thyroid function tests showing euthyroidism one month apart). In addition, they should be informed about the low risk of fetal malformations associated with ATD treatment and advised to switch from methimazole to propylthiouracil until the sixteenth week of pregnancy, and to switch back to methimazole thereafter. In methimazole-treated women with unplanned pregnancy, therapeutic abortion is not warranted (23). If, after a shared decision-making process, RAI treatment is selected prior to pregnancy, the patient should be informed that a negative pregnancy test performed no more than 48 hours prior to RAI administration is required to exclude unexpected pregnancy (16), and pregnancy should be avoided for at least six months after RAI treatment (23). Finally, the patient should be advised that post-RAI or post-thyroidectomy hypothyroidism needs to be stably corrected by levothyroxine (LT4) treatment before seeking pregnancy.

13.3 Hypothyroidism in Pregnancy

13.3.1 Definition, Epidemiology, and Etiology

Hypothyroidism is defined as the reduced secretion or effect of thyroid hormones, the latter being rare and related to resistance to thyroid hormone at the receptor level in peripheral tissues. In turn, a decrease in thyroid hormone secretion may be due to abnormalities at the hypothalamus-pituitary level (central hypothyroidism) or at the thyroid level (primary hypothyroidism). Primary hypothyroidism is by far more frequent than central hypothyroidism. Primary hypothyroidism may be overt (presence of symptoms and signs associated with decreased serum FT4 and FT3 concentrations and increased serum TSH levels) or subclinical (absent/limited clinical manifestations, normal serum FT4 and FT3 concentrations, but increased serum TSH). The prevalence of overt hypothyroidism in the general population widely varies across the world (0.3–5 percent) depending on the definition used (particularly, serum TSH threshold), the iodine intake, and the population enrolled, while the prevalence of subclinical hypothyroidism is several-fold higher (2). In pregnancy, in iodine-sufficient areas and based on gestation-specific normal ranges for serum TSH and FT4, the prevalence of overt hypothyroidism and subclinical hypothyroidism ranges between 0.2–0.9 percent and 2.3–4 percent, respectively (29).

The most common cause of hypothyroidism amongst pregnant women in iodine-sufficient areas is chronic autoimmune thyroiditis, which can associated with both overt and subclinical hypothyroidism (30) (Table 13.1). Iodine intake is also essential, as both iodine deficiency and (marked) iodine excess may responsible for maternal hypothyroidism. Based on the essential role of iodine for thyroid hormone synthesis and the increased requirements during pregnancy, an adequate iodine supplementation during pregnancy is recommended both in iodine-sufficient and iodine deficient areas (30). A daily intake of 250 µg in pregnancy and 250–290 µg during breastfeeding is recommended, but sustained iodine intake exceeding 500–1,100 µg/day should be avoided (16). Likewise, iron deficiency should be corrected, because depletion of iron stores increases the risk of maternal hypothyroxinemia (31). Hypothyroidism in pregnant women may then be due to previous thyroidectomy or RAI treatment, or to inadequate levothyroxine replacement therapy (Table 13.4).

13.3.2 Clinical Features and Diagnosis

Hypothyroidism can be overt when associated with symptoms and signs (somnolence, constipation, tiredness, cold intolerance, weight gain, puffiness, bradycardia, cognitive or memory disorders), or, more commonly, subclinical, when clinical signs and symptoms are limited or absent.

At laboratory level, serum TSH levels are increased in both conditions, whereas serum FT4 and FT3 concentrations are decreased in overt hypothyroidism, but normal in subclinical hypothyroidism. It should, however, be noted that these definitions should be based on pregnancy trimester specific TSH (and FT4) reference range, rather than on general population range. In the absence of trimester-specific reference ranges for each hospital setting, the 2014 European guidelines recommended a fixed upper normal TSH limit of 2.5 mU/liter for the first trimester, 3.0 mU/liter in the second trimester, and 3.5 mU/liter in the third trimester (32). This probably led to an overdiagnosis of subclinical hypothyroidism. More recently, the American guidelines still recommended the use of trimester-specific TSH reference ranges, but, in their absence, advocated the use of an upper normal TSH limit equal to that of the general population minus 0.5 mU/liter (usually around 4 mU/liter)(16).

An additional situation encountered in pregnancy is isolated hypothyroxinemia, in which serum TSH is normal, but serum FT4 is in the lowest 2.5–5 percentile of normal reference test (33), possibly due to marginal iodine deficiency (30), but also to other contributing factors, including iron status, placental angiogenic factors, body mass index, and age (11).

Because primary hypothyroidism is most commonly due to chronic autoimmune thyroiditis, search for anti-thyroglobulin (anti-Tg) and anti-thyroperoxidase (anti-TPO) autoantibodies is useful to establish the etiology of both overt hypothyroidism and subclinical hypothyroidism, but it is useless in the followup of patients, either treated or untreated, although thyroid autoantibody titers tend to decrease during the course of pregnancy. Thyroid ultrasonography is useful at diagnosis to show the typical features of the gland which in chronic autoimmune thyroiditis appears hypoechoic, inhomogeneous, often irregular in shape, and to unveil the presence of thyroid nodules. In the absence of nodular disease and/or changes in the palpatory features of the gland, ultrasonography is useless in the followup of patients.

13.3.3 Maternal-Fetal Consequences of Hypothyroidism

Substantial evidence supports the concept that overt undiagnosed or uncontrolled hypothyroidism of the mother is bound to increase risk of complications (11,30). As illustrated in Table 13.3, these include miscarriage, pre-term delivery, placental abruption, preeclampsia, postpartum hemorrhage, low birth weight, and neonatal respiratory distress (11,30). In addition, children born to hypothyroid women may later show a reduction in the IQ, as well as a delay in language development and motor skill development, compared to those born to euthyroid mothers (34). A recent meta-analysis of 29 studies showed an association of maternal hypothyroidism with an increased risk of attention deficit hyperactivity disorder, autism spectrum disorders, and epilepsy (35) (Table 13.3). Women whose hypothyroidism is adequately treated by LT4 replacement therapy have no increased risk of maternal, obstetrical, and offspring complications (11).

Subclinical hypothyroidism may also be associated with multiple adverse maternal and neonatal outcomes, including pregnancy loss, placental abruption, premature rupture of membranes, and neonatal death (36) (Table 13.3). A recent systematic review and individual-participant data meta-analysis showed that maternal subclinical hypothyroidism in pregnancy is associated with a higher risk of small for gestational age and lower birth weight, while isolated hypothyroxinemia is associated with a lower risk of small for gestational age and higher birth weight (37), but also with some adverse neurobehavioral outcomes in the newborns (11).

13.3.4 Treatment of Hypothyroidism in Pregnancy

As several studies have documented the detrimental effects of overt hypothyroidism, this condition should be adequately treated to achieve normalization of thyroid status. Since T4, rather than T3, plays a fundamental role in fetal brain development, LT4 is the preferred treatment for hypothyroidism in pregnancy (29). At variance, desiccated thyroid preparations – which contain a relative excess of T3, or T4+T3 combination therapy – may expose the mother to supraphysiologic T3 levels and be associated with an inadequate transfer to T4 to the fetus, and therefore should not be used in pregnancy (16). The aim of treatment is to maintain serum TSH within the trimester-specific normal range, or, if this is not available, around 2.5 mU/liter (16). Because of the increased thyroid hormone demand physiologically associated with pregnancy, a large proportion of pregnant will require an increase of the LT4 dose they were taking in the preconception period (29). This adjustment, usually about a 25–30 percent increase with respect to the preconception period, should be made as early as possible and monitored throughout pregnancy for possible

further adjustments (16). The therapeutic window is probably smaller than previously believed, as high-normal serum FT4 concentration may be associated with impaired fetal growth and lower birth weight (17); therefore, close monitoring of thyroid status is required. In the postpartum period, LT4 daily dose can be reduced to the preconception daily dose, but thyroid status should be checked six weeks after delivery (29).

Treatment of subclinical hypothyroidism is more controversial. Previous cut-off values of TSH during pregnancy (32) were probably too low and led to overdiagnosis and overtreatment of subclinical hypothyroidism (38). The more recent American guidelines recommend LT4 treatment for (1) pregnant women with TSH levels higher than pregnancy-specific reference range and positive anti-TPO autoantibody tests; (2) serum TSH >10 mU/liter and negative anti-TPO autoantibody tests (16); treatment may be considered in (3) anti-TPO-positive women whose TSH is higher than 2.5 mU/l and lower than the pregnancy-specific upper limit of normal; and (4) anti-TPO-negative women with serum TSH higher than the pregnancy-specific upper limit of normal and lower than 10 mU/liter (16). LT4 treatment is not recommended when serum TSH is within the pregnancy-specific normal range (or, in its absence, is <4 mU/liter) (16). Because thyroid autoantibodies may be negative in pregnant women with chronic autoimmune thyroiditis (38), and studies reporting a lack of benefit on maternal and fetal outcomes in women treated with LT4 had the major limitation that treatment was initiated too late (between thirteenth and sixteenth weeks of gestation) (39,40), a recent Italian consensus recommends treating pregnant anti-TPO-negative women with serum TSH higher than the pregnancy-specific upper limit of normal and lower than 10 mU/liter (38). The use of small doses of LT4 (e.g., 25–50 μg/day, checking hormone levels after 2–3 weeks) is highly unlikely to have detrimental effect and may be useful to reduce the potential risks of borderline thyroid insufficiency in a condition, such as pregnancy, associated with an increased thyroid hormone demand. Close monitoring of therapy is, however, recommended to avoid overtreatment.

According to the American guidelines (16), treatment of isolated hypothyroxinemia is not routinely recommended. However, this condition may be associated with some negative neurobehavioral outcomes in the offspring (11). On the other hand, interventional studies showing the benefit of LT4 replacement are missing. Thus, for the time being, the question of whether isolated hypothyroxinemia should be untreated is unsettled, although some physicians use LT4 in the first trimester of pregnancy (41).

13.3.5 Universal Screening for Thyroid Dysfunction in Pregnancy?

It is a matter of argument whether, given the frequency of clinical and subclinical thyroid dysfunction (particularly subclinical hypothyroidism) during pregnancy, the latter should be actively looked for in all women who are planning pregnancy or are already pregnant. Not only the high frequency of thyroid dysfunction, but also the negative maternal, obstetrical, and fetal outcomes would imply that universal screening be advisable. In addition, screening for thyroid dysfunction by measuring serum TSH and free thyroid hormones (mainly FT4) is not expensive and widely available. Nonetheless, the American guidelines concluded that "there is insufficient evidence to recommend for or against universal screening for abnormal TSH concentrations in early pregnancy" (Recommendation 93) or " . . . preconception, with the exception of a number of women planning assisted reproduction or known to have anti-TPO positivity" (Recommendation 94) (16). In addition, universal screening for detecting low FT4 was not recommended either (Recommendation 95) (43). All these negative recommendations were justified by the insufficient evidence that LT4 treatment is associated with improved outcomes. Accordingly, thyroid function testing should be targeted, including women with previous history of either hyper- or hypothyroidism, type 1 diabetes or other autoimmune diseases, history of pregnancy loss, pre-term delivery or infertility, older age, morbid obesity, family history of autoimmune thyroid disease, and residing in geographical areas with moderate to severe iodine deficiency (16). This targeted testing in not shared by a number of providers who are performing universal screening contrary to society guidelines recommendations, because it is cost-effective in diagnosing and treating overt thyroid disease (42).

13.4 Euthyroid Autoimmune Thyroid Disease in Pregnancy

Thyroid autoimmunity is very frequent in the general population. The prevalence of thyroid autoantibodies increases with age, ranging in women of childbearing age from around 10 percent in women aged 20–29 years, to 14 percent in women aged 30–39 years, and around 17 percent in women aged 40–49 years (43). Amongst pregnant women, prevalence of anti-TPO and anti-Tg autoantibodies ranges 5–14 percent and 3–18 percent respectively, although a decrease in autoantibody prevalence and titer has been often reported, possibly owing to a state of pregnancy-related immune tolerance (44).

An association between thyroid autoimmunity and both spontaneous sporadic and recurrent miscarriage seems to be evident, although results of studies are not unequivocal (44). Association does not mean causality and might reflect the association of thyroid autoimmunity with other autoimmune disorders (e.g., the antiphospholipid antibody syndrome). Whether LT4 treatment may be beneficial to reduce miscarriage in euthyroid thyroid antibody-positive women is unclear. The American guidelines do not recommend in favor or against (16), but a recent systematic review and meta-analysis of randomized clinical trials concluded that there is no current evidence of benefit for LT4 use in euthyroid women with thyroid autoimmunity who are pregnant or planning pregnancy, not only in terms of miscarriage, but also of pre-term delivery or live birth (45). However, a strict control of thyroid function seems advisable in this clinical setting. In view of inconclusive and conflicting results from available studies, selenium supplementation is not recommended for the treatment of euthyroid thyroid antibody-positive pregnant women (16).

The relation between thyroid autoimmunity and infertility remains uncertain, although a meta-analysis of four studies showed that euthyroid thyroid antibody-positive women had a slight, but significantly increased risk of unexplained infertility compared to thyroid antibody-negative women (46). The American guidelines do not recommend LT4 treatment in euthyroid thyroid antibody-positive women in an attempt to improve fertility (16).

The relation between thyroid autoimmunity and assisted reproductive technology (ART)

147

outcomes is also uncertain (44). Although results are conflicting, most studies seem to indicate an absence of association between the presence of thyroid autoimmunity and the likelihood of pregnancy in euthyroid thyroid antibody-positive women submitted to ART cycles (44). On the other hand, it would appear that the presence of thyroid autoimmunity might increase the risk of miscarriage after ART treatment (47).

The recent European Thyroid Association guidelines on thyroid disorders prior to and during assisted reproduction recommend or suggest that: (1) women seeking medical advice for fertility problems should be screened for TSH and thyroid autoantibodies; (2) women with/without thyroid autoimmunity and TSH >4 mU/liter should be treated to maintain serum TSH levels <2.5 mU/liter; (3) women already receiving LT4 replacement therapy should have their dose adjusted as to maintain serum TSH levels <2.5 mU/liter; (4) women with thyroid autoimmunity and serum TSH >2.5 mU/liter and <4 mU/liter before ovarian stimulation may be given a low dose of LT4 25–50 μg/day if they have a history of recurrent miscarriage, age is >35 years, or there are ovarian causes of subfertility; and (5) serum TSH concentration should be checked after ovarian stimulation in women with thyroid autoimmunity and treated with LT4 (48). The same guidelines suggest that euthyroid thyroid antibody-positive women undergoing in vitro fertilization/intracytoplasmic sperm injection should not be treated systematically with LT4 (48).

13.5 Postpartum Thyroid Thyroiditis

Postpartum thyroiditis (PPT) is an autoimmune condition causing thyroid dysfunction in the postpartum period (between 6 weeks and 12 months after delivery) in women who were euthyroid before pregnancy (44). The classic form is characterized by a self-limiting phase of thyrotoxicosis due to painless destructive thyroiditis, followed by a transient phase of hypothyroidism and subsequent restoration of euthyroidism, but PPT may present as isolated thyrotoxicosis or isolated hypothyroidism (44). At the end of the postpartum period, about half of the patients have persistent hypothyroidism (49). PPT occurs in about 8 percent of pregnancies, and thyroid antibody-positive pregnant women have about a six-fold higher risk of developing PPT (50). If the thyrotoxic phase is identified, Graves' hyperthyroidism should be excluded. In this regard, presence of detectable TSHR-Abs in the circulation, a bruit over the thyroid gland, and/or ocular involvement (Graves' orbitopathy) help to establish the diagnosis of Graves' disease. During the thyrotoxic phase, ATDs are not indicated, because this is a thyroid destructive process; in symptomatic patients, low doses of β-blockers may be used for a short period of time in lactating women (16). In the hypothyroid phase, usually no treatment is required, but symptomatic patients may be given LT4. The need for permanent LT4 replacement should be assessed by gradually tapering LT4 within the first year postpartum.

References

1. Moleti M, Trimarchi F, and Vermiglio F. Thyroid physiology in pregnancy. *Endocr Pract.* 2014, 6: 589–596.

2. Taylor PN, Albrecht D, Scholz A, et al. Global epidemiology of hyperthyroidism and hypothyroidism. *Nat Rev Endocrinol.* 2018, 14: 301–316.

3. Garmendia Madariaga A, Santos Palacios S, Guillén-Grima F, et al. The incidence and prevalence of thyroid dysfunction in Europe. *J Clin Endocrinol Metab.* 2014, 99: 923–931.

4. Carlé A, Andersen SL, Boelaert K, et al. Subclinical thyrotoxicosis: Prevalence, causes and choice of therapy. *Eur J Endocrinol.* 2017, 176: R325–37.

5. Bartalena L. Diagnosis and management of Graves' disease: A global overview. *Nat Rev Endocrinol.* 2013, 9: 724–734.

6. Carlé A, Bulow Pedersen I, Knudsen N, et al. Epidemiology of subtypes of hyperthyroidism in Denmark: A population-based study. *Eur J Endocrinol.* 2011, 164: 801–809.

7. Cooper DS, and Laurberg P. Hyperthyroidism in pregnancy. *Lancet Diabetes Endocrinol.* 2013, 1: 238–249.

8. Kahaly GJ. Management of Graves thyroidal and extrathyroidal disease: An update. *J Clin Endocrinol Metab.* 2020, 105: 3704–3720.

9. Abraham-Nordling M, Bystrom K, Torring O, et al. Incidence of hyperthyroidism in Sweden. *Eur J Endocrinol.* 2011, 165: 899–905.

10. Korelitz JJ, McNally DN, Masters MN, et al. Prevalence of thyrotoxicosis, antithyroid

medication use, and complications among pregnant women in the United States. *Thyroid.* 2013, 23: 758–765.

11. Korevaar TIM, Medici M, Visser TJ, et al. Thyroid disease in pregnancy: new insights in diagnosis and clinical management. *Nat Rev Endocrinol.* 2017, 13: 610–622.

12. Rodien P, Bremont C, Sanson ML, et al. Familial gestational hyperthyroidism caused by a mutant thyrotropin receptor hypersensitive to human chorionic gonadotropin. *N Engl J Med.* 1998, 339: 1823–1826.

13. Lee RH, Spencer CA Mestman JH, et al. Free T4 immunoassays are flawed during pregnancy. *Am J Obstet Gynecol.* 2009; 200: 260. e1–6.

14. Bartalena L, and Fatourechi V. Extrathyroidal manifestations of Graves' disease: a 2014 update. *J Endocrinol Invest.* 2014, 37: 691–700.

15. Yoshihara A, Noh JY, Mukasa K, et al. Serum human chorionic gonadotropin levels and thyroid hormone levels in gestational transient thyrotoxicosis: Is the serum hCG level useful for differentiating between active Graves' disease and GTT? *Endocr J.* 2015, 62: 557–560.

16. Alexander EK, Pearce EN, Brent GA, et al. 2017 Guidelines of the American Thyroid Association for the diagnosis and management of thyroid disease during pregnancy and post-partum. *Thyroid.* 2017, 27: 315–389.

17. Medici M, Timmermans M, Visser W, et al. Maternal thyroid hormone parameters during early pregnancy and birth weight: the Generation R Study. *J Clin Endocrinol Metab.* 2013, 98: 59–66.

18. Korevaar TIM, Muetzel R, Medici M, et al. Association of maternal thyroid function during early pregnancy with offspring IQ and brain morphology in childhood: a population-based prospective cohort study. *Lancet Diabetes Endocrinol.* 2016, 4: 35–43.

19. Mannisto T, Mendola P, Grewal J, et al. Thyroid diseases and adverse pregnancy outcomes in a contemporary US cohort. *J Clin Endocrinol Metab.* 2013, 98: 2725–2733.

20. Andersen SL, Laurberg P, Wu CS, et al. Attention deficit hyperactivity disorder and autism spectrum disorder in children born to mothers with thyroid disorders: A Danish nationwide cohort study. *BJOG.* 2014, 121: 1365–1374.

21. Andersen SL, Olsen J, Wu CS, et al. Spontaneous abortion, stillbirth and hyperthyroidism: A Danish population-based study. *Eur Thyroid J.* 2014, 3: 164–172.

22. Andersen Sl, Olsen J, and Laurberg P. Foetal programming by maternal thyroid disease. *Clin Endocrinol (Oxf).* 2015, 83: 751–758.

23. Kahaly GJ, Bartalena L, Hegedus L, et al. 2018 European Thyroid Association guideline for the management of Graves' hyperthyroidism. *Eur Thyroid J.* 2018, 7: 167–186.

24. Bartalena L, Chiovato L, and Vitti P. Management of hyperthyroidism due to Graves' disease: Frequently asked questions and answers (if any). *J Endocrinol Invest.* 2016, 39: 1105–1114.

25. Andersen SL, Olsen J, and Laurberg P. Antithyroid drug side effects in the population and in pregnancy. *J Clin Endocrinol Metab.* 2016, 101: 1606–1614.

26. Andersen SL, Olsen J, Wu CS, et al. Birth defects after early pregnancy use of antithyroid drugs: A Danish nationwide study. *J Clin Endocrinol Metab.* 2013, 98: 4373–4381.

27. Tonacchera M, Chiovato L, Bartalena L, et al. Treatment of Graves' disease with thionamides: A position paper on indications and safety in pregnancy. *J Endocrinol Invest.* 2020, 43: 257–265.

28. Rotondi M, Cappelli C, Pirali B, et al. The effect of pregnancy on subsequent relapse from Graves' disease after a successful course of antithyroid drug therapy. *J Clin Endocrinol Metab.* 2008, 93: 3985–3988.

29. Shan Z, and Teng W. Thyroid hormone therapy of hypothyroidism in pregnancy. *Endocrine.* 2019, 66: 35–42.

30. Teng W, Shan Z, Patil-Sisodia K, et al. Hypothyroidism in pregnancy. *Lancet Diabetes Endocrinol.* 2013, 1: 228–237.

31. Zimmermann MB, Burgi H, and Hurrell R. Iron deficiency predicts poor maternal thyroid status during pregnancy. *J Clin Endocrinol Metab.* 2007, 92: 3436–3440.

32. Lazarus JH, Brown RS, Daumerie C, et al. 2014 European Thyroid Association guidelines for the management of subclinical hypothyroidism in pregnancy and in children. *Eur Thyroid J.* 2014, 3: 76–94.

33. Stagnaro-Green A, Abalovich M, Alexander E, et al. Guidelines of the American Thyroid Association for the diagnosis and management of thyroid disease during pregnancy and postpartum. *Thyroid.* 2011, 21: 1081–1125.

34. Haddow JE, Palomaki GE, Allan WC, et al. Maternal thyroid deficiency during pregnancy and subsequent neuropsychological development of the child. *N Engl J Med.* 1999, 341: 549–555.

35. Ge GM, Leung MTY, Man KKC, et al. Maternal thyroid dysfunction during pregnancy

and the risk of adverse outcomes in the offspring: A systematic review and meta-analysis. *J Clin Endocrinol Metab.* 2020, 105(12): dgaa555. https://doi.org/10.1210/clinem/dgaa555.

36. Maraka S, Singh Ospina NM, O'Keefe DT, et al. Subclinical hypothyroidism in pregnancy: A systematic review and meta-analysis. *Thyroid.* 2016, 26: 580–590.

37. Derakhshan A, Peeters RP, Taylor PN, et al. Association of maternal thyroid function with birthweight: A systematic review and individual-participant data meta-analysis. *Lancet Diabetes Endocrinol.* 2020, 8: 501–510.

38. Rotondi M, Chiovato L, Pacini F, et al. Management of subclinical hypothyroidism in pregnancy: A comment from the Italian Society of Endocrinology and the Italian Thyroid Association to the 2017 American Thyroid Association guidelines- "The Italian way". *Thyroid.* 2018, 551–555.

39. Lazarus JH, Bestwick JP, Channon S, et al. Antenatal thyroid screening and childhood cognitive function. *N Engl J Med.* 2012, 366: 493–501.

40. Casey BM, Thom EA, Peaceman AM, et al. Treatment of subclinical hypothyroidism or hypothyroxinemia in pregnancy. *N Engl J Med.* 2017, 376: 815–825.

41. Taylor PN, Muller I, Nana M, et al. Indications for treatment of subclinical hypothyroidism and isolated hypothyroxinemia in pregnancy. *Best Pract Res Clin Endocrinol Metab.* 2020. https://doi.org/10.1016/j.beem.2020.101436.

42. Stagnaro-Green A, Dong A, and Stephenson MD. Universal screening for thyroid disease during pregnancy should be performed. *Best Pract Res Clin Endocrinol Metab.* 2019. https://doi.org/10.1016/j.beem.2019.101320.

43. Hollowell JG, Staehling NW, Flanders WD, et al. Serum TSH, T4, and thyroid antibodies in the United States population (1988 to 1994): National Health and Nutrition Examination Survey (NHANES III). *J Clin Endocrinol Metab.* 2002, 87: 489–499.

44. De Leo S, and Pearce EN. Autoimmune thyroid disease during pregnancy. *Lancet Diabetes Endocrinol.* 2018, 6: 575–586.

45. Lau L, Benham JL, Lemieux P, et al. Impact of levothyroxine in women with thyroid antibodies on pregnancy outcomes: A systematic review and meta-analysis of randomised controlled trials. *BMJ Open.* 2021, 11(2): e043751. https://doi.org/10.1136/bmjopen-2020-043751.

46. van den Boogard E, Vissenberg R, Landa JA, et al. Significance of (sub)clinical thyroid dysfunction and thyroid autoimmunity before conception and in early pregnancy: A systematic review. *Hum Reprod Update.* 2011, 17: 605–619.

47. Busnelli A, Paffoni A, Fedele L, and et al. The impact of thyroid autoimmunity on IVF/ICSI outcome: A systematic review and meta-analysis. *Hum Reprod Update.* 2016, 22: 793–794.

48. Poppe K, Bisschop P, Fugazzola L, et al. 2021 European Thyroid Association guideline on thyroid disorders prior to and during assisted reproduction. *Eur Thyroid J.* 2020; 9: 281–295.

49. Stagnaro-Green A, Schwartz A, Gismondi R, et al. High rate of persistent hypothyroidism in a large-scale prospective study of postpartum thyroiditis in Southern Italy. *J Clin Endocrinol Metab.* 2011; 96: 652–657.

50. Stagnaro-Green A. Approach to the patient with postpartum thyroiditis. *J Clin Endocrinol Metab.* 2012, 97: 334–342.

Chapter

14

The Role of Hormones in Hypertensive Disorders of Pregnancy

Leslie Myatt and James M. Roberts

14.1 Introduction

The hypertensive disorders of pregnancy including preeclampsia affect 5–7 percent of pregnancies worldwide and are responsible for 500,000 fetal deaths and 75,000 maternal deaths worldwide a year. In addition, these pregnancies cause significant maternal and fetal morbidity. While delivery of the placenta and fetus is the definitive treatment to prevent progression of hypertension or preeclampsia, the effects of being exposed to hypertension or preeclampsia are not confined to pregnancy *per se*. We are now aware that the long term consequences of hypertensive disorders or preeclampsia for the mother include an increased risk for cardiovascular disease in later life (1) but also that the offspring of women affected by hypertensive disorders are exposed to an adverse intrauterine environment that programs them to display cardiovascular disease and metabolic syndrome in later life (2). While the continuous and extensive investigation of the preeclampsia syndrome, we still do not understand the underlying pathophysiology. There have been many studies of changes in hormone concentrations in normal pregnancy and in women with pree-clampsia. Earlier studies were predominantly cross-sectional in women diagnosed with preeclampsia versus those who remained normotensive while latterly longitudinal prospective studies have been performed. In addition, definitions of preeclampsia, particularly those used in clinical practice, have evolved over time such that the patient populations under study may have changed.

14.2 The "Hormonal Origin" of Preeclampsia

For many years it has been evident that the presence of the placenta is mandatory for the development of preeclampsia. Acute manifestations of preeclampsia begin to abate only with the delivery of the placenta. Conversely, when the placenta was maintained *in situ* with abdominal pregnancy, preeclampsia persisted for weeks postpartum (3). Furthermore, other relevant reproductive components are not mandatory for the disorder. Preeclampsia with abdominal pregnancy indicates that uterine distension is not needed, and the even higher incidence of preeclampsia with hydatidiform mole than with usual pregnancies indicates the presence of the fetus *per se* is also not necessary (4). What differentiated the placenta of a woman with preeclampsia from that of a woman without preeclampsia was suggested by Ernest Page years ago, who proposed that hypoxia could be the common insult.

The thought was that the abnormal placenta produced "toxins" that led to the maternal syndrome. This was supported by the adverse effects of "grinding up" placentas or placental components and injecting these into various animal recipients, ignoring the adverse consequences of injecting foreign proteins (5). The concept of unique placental toxins has largely been abandoned. In the late 1980's, the concept of the relevance of placental products was revised and revived with the concept that materials secreted from the abnormal placenta could act preferentially on endothelium (6). This concept later was more appropriately expanded to indicate endothelial targeting as a component of a generalized inflammatory cascade with preeclampsia (7). The concept of unknown toxins was abandoned in favor of a release or failure to release usual placental products.

It is evident with this thought process that toxins or usual placental products are acting as hormones signaling changes in maternal physiology. In our current thinking hypoxia and failed nutrient delivery to the placenta are proposed to act preferentially on syncytiotrophoblast (i.e., syncytiotrophoblast stress). This results in endoplasmic reticulum and oxidative stress with the subsequent release of the products of these pathologies (e.g., misfolded proteins, reactive oxygen species) as well as increased or reduced placental products (cytokines, angiogenic and antiangiogenic materials, etc.) (8). This is also accompanied by a unique type of "hormonal" activity. In addition to humoral placental products, syncytial fragments from damaged (damage vesicles) or produced by normal cellular processes (apoptotic vesicles or endosomes) are continuously released into the maternal circulation (8). These fragments change in character, content, and quantity with syncytiotrophoblast stress and preeclampsia (8). Information is carried not only on, but within these fragments. The vesicle has the capacity to bind to and enter maternal tissues with the consequent transfer of a complex combination of humoral and particulate components including fetal RNA, all of which can alter maternal tissue function.

These long held concepts of placental production and release of products altering maternal physiology would posit that the abnormal placenta of preeclampsia is the source of materials initiating the maternal preeclampsia syndrome. In this presentation we favor this concept, but also consider the role of hormones from maternal sources in all cases considering as best possible, changes – whether placental or maternal – are causal, adaptive, due to damage, or perhaps a combination of these possibilities.

14.3 Role of Hormones in the Metabolic and Cardiovascular Adaptations of Pregnancy

Obviously in the non-pregnant state the hormones that regulate metabolism and cardiovascular function are from maternal tissues themselves. However, in pregnancy these are joined by the prodigious amounts of peptide and steroid hormones produced by the developing placenta. Steroid and polypeptide hormones produced by the mother herself and by the placenta, change dramatically during pregnancy and have a key role in controlling the changes in many aspects of maternal physiology during pregnancy. These include overall metabolism and renal and pulmonary function, as well as cardiovascular function, including heart rate, blood volume, vascular reactivity, and blood pressure. With hypertensive disorders and preeclampsia, the vascular adaptations do not occur normally and are associated with differences in steroid and peptide hormone levels. Women with preeclampsia at term have reduced volume expansion, decreased cardiac output, and increased total peripheral vascular resistance compared with women who remained normotensive in pregnancy (9). These changes are apparent at the beginning of the second trimester of pregnancy antedating clinical preeclampsia. It is suggested that this could be secondary to changes in placental hormones estradiol, progesterone and atrial (ANF) or brain (BNF) naturietic factors. It is, however, unclear if the changes in hormone levels are causative factors in the altered cardiovascular function seen with hypertensive disorders or whether they are a result of altered synthesis by a damaged/dysfunctional placenta.

Pregnancy is further characterized by plasma volume expansion, an increase in heart rate and cardiac output (50 percent), and a decrease in peripheral resistance and in blood pressure that reaches a nadir in the second trimester before increasing again towards term. The fall in systemic vascular resistance may lead to plasma volume expansion by activation of volume restoration by renal vasodilation and activation of the renin-angiotensin-aldosterone system early in gestation (10). The renin-angiotensin system can be stimulated by estrogen from the placenta (11) which also stimulates endothelial nitric oxide synthase (e-NOS) expression and vasodilation (12). Estrogen stimulation of NO synthase in the uterine vasculature (12) and of angiogenic factors (13) plays a large role in increasing blood flow across gestation. Progesterone may not have a direct effect on vascular reactivity in pregnancy but may antagonize the effects of estrogen; for example, on NO production by endothelium (14). In women who subsequently develop PE lower plasma volumes, caused by failure of expansion, are seen by the beginning of the second trimester of pregnancy but which predates changes in estradiol concentrations (9) again suggesting the reduced estrogen is a consequence of reduced volume expansion and the development of PE.

14.4 Placental Hormones in Preeclampsia

14.4.1 Placental Steroid Hormones

The placenta is a veritable factory for production of steroid and peptide hormones. In early gestation estrogens are mainly synthesized in the corpus luteum, but at about 9 weeks' gestation synthesis switches to the placenta. To produce estrogen and progesterone, the placenta functions in concert with the fetus (15) and can convert DHEAS and 16OH DHEAS derived from the fetus to DHEA and 16OH DHEA via sulfatase. DHEA is subsequently metabolized via type 1 3β hydroxysteroid dehydrogenase (3βHSD) to androstenedione which is then converted by aromatase (CYP19A1) to estrone and via 17βHSD1 to estradiol, exclusively in the placenta. 16OH DHEA is metabolized via 3βHSD and aromatase to estriol. Estrone and estradiol from the placenta can be converted to estriol, the major estrogen in pregnancy, or estetrol and to catecholestrogens by hydroxylation and to methoxyestrogens via catechol-O-methyltransferase in the placenta. Androstenedione can also be converted to testosterone in the placenta by aldo keto reductase family 1 member C3 enzyme (AKR1C3), the testosterone then being converted to estradiol by aromatase.

14.4.1.1 Estrogens

Estrogens are potent systemic and uterine artery vasodilators. In the uterine artery, estrogens act via stimulation of eNOS activity to produce nitric oxide (NO) (16,17) but may also have nongenomic vasodilator effects via action on vascular smooth muscle ion channels (18). Additionally, estrogens may promote angiogenesis via stimulation of the angiogenic factors VEGF and PLGF in the uterus (19,20). The catechol estrogens 2-OHE2 and 4-OHE2 and the methoxyestrogen 2-ME2 are also uterine vasodilators (15).

There have been several studies, usually cross-sectional, of estrogen concentrations in preeclampsia. These data were summarized (15) with the consensus being that plasma estradiol concentrations are lower in women with preeclampsia and that this is related to decreased aromatase activity both in plasma and in the placenta (21) with increased androstenedione being found (22). Paradoxically, however, women with placental CYP19 deficiencies have not been reported to present with preeclampsia (15). Interestingly polymorphisms associated with impaired aromatase expression and activity (21) and increased levels of microRNAs (23) that decrease aromatase expression are found in women with PE versus those that are normotensive. These data may be taken to infer that the decreased estrogen is a consequence of altered placental function in PE and not a cause of the condition. It still remains to be definitively determined if the reduction in estrogens seen with preeclampsia are a cause or a consequence of placental dysfunction associated with the condition as most data are generated by cross-sectional studies in women with preeclampsia, although prospective studies suggest estriol may be reduced prior to the clinical appearance of preeclampsia (24).

14.4.1.2 Testosterone

There is evidence that the placenta can synthesize testosterone from androstenedione (25). Increased plasma testosterone has been reported in pregnancies complicated by preeclampsia (26), which correlates with the severity, and suggested to be associated with a reduction in placental aromatase activity, that redirects androstenedione to testosterone. Indeed, increased testosterone in trophoblast has been shown to decrease aromatase mRNA via mir 22 (27). There also appears to be a sexual dimorphism with higher testosterone production by the placenta of a male fetus (25). Further evidence for a role of testosterone in development of preeclampsia is provided by the increased risk of development of preeclampsia in women who overproduce testosterone due to PCOS or with obesity and insulin resistance and in women of African American origin, who have 20–30 percent higher testosterone levels in pregnancy (26). There is an association of testosterone levels with both systolic and diastolic blood pressure (28) in women with prior preeclampsia. Infusion of testosterone in pregnant rats increases vascular reactivity and blood pressure, blocked by an AT1 receptor antagonist, and increases uterine vascular resistance and decreases flow. Together with increases seen in the renin angiotensin system, renal hypertrophy, and proteinuria, as well as alterations in eicosanoid synthesis and platelet aggregation, this makes testosterone attractive as a potential mediator of preeclampsia (26). It also emphasizes the sexual dimorphism of preeclampsia directed by the fetus/placenta.

14.4.1.3 Progesterone

Progesterone is synthesized in the placenta from cholesterol via pregnenolone. Unlike animal species, the placenta cannot convert progesterone to estrogen as it lacks 17α hydroxylase-17,20 lyase

153

activity (29). The major site of estrogen and progesterone synthesis is the syncytiotrophoblast layer of the placenta, with progesterone being produced in much greater amounts. Progesterone concentrations increase across gestation, being initially produced by the corpus luteum with synthesis then switching to the placenta and increasing in an exponential manner which parallels the increasing syncytiotrophoblast volume. Surprisingly there have been fewer studies of progesterone production with preeclampsia. While earlier studies reported no association of progesterone with preeclampsia (30), later studies have found an increase in progesterone with preeclampsia (9) and that concentrations increase before clinical appearance of the disorder (31).

14.4.1.4 Cortisol

Cortisol is produced by the mother but is prevented from crossing the placenta in appreciable amounts by the activity of 11b HSD2 in the placenta itself which converts cortisol to inactive cortisone (32). Placental mRNA (32), protein, and activity (33) of 11bHSD2 are reduced in preeclampsia, allowing increased cortisol to reach the fetus resulting in growth restriction, prematurity, and fetal programming.

14.4.2 Placental Peptide Hormones

In addition to acting in concert with the fetus to produce steroid hormones in pregnancy, the placenta produces prodigious amounts of a wide variety of peptide hormones. Indeed, the placenta is second only to the brain in the number of transcripts it expresses. Certain of these peptides (e.g., human chorionic somatomammotropin [hCS or hPL]) play prominent roles in regulation of maternal metabolism to ensure nutrient supply to the placenta and developing fetus. Human chorionic gonadotropin (hCG) is produced by trophoblast and regulates progesterone production, implantation, uterine growth, and immune cell function (34) in addition to roles in regulation of placental development, angiogenesis, and vasculogenesis acting via VEGF (35). It has been suggested that high or low hCG concentrations are a marker of subsequent development of preeclampsia, although variation in study design make it difficult to reconcile these findings. A recent prospective population-based cohort study has shown high total hCG in early

pregnancy to be associated with an increased risk of preeclampsia and with a higher risk with high hCG and a male fetus (36). There was also an association of high hCG with high sFlt-1/PlGF ratios in the same women, suggesting the effect of hCG might be mediated via effects on these angiogenic factors.

Other peptide hormones (e.g., corticotropin releasing hormone [CRH]), insulin-like growth factors [IGF's], placental growth factor [PGF], soluble fms-like tyrosine kinase-1 [sFlt-1], and s-endoglin) participate in regulation of the maternal cardiovascular system, control of fetal growth and development, and maturation of fetal systems. The pattern of production and secretion of these peptides into the maternal circulation parallels the size of the syncytiotrophoblast surface area and the number of transcriptionally active nuclei in syncytiotrophoblast. Hence maternal plasma concentrations of peptides such as CRH, sFLT-1, and s-endoglin increase exponentially across gestation (37–39). An exception to this is synthesis and release into the maternal circulation of PlGF, which reach a maximum at 30 weeks' gestation and falls thereafter (38). This may relate to the functional role of pro-angiogenic PlGF in the placenta as the initial increase and subsequent decline matches the switch from branching to nonbranching angiogenesis seen in the villous vasculature from the second to the third trimester of pregnancy.

The angiogenic factors including PlGF, sFlt-1, and s-endoglin appear to have roles in the cardiovascular adaptations of pregnancy and the changes in their synthesis by placenta and hence their maternal plasma level may have a role in the etiology of PIH and preeclampsia. What then are the roles of these peptide hormones? PlGF is proangiogenic and displaces VEGF from the VEGFR1 on to the VEGFR2 receptor where it exerts a vasodilator effect hence participating in the systemic decrease in vascular resistance and blood pressure seen in the first two trimesters (40). The fall in PlGF in the third trimester may then be related to the normal increase in resistance and blood pressure seen in the third trimester. However, sFlt-1 is anti-angiogenic by virtue of binding to PlGF, thereby reducing its bioactivity and causing vasoconstriction. In pregnancies with adverse outcomes, including preeclampsia, IUGR, and pre-term birth, the pattern of peptide hormone synthesis by the placenta is altered. For example,

CRH, sFlt-1, and s-endoglin synthesis increases earlier and to a greater extent than in normotensive pregnancy (37,39), and the SFlt-1/PlGF ratio is increased (37). This appears to occur in parallel with the increased rate of apoptosis and turnover of syncytiotrophoblast seen with preeclampsia. The net result though is a further increase in sFlt-1 in late gestation with preeclampsia, further binding to PlGF, reducing its bioactivity and preventing the vasodilator activity and promoting hypertension. This is reflected by plasma PlGF not appearing to increase to the same extent as that seen in normotensive gestation and beginning to fall sooner in the third trimester in women with preeclampsia (38). Interestingly, lowering of elevated sFlt-1 by apheresis in individuals with very pre-term preeclampsia was able to decrease proteinuria and prolong pregnancy (41).

While there is now abundant evidence of altered placental production of such hormones in preeclampsia, it is still unclear whether this is causative in the pathophysiology of preeclampsia, or a consequence of preeclampsia induced placental damage/dysfunction.

14.5 Maternal Hormones in Preeclampsia

Despite the obviously important role of the placenta in preeclampsia, hormones of maternal origin have long been thought to be involved in the maternal syndrome of preeclampsia as either primary, or more likely, as pathophysiologically relevant responses to the placental insult. A multitude of maternal hormones that play a role in pregnancy have been suggested to be involved in the pathogenesis of preeclampsia. These include relaxin, thyroid hormones, the renin-angiotensin system, adrenal gland products, cortisol, aldosterone, epinephrine and norepinephrine, melatonin from the pineal gland, arginine vasopressin, ANP, and BNP (42). However, despite their effects on maternal physiology and changes observed in women with PE, it remains to be determined if the alterations seen are a cause or consequence of PE.

14.5.1 Role of the Corpus Luteum – Relaxin

Hormones that regulate the early maternal adaptations to pregnancy in particular vasodilation and volume expansion are of particular interest in relation to the pathophysiology, especially as there is evidence that failure of these adaptations precedes the development of PE. Relaxin, produced by the corpus luteum, is a potent vasodilator, and circulating concentrations are highest in early gestation (43). Elevated first trimester relaxin is associated with increased blood pressure in the third trimester, and women who have no circulating relaxin due to lack of a corpus luteum with oocyte donation are at increased risk for preeclampsia (44). However, first trimester relaxin concentrations do not appear to be a good biomarker for early prediction of the development of preeclampsia (45), although this study suggested low relaxin levels in pregnancy may have a pathophysiologic role in development of late onset PE.

14.5.2 Thyroid Hormones

The physiologic changes of pregnancy include increased uptake of iodine, synthesis of thyroid hormones, fetal consumption of maternal thyroid hormone, synthesis of thyroxine-binding globulins, and increased degradation of thyroid hormone by placental type 3 deiodinase (46). Human chorionic gonadotropin produced by trophoblast is a weak agonist of the TSH receptor and increases thyroid hormone production (46). Estrogen production by the placenta stimulates maternal hepatocytes to increase thyroid binding globulin in the circulation leading to increased T3 and T4 in plasma. Further, angiogenic factors produced by the placenta can alter thyroid vascular density. Indeed, high sFLT-1 and PlGF can increase the risk of subclinical hypothyroidism and hypothyroxemia and also influence the thyroid response to hCG stimulation (46). Hence the placenta influences thyroid function in several ways. Thyroid dysfunction, both hypo and hyperthyroidism, appears to increase the risk of hypertension (47). Both overt (0.2–0.6 percent of pregnancies) and subclinical (3.5–18 percent of pregnancies) hypothyroidism are associated with hypertension, dyslipidemia, and atherosclerosis and alteration in coagulation parameters leading to hypercoagulability (47), all features of preeclampsia. Indeed, women with subclinical hypothyroidism were found to have an increased incidence of severe preeclampsia (48). Several subsequent cross-sectional studies have shown significant increases in TSH (hypothyroidism), but no alteration in T3 and T4, in women with preeclampsia, and suggested thyroid disorders are a predisposing feature for preeclampsia (46)

14.5.3 Renin – Angiotensin Aldosterone System (RAAS) and Prorenin

The attention to the obvious renal and volume changes in preeclampsia directed attention to the renin, angiotensin, aldosterone system (RAAS). This system historically was considered to be of primary importance in regulating volume and vasoconstrictor responses. Although data was not totally unambiguous, there was evidence of increased sensitivity to angiotensin infusion (49), differences in circulating or tissue concentrations of components of the RAAS (50), association with relevant gene polymorphisms (50), and more recently the interesting finding of stimulatory autoantibodies to the angiotensin subtype 1 receptor (AT1R) present in women with preeclampsia (51). Although there is some conflicting information regarding genetic changes (50), the other findings have been more consistent.

However, the RAAS system is considerably more complex than simply a regulator of volume and vascular response. Angiotensin II has effects on many systems beyond its renal and vascular effects. It is an activator of inflammatory responses with receptors on several types of immune modulatory cells (52). It has the capacity to directly stimulate HIF-1 alpha activating "hypoxic responses" (53) as well as leading to sFlt release (54) with subsequent angiogenic inhibition. The effects of angiotensin II to increase blood pressure and stimulate sodium retention are countered by interaction of a breakdown product of angiotensin II – angiotensin III – with a second angiotensin receptor, the angiotensin II subtype 2 receptor (AT2R), which is vasodilatory and prevents sodium retention (55). Furthermore, the breakdown of the angiotensin II precursor, angiotensinogen, results in several different peptides with very different effects than angiotensin II (56). In addition, there is evidence that angiotensinogen itself may have biological activities even without degradation. Effects of genetically induced angiotensinogen depletion include cardiac and renal functional and morphological changes that cannot be restored by angiotensin 2 administration (56).

However, perhaps the finding which has most modified thinking about the system is the diverse biological activity of prorenin, which had been considered an inactive precursor to the proteolytic enzyme renin. A prorenin receptor ([P]RR) was discovered in 2002 as a transmembrane receptor that bound renin and prorenin (57). The initial role of the receptor was proposed to be enhanced activation of the renin angiotensin system. Binding of prorenin to the (P)RR induces a conformational change in prorenin that exposes the active site of renin, usually exposed by proteolytic modification. This allows renin to augment RAAS activity by generating angiotensin 1 from angiotensinogen without degradation of the molecule. However, this turns out be only a small component of the function of (P)RR activation, which influences a multitude of physiological processes, including cell cycle, autophagy, acid base balance, energy balance, embryonic development, T cell homeostasis, cardiac remodeling, and podocyte structure. (P)RR can be degraded to a soluble form (s[P]RR) which is biologically active and released into extracellular fluid (57).

Not surprisingly the role of the RAAS in pregnancy and preeclampsia has not been definitively delineated. There is clearly a relationship, based on reasonably consistent findings of reduction in most of the components of the RAAS system compared to normal pregnancy (50,58). However, the net result of these changes coupled with increased angiotensin sensitivity and circulating stimulatory antibodies to the AT-R1 receptors has not been established. Information on the prorenin receptor component of the system indicates an increase in the soluble activating receptor s(P)RR in preeclampsia, perhaps due to placental hypoxia, which correlates with increased blood pressure and reduced GFR (57). Whether this is actually due to effects of the RAAS or other of the myriad responses to s(P)RR activation is not known. Further, this receptor activation may be beneficial since increased concentrations of cord blood s(P)RR are associated with a reduced risk of fetal growth restriction (57). Genetic variants in virtually every component of the RAAS have been reported. Yang and his colleagues present an extensive detailed review of these changes, as well as changes in relevant micro-RNAs (50). Unfortunately, they conclude that " … controversial results hinder research from a definitive conclusion on the influence of genetic polymorphisms due to variations in ethnic population, genetic basis, genetic misclassification, preeclampsia criteria, sample sizes, defective methods, and so on."

In summary, although not completely resolved, there are differences in the RAAS system of women with preeclampsia compared to nonhypertensive pregnant women. The important question is whether these are causal, compensatory, or facilitatory. The possibility that all or some cases of preeclampsia can be caused by RAAS cannot be resolved until longitudinal studies demonstrate relevant changes prior to clinical preeclampsia. Such studies are not currently available. It is also highly unlikely that the differences of the RAAS measured in preeclampsia indicate compensatory changes since most changes in preeclampsia are in a direction opposite to what would be predicted to occur with volume depletion or hypertension. However, it is possible that they might be an appropriate response to any of the myriad of other responses regulated by the RAAS that is not appropriate for blood pressure and volume control. The interesting observation of increased sensitivity to angiotensin persisting postpartum (59,60) raises the possibility that this sensitivity might be facilitatory to the maternal preeclampsia. The last possibility cannot be supported until information that the sensitivity precedes preeclampsia, rather than being a residual effect of the disorder.

14.5.4 Naturietic Factors and Corin

Other volume regulatory hormones, the natriuretic factors, have also been implicated in preeclampsia (61). Their effects are opposite to those of the conventional RAAS system. Atrial naturietic factor (or peptide ANP) is released by the atrium and brain naturietic factor (or peptide BNP) from the cardiac ventricle with increased stretch. They function to overcome volume overload, reducing blood volume and dilating vessels (61). It would seem likely that in pregnancy with the normally occurring profound changes in volume, they would be activated. However, this does not appear to be the case. In most studies, ANP and BNP are not different in pregnancy when compared to nonpregnant women (62). In longitudinal studies ANP has been reported as increased (63) or decreased (62) with term pregnancies. The authors of both studies suggested that this implied that pregnancy related volume

changes might be due to ANP. However, since the major volume changes of pregnancy occur earlier than this time in pregnancy, this does not seem likely. Interestingly, both ANP (64) and BNP (65) are increased in women with preeclampsia, which is paradoxical in light of the reduced plasma volume that characterizes preeclampsia.

An additional complexity in the relationship of naturietic factors to preeclampsia was introduced by the discovery of the corin (66), a serine protease that converts the inactive precursors of ANP and BNP to their biologically active forms. Although corin is located primarily in the heart, it was found that corin was present in mouse uteri but only during pregnancy (67). Mice in which all corin genes have been knocked out are hypertensive. (68). However, if corin is specifically knocked out in the uterus but not the heart, mice are normotensive until pregnancy when they develop hypertension and proteinuria in late gestation, and also manifest failed remodeling of the spiral arteries. In keeping with this, ANP stimulates trophoblast invasion in vitro (68). Human genetic variants that alter corin activity are present more commonly in preeclamptic women (69). Furthermore, as in preeclamptic women (70), circulating corin was increased in the uterine corin knockout mice, suggesting increased cardiac corin production which cannot alter uterine pro-ANP activation (71). The question is far from settled as other investigators have found that syncytiotrophoblast from women with preeclampsia produces more corin (70,72). Another interesting finding is that in animal experiments with corin the effect seems greater as the animal ages (73). Currently, these findings, although complex, suggest a potential causal role for corin and consequently naturietic factors in a subset of women with preeclampsia.

14.5.5 Arginine Vasopressin and Copeptin

Arginine vasopressin (AVP), a hypothalamic hormone now recognized to have a myriad of effects, was originally considered as relevant to preeclampsia because of the duo of its originally recognized effects, vasoconstriction, and the regulation of volume and osmolality. In recent years several receptors for AVP have been recognized and its knowledge of its activities expanded. Additional functions relevant to preeclampsia have been identified, including platelet aggregation, activation of the inflammatory and stress responses, and immunomodulation (74).

The role of AVP has been difficult to establish due to several challenges to measurement including very high vasopressinase activity in the blood pf pregnant women (75). An alternative strategy for estimation of AVP is the measurement of copeptin, a glycoprotein that is part of the vasopressin precursor, and which is released stoichiometrically with AVP. Copeptin is stable and, in many studies, has been used as a surrogate for AVP. Based on the myriad of AVP activities relevant to preeclampsia, these include measures of copeptin before and during preeclampsia. A seminal study by Santillan et al. in 2014 demonstrated that copeptin levels were significantly elevated as early as the first trimester (76). These same authors also showed that infusion of a low dose of AVP to mice from early pregnancy resulted in many changes, including immunological changes, consistent with preeclampsia (77). In a meta-analysis, copeptin was elevated in all trimesters, with early and late and mild and severe preeclampsia (78). Interestingly, unlike most biomarkers associated with preeclampsia, copeptin was not increased with fetal growth restriction or pre-term birth, suggesting that the copeptin increase is not a marker of placental dysfunction (78). In the Santillan study, sFlt-1 was also measured. sFlt has consistently been found to be elevated in fetal growth restriction (79), as well as preeclampsia. However, in the Santillan study, the women with preeclampsia did not have elevated concentrations of sFlt (76).

Thus, it would appear that increased AVP as measured by circulating copeptin is associated in particular with the maternal syndrome of preeclampsia. The question which must be answered is – why does this occur? Despite the significant relationship of first, second, and third trimester copeptin and preeclampsia, there is still considerable overlap of the results in control and preeclamptic women. Thus, high AVP does not explain all preeclampsia and a search for relevant genetic, demographic, pathophysiological, and immunological relations associated with high AVP concentrations may help decipher this effect. Presently, it seems likely that the association of AVP is due to a maternal predisposition. (But a predisposition to what?) In animal experiments, pregnant rats subjected to reduced uterine perfusion (RUPP) do not have increased copeptin

despite the usual preeclampsia-like findings (80). However, RUPP-treated animals demonstrated AVP dependent (81) high salt hypertension and elevated copeptin three weeks postpartum. Currently the exciting findings related to AVP require more attention, including the possibility that copeptin itself may have as yet unknown biological activities.

14.5.6 Other Maternal Hormones

It is evident that we have touched minimally on the myriad of hormonal changes in pregnancy and their relevance to preeclampsia. We have concentrated on maternal hormones about which most has been learned recently. For many years sympathetic activity– humoral and neural– has been a target of study with no clear resolution. However, a recent meta-analysis assessing newer, less invasive techniques concluded autonomic dysfunction could be detected in many preeclamptic women (82). There is of course no determination of whether this is causal, adaptive, or a pathological effect. Further inquiry is warranted to make such demonstrations. More recently epidemiological relationship to reduced vitamin D have been emphasized, but thus far with at best a modest affect with interventions (83). There is also interest in melatonin (84), kisspeptin (85), gluco and mineralocorticoids, among others. Unfortunately, an in-depth discussion of these and other hormones is not possible within a brief chapter.

14.6 Conclusion

The hormonal changes of pregnancy and preeclampsia are complex (Figure 14.1). Perhaps even more complex is whether these are primarily causal to alter pathophysiology or secondary to other pathological changes. Clearly central to all is the placenta, which drives the physiology of pregnancy and the pathophysiology of preeclampsia. It is also likely that organ pathophysiology also affects placental function. It is very difficult to extract the placental pathology and its "hormonal" products from the other pathophysiology. It is possible that some women may have specific physiological changes antedating pregnancy making them more sensitive to any of these signals. The complexity of these interactions is an important reminder that there are many routes to preeclampsia, and the importance of any of these pathways in a particular woman may vary (86).

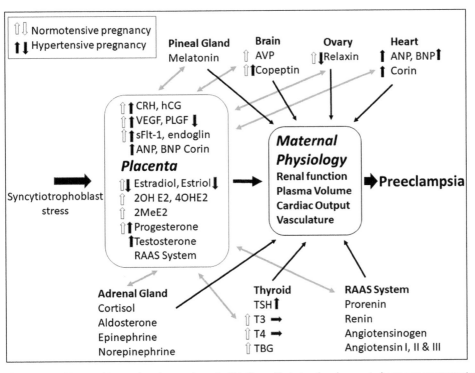

Figure 14.1 Hormonal interactions in preeclampsia. This figure illustrates the changes in hormone concentrations in normal pregnancy and with preeclampsia where established. The root of preeclampsia is the placenta whose function is altered by syncytiotrophoblast stress (8). The dysfunctional placenta has direct influences on maternal physiology. However, it also influences the physiology of other organs but in turn is also influenced by them (gray arrows). It is also possible in some women that the route to syncytiotrophoblast stress may actually be influenced by preexisting functional differences in other organs.

References

1. Staff AC, Redman CW, Williams D, et al. Pregnancy and long-term maternal cardiovascular health: Progress through harmonization of research cohorts and biobanks. *Hypertension*. 2016, 67:251–260.

2. Stojanovska V, Scherjon SA, and Plosch T. Preeclampsia as modulator of offspring health. *Biol Reprod*. 2016, 94:53.

3. Piering WF, Garancis JG, Becker CG, et al. Preeclampsia related to a functioning extrauterine placenta: Report of a case and 25-year follow-up. *Am J Kidney Dis*. 1993, 21:310–313.

4. Brittain PC, and Bayliss P. Partial hydatidiform molar pregnancy presenting with severe preeclampsia prior to twenty weeks gestation: A case report and review of the literature. *Mil Med*. 1995, 160:42–44.

5. Chesley LC. Hypertensive disorders of pregnancy. In. New York: Appleton-Century-Crofts, 1978.

6. Roberts JM, Taylor RN, Musci TJ, et al. Preeclampsia: An endothelial cell disorder. *Am J Obstet Gynecol*. 1989, 161:1200–1204.

7. Redman CW, Sacks GP, and Sargent IL. Preeclampsia: An excessive maternal inflammatory response to pregnancy. *Am J Obstet Gynecol*. 1999, 180:499–506.

8. Redman CWG, Staff AC, and Roberts JM. Syncytiotrophoblast stress in preeclampsia: The convergence point for multiple pathways. *Am J Obstet Gynecol*. 2020, 08:08.

9. Salas SP, Marshall G, Gutierrez BL, et al. Time course of maternal plasma volume and hormonal changes in women with preeclampsia or fetal growth restriction. *Hypertension*. 2006, 47:203–208.

10. Duvekot JJ, Cheriex EC, Pieters FA, et al. Early pregnancy changes in hemodynamics and volume homeostasis are consecutive adjustments triggered by a primary fall in systemic vascular tone. *Am J Obstet Gynecol*. 1993, 169:1382–1392.

11. Oelkers WK. Effects of estrogens and progestogens on

the renin-aldosterone system and blood pressure. *Steroids.* 1996, 61:166–171.

12. Van Buren GA, Yang DS, and Clark KE. Estrogen-induced uterine vasodilatation is antagonized by L-nitroarginine methyl ester, an inhibitor of nitric oxide synthesis. *Am J Obstet Gynecol.* 1992, 167:828–833.

13. Johnson ML, Grazul-Bilska AT, Redmer DA, et al. Effects of estradiol-17beta on expression of mRNA for seven angiogenic factors and their receptors in the endometrium of ovariectomized (OVX) ewes. *Endocrine.* 2006, 30:333–342.

14. Miller VM, and Vanhoutte PM. Progesterone and modulation of endothelium-dependent responses in canine coronary arteries. *Am J Physiol.* 1991, 261:R1022–1027.

15. Berkane N, Liere P, Oudinet JP, et al. From pregnancy to preeclampsia: A key role for estrogens. *Endocr Rev.* 2017, 38:123–144.

16. Magness RR, Sullivan JA, Li Y, et al. Endothelial vasodilator production by uterine and systemic arteries. VI. Ovarian and pregnancy effects on eNOS and NO(x). *Am J Physiol Heart Circ Physiol.* 2001, 280: H1692–1698.

17. Nelson SH, Steinsland OS, Wang Y, et al. Increased nitric oxide synthase activity and expression in the human uterine artery during pregnancy. *Circ Res.* 2000, 87:406–411.

18. Salom JB, Burguete MC, Perez-Asensio FJ, et al. Relaxant effects of 17-beta-estradiol in cerebral arteries through Ca(2+) entry inhibition. *J Cereb Blood Flow Metab.* 2001, 21:422–429.

19. Bausero P, Ben-Mahdi M, Mazucatelli J, et al. Vascular endothelial growth factor is modulated in vascular muscle cells by estradiol, tamoxifen, and hypoxia. *Am J Physiol Heart Circ Physiol.* 2000, 279: H2033–2042.

20. Mueller MD, Vigne JL, Minchenko A, et al. Regulation of vascular endothelial growth factor (VEGF) gene transcription by estrogen receptors alpha and beta. *Proc Natl Acad Sci U S A.* 2000, 97:10972–10977.

21. Shimodaira M, Nakayama T, Sato I, et al. Estrogen synthesis genes CYP19A1, HSD3B1, and HSD3B2 in hypertensive disorders of pregnancy. *Endocrine.* 2012, 42: 700–707.

22. Sharifzadeh F, Kashanian M, and Fatemi F. A comparison of serum androgens in pre-eclamptic and normotensive pregnant women during the third trimester of pregnancy. *Gynecol Endocrinol.* 2012, 28:834–836.

23. Kumar P, Luo Y, Tudela C, et al. The c-Myc-regulated microRNA-17~92 (miR-17~92) and miR-106a~363 clusters target hCYP19A1 and hGCM1 to inhibit human trophoblast differentiation. *Mol Cell Biol.* 2013, 33:1782–1796.

24. Stamilio DM, Sehdev HM, Morgan MA, et al. Can antenatal clinical and biochemical markers predict the development of severe preeclampsia? *Am J Obstet Gynecol.* 2000;182:589–594.

25. Steier JA, Ulstein M, and Myking OL. Human chorionic gonadotropin and testosterone in normal and preeclamptic pregnancies in relation to fetal sex. *Obstet Gynecol.* 2002, 100:552–556.

26. Kumar S, Gordon GH, Abbott DH, et al. Androgens in maternal vascular and placental function: implications for preeclampsia pathogenesis. *Reproduction.* 2018, 156: R155–R167.

27. Shao X, Liu Y, Liu M, et al. Testosterone represses estrogen signaling by upregulating miR-22: A mechanism for imbalanced steroid hormone production in preeclampsia. *Hypertension.* 2017, 69:721–730.

28. Laivuori H, Kaaja R, Rutanen EM, et al. Evidence of high circulating testosterone in women with prior preeclampsia. *J Clin Endocrinol Metab.* 1998, 83:344–347.

29. Pion R, Jaffe R, Eriksson G, et al. Studies on the metabolism of C-21 steroids in the human foeto-placental unit. I. Formation of a beta-unsaturated 3-ketones in midterm placentas perfused in situ with pregnenolone and 17-alpha-hydroxypregnenolone. *Acta Endocrinol (Copenh).* 1965, 48:234–248.

30. Rosing U, and Carlstrom K. Serum levels of unconjugated and total oestrogens and dehydroepiandrosterone, progesterone and urinary oestriol excretion in pre-eclampsia. *Gynecol Obstet Invest.* 1984, 18:199–205.

31. Tamimi R, Lagiou P, Vatten LJ, et al. Pregnancy hormones, pre-eclampsia, and implications for breast cancer risk in the offspring. *Cancer Epidemiol Biomarkers Prev.* 2003, 12:647–650.

32. Schoof E, Girstl M, Frobenius W, et al. Course of placental 11beta-hydroxysteroid dehydrogenase type 2 and 15-hydroxyprostaglandin dehydrogenase mRNA expression during human gestation. *Eur J Endocrinol.* 2001, 145:187–192.

33. Aufdenblatten M, Baumann M, Raio L, et al. Prematurity is related to high placental cortisol in preeclampsia. *Pediatr Res.* 2009, 65:198–202.

34. Cole LA. Biological functions of hCG and hCG-related molecules. *Reprod Biol Endocrinol.* 2010, 8:102.

35. Zygmunt M, Herr F, Keller-Schoenwetter S, et al. Characterization of human chorionic gonadotropin as a novel angiogenic factor. *J Clin Endocrinol Metab.* 2002, 87:5290–5296.

36. Barjaktarovic M, Korevaar TIM, Jaddoe VWV, et al. Human chorionic gonadotropin and risk of pre-eclampsia: prospective population-based cohort study. *Ultrasound Obstet Gynecol.* 2019, 54:477–483.

37. Levine RJ, Lam C, Qian C, et al. Soluble endoglin and other circulating antiangiogenic factors in preeclampsia. *N Engl J Med.* 2006, 355:992–1005.

38. Levine RJ, Maynard SE, Qian C, et al. Circulating angiogenic factors and the risk of preeclampsia. *N Engl J Med.* 2004, 350:672–683.

39. Campbell EA, Linton EA, Wolfe CD, et al. Plasma corticotropin-releasing hormone concentrations during pregnancy and parturition. *J Clin Endocrinol Metab.* 1987, 64:1054–1059.

40. Chau K, Hennessy A, and Makris A. Placental growth factor and pre-eclampsia. *J Hum Hypertens.* 2017, 31:782–786.

41. Thadhani R, Hagmann H, Schaarschmidt W, et al. Removal of soluble fms-like tyrosine kinase-1 by dextran sulfate apheresis in preeclampsia. *J Am Soc Nephrol.* 2016, 27: 903–913.

42. Salustiano EM, De Pinho JC, Provost K, et al. Maternal serum hormonal factors in the pathogenesis of preeclampsia. *Obstet Gynecol Surv.* 2013, 68:141–150.

43. Conrad KP. Emerging role of relaxin in the maternal adaptations to normal pregnancy: Implications for preeclampsia. *Semin Nephrol.* 2011, 31:15–32.

44. Conrad KP, and Baker VL. Corpus luteal contribution to maternal pregnancy physiology and outcomes in assisted reproductive technologies. *Am J Physiol Regul Integr Comp Physiol.* 2013, 304:R69–72.

45. Post Uiterweer ED, Koster MPH, Jeyabalan A, et al. Circulating pregnancy hormone relaxin as a first trimester biomarker for preeclampsia. *Pregnancy Hypertens.* 2020, 22:47–53.

46. Korevaar TIM, Medici M, Visser TJ, et al. Thyroid disease in pregnancy: New insights in diagnosis and clinical management. *Nat Rev Endocrinol.* 2017, 13:610–622.

47. Berta E, Lengyel I, Halmi S, et al. Hypertension in thyroid disorders. *Front Endocrinol.* 2019, 10:482.

48. Wilson KL, Casey BM, McIntire DD, et al. Subclinical thyroid disease and the incidence of hypertension in pregnancy. *Obstet Gynecol.* 2012, 119:315–320.

49. Gant NF, Daley GL, Chand S, et al. A study of angiotensin II pressor response throughout primigravid pregnancy. *J Clin Invest.* 1973, 52:2682–2689.

50. Yang J, Shang JY, Zhang SL, et al. The role of the renin-angiotensin-aldosterone system in preeclampsia: genetic polymorphisms and microRNA. *J Mol Endocrinol.* 2013, 50:R53–R66.

51. Xia Y, Kellems RE, Xia Y, et al. Angiotensin receptor agonistic autoantibodies and hypertension: Preeclampsia and beyond. *Circ Res.* 2013, 113:78–87.

52. Chang Y, and Wei W. Angiotensin II in inflammation, immunity and rheumatoid arthritis. *Clin Exper Immunol.* 2015, 179:137–145.

53. Chen T-H, Wang J-F, Chan P, et al. Angiotensin II stimulates hypoxia-inducible factor 1alpha accumulation in glomerular mesangial cells. *Ann NY Acad Sci.* 2005, 1042:286–293.

54. Zhou CC, Ahmad S, Mi T, et al. Angiotensin II induces soluble fms-Like tyrosine kinase-1 release via calcineurin signaling pathway in pregnancy. *Circ Res.* 2007, 100:88–95.

55. Carey RM. Update on angiotensin AT2 receptors. *Curr Opin Nephrol Hypertens.* 2017, 26:91–96.

56. Wu C, Lu H, Cassis LA, et al. Molecular and pathophysiological features of angiotensinogen: A mini review. *N Am J Med Sci.* 2011, 4:183–190.

57. Ichihara A, and Yatabe MS. The (pro)renin receptor in health and disease. *Nat Rev Nephrol.* 2019, 15:693–712.

58. Gathiram P, and Moodley J. The role of the renin-angiotensin-aldosterone system in preeclampsia: A review. *Curr Hypertens Rep.* 2020, 22:89.

59. Hladunewich MA, Kingdom J, Odutayo A, et al. Postpartum assessment of the renin angiotensin system in women with previous severe, early-onset preeclampsia. *J Clin*

Endocrinol Metab. 2011, 96:3517–3524.

60. Saxena AR, Karumanchi SA, Brown NJ, et al. Increased sensitivity to angiotensin II is present postpartum in women with a history of hypertensive pregnancy. *Hypertension.* 2010, 55:1239–1245.

61. Vinnakota S, and Chen HH. The importance of natriuretic peptides in cardiometabolic diseases. *J Endocr Soc.* 2020, 4: bvaa052.

62. Thomsen JK, Fogh-Andersen N, and Jaszczak P. Atrial natriuretic peptide, blood volume, aldosterone, and sodium excretion during twin pregnancy. *Acta Obstet. Gynecologica Scand.* 1994, 73:14–20.

63. Yoshimura T, Yoshimura M, Yasue H, et al. Plasma concentration of atrial natriuretic peptide and brain natriuretic peptide during normal human pregnancy and the postpartum period. *J Endocrinol.* 1994, 140:393–397.

64. Adam, Malatyalio, Gbreve, lu, Alvur, Kokcu, et al. Plasma atrial natriuretic peptide levels in preeclampsia and eclampsia. *J Matern Fetal Investig.* 1998, 8:85–88.

65. Franz MB, Andreas M, Schiessl B, et al. NT-proBNP is increased in healthy pregnancies compared to non-pregnant controls. *Acta Obstet Gynecol Scand.* 2009, 88:234–237.

66. Li H, Zhang Y, and Wu Q. Role of corin in the regulation of blood pressure. *Curr Opin Nephrol Hyperten.* 2017, 26:67–73.

67. Yan W, Sheng N, Seto M, et al. Corin, a mosaic transmembrane serine protease encoded by a novel cDNA from human heart. *J Biol Chem.* 1999, 274:14926–14935.

68. Cui Y, Wang W, Dong N, et al. Role of corin in trophoblast invasion and uterine spiral artery remodelling in pregnancy. *Nature.* 2012, 484:246–250.

69. Stepanian A, Alcais A, de Prost D, et al. Highly significant association between two common single nucleotide polymorphisms in CORIN gene and preeclampsia in caucasian women. *PLoS ONE.* 2014, 9.

70. Degrelle SA, Chissey A, Stepanian A, et al. Placental overexpression of soluble CORIN in preeclampsia. *Am J Pathol.* 2020, 190:970–976.

71. Jadli A, Ghosh K, and Shetty S. Is peripheral blood corin level clinically relevant for prediction of pre-eclampsia? *Ultrasound Obstet Gynecol.* 2015, 46:380.

72. Degrelle SA, Chissey A, Stepanian A, et al. Placental overexpression of soluble CORIN in preeclampsia. *Am J Pathol.* 190:970–976.

73. Baird RC, Li S, Wang H, et al. Pregnancy-associated cardiac hypertrophy in corin-deficient mice: Observations in a transgenic model of preeclampsia. *Can J Cardiol.* 2019, 35:68–76.

74. Rotondo F, Butz H, Syro LV, et al. Arginine vasopressin (AVP): A review of its historical perspectives, current research and multifunctional role in the hypothalamo-hypophysial system. *Pituitary.* 2016, 19:345–355.

75. Christ-Crain M. Vasopressin and Copeptin in health and disease. *Rev Endocr Metab Disord.* 2019, 20:283–294.

76. Santillan MK, Santillan DA, Scroggins SM, et al. Vasopressin in preeclampsia: A novel very early human pregnancy biomarker and clinically relevant mouse model. *Hypertension.* 2014, 64:852–859.

77. Scroggins SM, Santillan DA, Lund JM, et al. Elevated vasopressin in pregnant mice induces T-helper subset alterations consistent with human preeclampsia. *Clin Sci.* 2018, 132:419–436.

78. Bellos I, Pergialiotis V, Papapanagiotou A, et al. Association between serum copeptin levels and preeclampsia risk: A meta-analysis. *Eur J Obstet Gynecol Reprod Biol.* 2020, 250:66–73.

79. Asvold BO, Vatten LJ, Romundstad PR, et al. Angiogenic factors in maternal circulation and the risk of severe fetal growth restriction. *Am J Epidemiol.* 2011, 173:630–639.

80. Palei AC, Warrington JP, and Granger JP. The effect of placental ischemia-induced hypertension on circulating copeptin levels of pregnant rats. *FASEB J.* 2016, 30.

81. Matsuura T, Shinohara K, Iyonaga T, et al. Prior exposure to placental ischemia causes increased salt sensitivity of blood pressure via vasopressin production and secretion in postpartum rats. *J Hyperten.* 2019, 37:1657–1667.

82. Yousif D, Bellos I, Penzlin AI, et al. Autonomic dysfunction in preeclampsia: A systematic review. *Front Neurol.* 2019, 10:816.

83. Palacios C, Kostiuk LK, and Peña-Rosas JP. Vitamin D supplementation for women during pregnancy. *Cochrane Database Syst Rev.* 2019, 7: Cd008873.

84. Langston-Cox A, Marshall SA, Lu D, et al. Melatonin for the management of preeclampsia:

A review. *Antioxidants*. 2021, 10:376.

85. Kapustin RV, Drobintseva AO, Alekseenkova EN, et al. Placental protein expression of kisspeptin-1 (KISS1) and the kisspeptin-1 receptor (KISS1R) in pregnancy complicated by diabetes mellitus or preeclampsia. *Arch Gynecol Obstet*. 2020, 301:437–445.

86. Roberts JM, Rich-Edwards JW, McElrath TF, et al. Subtypes of preeclampsia: Recognition and determining clinical usefulness. *Hypertension*. 2021, 77:1430–1441.

Chapter 15

Adrenal Disease in Pregnancy

Jack Lockett, Warrick Inder, David H. McIntyre, Helen L. Barrett, Sailesh Kumar, and Vicki Lee Clifton

15.1 Adrenal Function in Pregnancy

The adrenal gland comprises two functionally distinct zones: the tri-layered cortex which produces corticosteroids, and the catecholamine secreting medulla (Figure 15.1). The former arises from the urogenital ridge, the latter the neural crest. Through hormonal secretion, the adrenal gland regulates cellular homeostasis, stress, inflammation, metabolism, salt and water balance, and reproductive function, amongst other systems. During pregnancy, significant changes

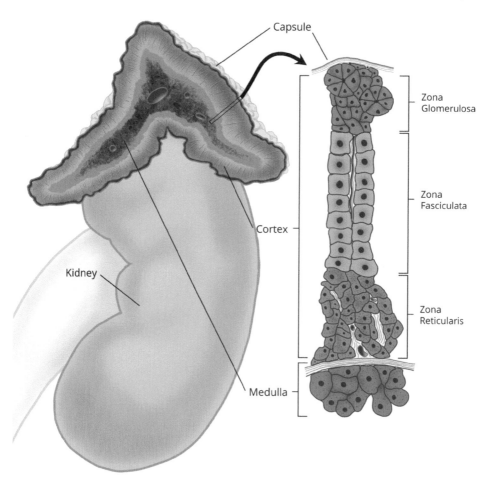

Figure 15.1 Anatomy and histology of the adrenal gland. The adrenals sit superior to the kidneys in the perinephric fat, enclosed by the renal fascia. The right is pyramidal, the left crescent-shaped. The fatty adrenal capsule encases the tri-layered adrenal cortex (corticosteroid-producing) and the medulla (catecholamine-producing). Functional zonation of the cortex into three distinct zones occurs through variable expression of the enzymes along the corticosteroid biosynthesis pathway. The zona glomerulosa secretes mineralocorticoids, fasciculata glucocorticoids, and reticularis sex steroids. Abundant arterial blood supply via the superior, middle, and inferior suprarenal arteries flows through capillary networks in the gland and drains via the adrenal veins directly into the inferior vena cava (right) or via the renal vein (left).

occur in adrenal hormonal homeostasis in the absence of significant adrenal morphological changes (1).

15.1.1 Glucocorticoids

Glucocorticoids are 21-carbon corticosteroid hormones secreted by the zona fasciculata under control of the hypothalamic-pituitary-adrenal (HPA) axis (Figure 15.2). These hormones, of which cortisol is the most important in humans, regulate the stress response, inflammation, and metabolism with pleiotropic effects in diverse tissues, acting via the glucocorticoid receptor. Corticotrophin-releasing hormone (CRH) is secreted by neurons of the hypothalamic paraventricular nucleus into the hypophyseal-portal system, stimulating adrenocorticotrophic hormone (ACTH) release from anterior pituitary corticotrophs (2,3). Additionally, ACTH secretion is stimulated by hypothalamic arginine vasopressin (AVP) (3). ACTH acts on adrenocortical cells

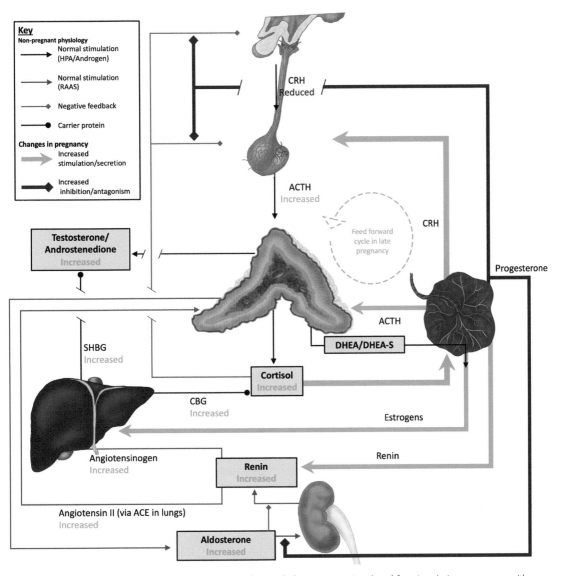

Figure 15.2 Adrenal function changes in pregnancy. Widespread changes occur in adrenal function during pregnancy with interactions between the hypothalamus/pituitary, feto-placental unit, kidney, and liver. See text for details. Abbreviations: ACE (angiotensin converting enzyme), ACTH (adrenocorticotrophic hormone), CBG (corticosteroid binding globulin), CRH (corticotrophin-releasing hormone), DHEA/-S (dehydroepiandrosterone/-sulphate), HPA (hypothalamic-pituitary-adrenal), RAAS (renin-angiotensin-aldosterone system), SHBG (sex hormone binding globulin).

Table 15.1. Reference ranges for adrenal hormones in pregnancy; trimester specific reference ranges of adrenal steroids reported in the literature

Steroid hormone	First trimester	Second trimester	Third trimester	Postpartum	Units
High-performance liquid chromatography-tandem mass spectrometry (LC/MS-MS) – reference ranges (2.5–97.5 percentiles) (7)					
Estradiol	1137.8–11010	7009.7–37911.11	7963.9–50829.5	<220.2–4550.8	pmol/L
Progesterone	23.56–111.80	50.18–244.35	110.85–440.11	<0.32–72.88	nmol/L
17α-hydroxyprogesterone	1.44–11.31	3.39–14.01	4.59–21.00	<0.3–14.85	nmol/L
Cortisol	133.25–1065.88	432.35–1670.41	315.47–1317.54	98.15–808.82	nmol/L
11-deoxycortisol	0.38–7.1	2.06–16.41	2.03–11.77	<0.29–4.23	nmol/L
DHEA	1.98–23.67	0.52–35.32	0.83–52.12	<0.35–19.92	nmol/L
DHEAS	2.70–67.53	1.96–38.97	1.47–29.48	3.48–78.27	nmol/L
Androstenedione	0.59–9.49	0.35–8.65	0.28–9.81	<0.35–4.45	nmol/L
Various cortisol measurements through pregnancy (LC/MS-MS) – mean ± SEM (8)					
Total plasma cortisol (LC/MS-MS)	577 ± 30	878 ±28	1043 ± 41	486 ± 38	nmol/L
Plasma free cortisol (LC/MS-MS)	14.5 ± 1.2	17.3 ± 1.4	19.6 ± 1.5	12.3 ± 2.0	nmol/L
24h urine free cortisol (LC/MS-MS)	135 ± 10	187 ± 13	242 ± 15	75 ± 9	nmol/d

to upregulate mitochondrial cholesterol transport and metabolism, and the enzymatic pathways responsible for the synthesis of cortisol (1,3). Circulating cortisol is predominantly bound to corticosteroid-binding globulin (CBG) with only free cortisol being bio-active. Free cortisol provides negative feedback at the hypothalamus and pituitary to regulate CRH and ACTH respectively (3) in turn regulating cortisol production. Plasma levels follow a diurnal rhythm in response to variations in ACTH secretory pulse frequency and amplitude, peaking in the morning, with a progressive decline to a nadir overnight (4).

Normal pregnancy is a state of increased HPA axis activity (5). Plasma total and free cortisol levels rise as gestation progresses, detectable as early as the eleventh week, reaching a two- to eight-fold elevation of total, and two- to four-fold elevation of free cortisol compared to non-pregnant controls by third trimester (Table 15.1) (1,2,5–8). Diurnal variation in cortisol levels is preserved, although the pattern may be blunted later in gestation (5,9). These changes are evident in plasma total and free cortisol, urinary free

cortisol, and salivary cortisol measurements (5), without definitive clinical evidence of hypercortisolism (1,6).

Elevated circulating estrogens stimulate hepatic production of CBG (5,6). It is presumed this initially causes a reduction in free cortisol, alleviating negative feedback on the hypothalamus-pituitary and increasing ACTH output to maintain normal free cortisol levels (2,5). The ensuing hypercortisolism may be in part due to the anti-glucocorticoid effects of elevated progestogens as significant correlations have been shown between salivary free cortisol and progesterone levels in later pregnancy (5). CRH increases exponentially through pregnancy from week 8, peaking at 40 weeks at a >1,000-fold elevation (5). CRH is secreted by the placenta in a nonpulsatile, non-diurnal fashion which increases in the third trimester (2,6). Additionally, during the final 12 weeks of gestation, CRH-binding protein levels fall, contributing to increased bioactive plasma CRH (3,6). The resultant rise in ACTH as gestation progresses peaks during delivery, consequently increasing cortisol in parallel (2,5).

Placental ACTH, secreted in response to CRH, may also contribute to circulating cortisol levels (5). Circulating cortisol is a secretagogue for placental CRH, creating a potent feed-forward mechanism towards the end of pregnancy (2). Placental CRH additionally stimulates fetal adrenal steroidogenesis, providing further positive feedback (6). These mechanisms combine to induce a state of hypercortisolism that downregulates hypothalamic CRH production as gestation proceeds, diminishing responsiveness of the HPA axis to both stress and exogenous steroids (2,5).

The fetus is protected from excessive maternal cortisol exposure throughout pregnancy by syncytial trophoblastic 11β-hydroxysteroid dehydrogenase 2 (11β-HSD 2) activity, an enzyme which converts cortisol to the inactive cortisone (2,5,6).

Postpartum, there is a rapid fall in CRH with delivery of the placenta, associated with reduced HPA axis responsiveness to exogenous glucocorticoids for up to three weeks and a return to normal CRH levels by twelve weeks. Plasma ACTH levels fall transiently, recovering by three to four days post-delivery. Cortisol levels fall gradually in the days postpartum to nonpregnant normal values, protected from falling below this range due to the elevated CBG (2).

15.1.2 Mineralocorticoids

The renin-angiotensin-aldosterone system (RAAS) governs mineralocorticoid secretion from the adrenocortical zona glomerulosa. Renin, produced in the juxta-glomerular apparatus of the nephron, catalyzes the conversion of hepatically synthesized angiotensinogen to angiotensin I. Angiotensin converting enzyme (ACE) further cleaves the product to angiotensin II (AngII) which in turn regulates glomerular blood flow, increases vascular tone, and stimulates aldosterone release. Aldosterone (21-carbon mineralocorticoid) acts in the nephron distal convoluted tubule and collecting duct to induce sodium (and hence water) retention and potassium excretion (5,6,10).

During early pregnancy, plasma renin activity is increased up to seven-fold through estrogen-stimulated angiotensinogen synthesis, and plasma renin mass (from ovarian/decidual renin release) increases from around the twentieth week of gestation (5,10,11). The resultant increase in AngII induces a progressive rise in serum aldosterone beginning in first trimester and peaking in the third at up to ten-fold nongravid levels (5). There is concurrent resistance to the vasopressor effect of AngII contributed to by progesterone and prostaglandin E2 (10). Despite the marked elevation in aldosterone, pregnant women display a normal diurnal variation and response to postural changes, salt restriction, and salt-loading, albeit at higher values (5,6). Deoxycorticosterone (DOC, another potent mineralocorticoid) concentrations parallel those of aldosterone. DOC is generated from extra-adrenal 21-hydroxylation of placentally derived progesterone and does not respond to the usual feedback mechanisms (6). Notwithstanding the excess mineralocorticoid, healthy pregnant women maintain normal or reduced blood pressure and normokalemia. This is due in part to the fact that these changes occur in response to the increased sodium requirement and vascular distensibility of pregnancy and are necessary to maintain adequate placental perfusion. Furthermore, progesterone antagonism of the mineralocorticoid receptor prevents hyperaldosteronism; aldosterone rises in unison with progesterone throughout gestation (5,10). By contrast, in Geller syndrome, a mutation of the mineralocorticoid receptor (MR) leads to enhanced MR affinity for progesterone and affected women develop severe hypertension during pregnancy (12).

15.1.3 Androgens

Adrenal 19-carbon steroid production from the zona reticularis increases during pregnancy (1). Production of dehydroepiandrosterone (DHEA) and DHEA-sulphate (DHEA-S) is doubled. However clearance is accelerated by placental metabolism to estrogens, providing 10–30 percent of the substrate (majority arising from the fetal adrenal) (6). This results in serum levels one third to one half of nongravid values (Table 15.1). Maternal levels of androstenedione and testosterone (adrenal or ovarian origin) increase through gestation secondary to estrogen-stimulated sex-hormone binding globulin release from the liver, but free androgen levels remain normal (1,4).

15.1.4 Catecholamines

The adrenal medulla is composed of chromaffin cells, migrated neural crest cells that differentiate under the control of cortisol (13). They produce and secrete catecholamines in concert with the sympathetic nervous system to adapt to, and protect against stress, including pregnancy- and parturition-induced (14). Adrenaline (epinephrine), noradrenaline (norepinephrine), and dopamine are catecholamine hormones and neurotransmitters, synthesized from tyrosine (14). They have numerous functions mediated via α-, β-adrenergic, and dopaminergic G-protein coupled receptors (14). During normal pregnancy, catecholamine levels are not consistently increased and are only slightly increased in women with preeclampsia (15). Maternal catecholamines have limited placental transit due to transporters and metabolic enzymes that impede delivery to the fetus (e.g., monoamine-oxidase and catechol-O-methyltransferase) (15); in fact, umbilical cord blood levels are <10 percent of maternal (15). The fetus has low circulating levels of catecholamines derived from the fetal adrenal which rise significantly during delivery and immediately postpartum (15).

15.1.5 The Fetal Adrenal Gland

The fetal adrenal develops at approximately eight weeks' gestation, and similar to the adult organ the fetal cortex is made up of an outer definitive zone, a middle transitional zone, and an inner fetal zone. The inner fetal zone predominates during gestation, accounting for 85–90 percent of the gland (16). It is the source of adrenal androgens (predominantly DHEA and DHEA-S) and grows significantly as gestation progresses. However, rapidly involutes and disappears in the post-natal period. The definitive and transitional zones only become hormonally active late in gestation, and within a few months after birth the definitive zone transforms into the zona glomerulosa, whilst the transitional zone develops into the zona fasciculata. The zona reticularis has no fetal counterpart and only develops until approximately six years after birth. In fetal life the adrenal medulla does not exist as a distinct region, islands of chromaffin cells migrate into the gland as early as nine weeks and are intermingled with adrenocortical cells. Soon after birth these coalesce centrally to form the adrenal medulla which only assumes a fully differentiated structure at the end of the first year of life (17). The two key functions of the fetal adrenal are to produce androgens which provide a major substrate for

placental estrogen production, and glucocorticoids, with fetal cortisol contributing to the feed-forward cycle stimulating placental CRH secretion towards the end of gestation (16). Both of these functions may contribute to the timing of delivery (1).

15.2 Adrenal Insufficiency: Primary and Secondary

15.2.1 Diagnosis

Adrenal insufficiency (AI) has been reported to occur at a prevalence of between 5–10/100,000 pregnancies (18). Most women with AI during pregnancy have a previously established diagnosis and therefore represent a management rather than a diagnostic problem. New onset AI is a rare presentation during pregnancy, and while the subject of multiple case reports, made up only 2 of 128 cases of AI in pregnancy in a large multi-center series (19). However, diagnosis of *de novo* AI in pregnancy is challenging as the symptoms may mimic other conditions such as hyperemesis gravidarum and the previously mentioned physiological changes in HPA axis function make interpretation of the standard diagnostic tests more difficult. Trimester-specific serum total and free cortisol concentrations in normal pregnancy have been quantified, allowing improved discrimination of what constitutes a low basal morning cortisol (8). The most frequently used dynamic test of HPA axis function is the $ACTH_{1-24}$ test. Reassuringly, $ACTH_{1-24}$ is considered safe in pregnancy, although there are few normative data (20). Recommendations regarding the 250 µg $ACTH_{1-24}$ test based on expert opinion suggest stimulated (60 min) total serum cortisol cutoffs of 700 nmol/L, 800 nmol/L and 900 nmol/L in the first, second, and third trimesters respectively (21). The known variability in serum cortisol measured with different immunoassays needs to be taken into consideration, and quantification by liquid chromatography-tandem mass spectrometry (LC-MS/MS) is the preferred method. Having identified a deficient cortisol response, the next step is determining whether the woman has primary (adrenal) or secondary (hypothalamic-pituitary) adrenal insufficiency. Plasma ACTH >22 pmol/L (100 ng/L) is considered as being consistent with primary AI during normal pregnancy (21). The RAAS is activated across pregnancy as described earlier which precludes using renin to aid in the differentiation between primary and secondary AI.

15.2.2 Etiology

Autoimmune adrenalitis is overall the commonest cause of primary AI. Other causes must also be considered, particularly bilateral adrenal hemorrhage if the presentation is of acute onset and in developing countries, tuberculous adrenalitis, and other infections. New onset secondary AI during pregnancy may be related to the development of lymphocytic hypophysitis which can present with isolated ACTH deficiency. Progression of a previously undiagnosed pituitary adenoma and the acute presentation of pituitary apoplexy are other possible causes of secondary AI during pregnancy. In the postpartum period, Sheehan's syndrome must be considered (pituitary infarction following intra/postpartum hemorrhage).

15.2.3 Chronic Corticosteroid Replacement

Glucocorticoid replacement is the cornerstone of management of AI in pregnancy, as in the nonpregnant state. In normal pregnancy, there is a progressive increase in both cortisol production and CBG (8). Historically, it was stated that no glucocorticoid dose adjustment was necessary during pregnancy – however, this reflects the supraphysiological dose regimens of around 30 mg hydrocortisone equivalent per day that were previously used. Increased appreciation of the normal cortisol production rate and of potential harm of high dose glucocorticoid regimens have led to lower physiological replacement doses, often less than 20 mg hydrocortisone equivalent per day in the nonpregnant state. Therefore, current recommendations for the management of AI in pregnancy are to increase the glucocorticoid dose by 20–40 percent in the third trimester (22,23). A large multicenter series however has shown that this recommendation is not invariably followed, with many women increasing the glucocorticoid dose as early as the first trimester and some not at all (19). Depending on the individual woman's usual maintenance dose in the nonpregnant state, the absolute dose increment generally ranges between 5–10 mg/day of hydrocortisone (19,21).

Hydrocortisone is the preferred glucocorticoid. Placental 11β-HSD 2 inactivates hydrocortisone (cortisol) to cortisone and thereby protects the fetus against excessive exposure to active glucocorticoids. Similarly, prednisolone is inactivated to prednisone via the same enzyme and can be used as an alternative (conversely, 11β-HSD type 1 activates the prodrug prednisone) (24). However, dexamethasone is not inactivated and freely crosses the placenta, potentially affecting the fetus. It should not be used for maintenance glucocorticoid replacement during pregnancy. For women with primary AI on mineralocorticoid replacement, adjustment in the fludrocortisone dose is required in a minority of cases (19,21,23).

15.2.4 Monitoring

There is no established role for routine monitoring of serum, urinary, or salivary cortisol levels in women with AI during pregnancy. Since an increase in renin is a normal finding in pregnancy, it cannot be used as an accurate indicator of mineralocorticoid replacement (21,23). The need for fludrocortisone dose increase should be made on clinical grounds such as presence of postural hypotension and hyperkalemia. The presence of hypokalemia, hypertension, or preeclampsia should lead to a fludrocortisone dose reduction and rarely, cessation (23). Clinical follow-up during pregnancy should be with an endocrinologist or obstetric physician who is experienced in the management of adrenal insufficiency.

15.2.5 Stress Dosing during Illness and Labor

As in the nonpregnant state, "stress" dosing during illness and surgery is crucial in the management of AI. Women and their partners should be instructed in the administration of parenteral hydrocortisone and when to use it (21). In particular, vomiting where the absorption of oral glucocorticoids is clearly compromised may lead to life threatening (both to mother and fetus) adrenal crisis if parenteral glucocorticoids are not promptly administered. During labor, some guidelines suggest a regimen of 50–100 mg intravenous (IV) hydrocortisone as a bolus, repeated 6-hourly. Recent evidence in the nonpregnant state demonstrates that a loading dose of hydrocortisone 50 mg IV followed by 200 mg infused over 24 hours provides superior stability of stress cortisol concentrations than intermittent IV injections (25). This protocol should be extrapolated to the management of AI during pregnancy and labor, as suggested in previous expert reviews (21,23). Given the high rates of HPA axis suppression in people treated with supraphysiological dosing of glucocorticoids for other indications (e.g. asthma, systemic lupus erythematosus) (26), stress dosing during parturition should be considered in these patients in the absence of a formal diagnosis of AI.

15.2.6 Summary

Women with established AI should be counselled that they can be safely managed during pregnancy. The diagnosis of new onset AI during pregnancy is challenging and requires a high index of suspicion, combined with knowledge of trimester-specific increases in normal cortisol production, to correctly interpret results of investigations. The treatment of choice is hydrocortisone, using standard replacement doses during the first trimester, increasing over the later second and third trimesters to mimic normal pregnancy. Cortisone acetate and prednisone/prednisolone may also be used, but dexamethasone should not. For women with primary adrenal insufficiency, mineralocorticoid replacement in the form of fludrocortisone may require dose adjustment on clinical grounds. During labor and delivery and if intercurrent illness, trauma, surgery, or major stress occur, parenteral "stress" dosing should be implemented, preferably by continuous IV infusion.

15.3 Congenital Adrenal Hyperplasia

Congenital adrenal hyperplasia (CAH) is a group of autosomal recessive disorders of adrenal steroidogenesis (Figure 15.3). The impaired function of a single enzyme in the cortisol biosynthesis pathway leads to corticosteroid deficiency. In the absence of negative feedback, ACTH-driven glucocorticoid precursors are diverted into alternate pathways, with enzyme-specific patterns of mineralocorticoid and androgen excess/deficiency. The most common cause is 21-hydroxylase deficiency (~95 percent) with an incidence of 1 in 10,000–20,000 live births (27,28).

Other forms result from deficiencies of 11β-hydroxylase, 3β-hydroxysteroid dehydrogenase, 17α-hydroxylase/17-20′lyase, steroidogenic acute regulatory protein, and cytochrome p450 oxidoreductase. The remainder of this section will refer to 21-hydroxylase deficiency with discussion of rarer forms following separately.

15.3.1 Diagnosis

The conversion of 17α-hydroxy progesterone (17α-OHP) to 11-deoxycortisol is the penultimate step in cortisol synthesis, catalyzed by 21-hydroxylase (27). The enzyme is also essential in aldosterone synthesis. The clinical spectrum of 21-hydroxylase deficiency is proportional to residual enzymatic function with strong genotype-phenotype correlations (29). Traditionally, three phenotypes of CAH due to 21-hydroxylase deficiency are described – classic salt-wasting (≤1 percent residual enzymatic activity), simple virilizing (2–20 percent activity), and nonclassic (late-onset; NCCAH) (30). The separation of the former two entities is no longer suggested due to the significant overlap in mineralocorticoid deficiency between the two, termed classic CAH (27). Due to the risk of salt wasting crisis and death engendered by severe 21-hydroxylase deficiency, many countries perform routine post-natal screening to diagnose CAH (28,31). If not diagnosed on routine screening, most cases of classic CAH will be diagnosed in childhood, presenting with salt-wasting crisis (neonate), varying degrees of virilization and ambiguous genitalia at birth (female fetuses), or with premature adrenarche (infancy/early childhood) (27,28,32). Nonclassic CAH may present with post-natal androgen excess or go undiagnosed until investigation of infertility (28). The clinical phenotype in adults is often similar to polycystic ovarian syndrome, including features of androgen excess and menstrual disturbance.

Diagnosis can be confirmed with measurement of 17α-OHP via radioimmunoassay following $ACTH_{1-24}$ stimulation. A basal (follicular phase if menstruating) level <6 nmol/L excludes the diagnosis and level of >30 nmol/L post-$ACTH_{1-24}$ is confirmatory (28).

15.3.2 Fertility

Early reports of fertility rates in patients with 21-hydroxylase CAH were low (33). However these

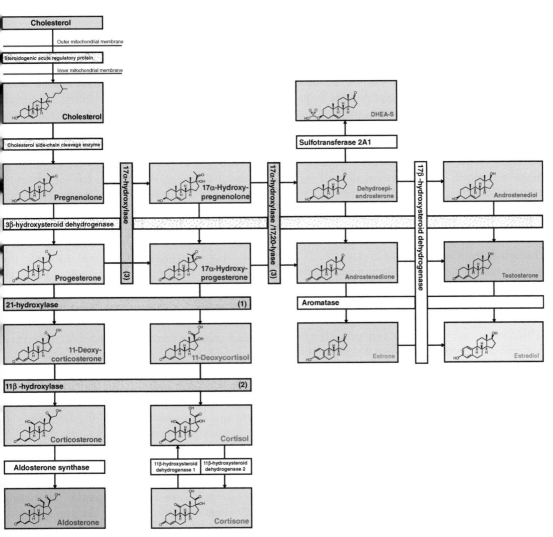

Figure 15.3 Adrenal corticosteroid biosynthesis pathway. Adrenal steroids are derived from cholesterol via a series of sequential enzymatic modifications to yield progestogens (magenta), mineralocorticoids (blue), glucocorticoids (green), androgens (orange), and estrogens (yellow). The main effector of each class is shaded in the respective color. The enzymatic defects in congenital adrenal hyperplasia are shaded with diagonal lines and numbered in ordered of frequency for the most common causes; rare causes are shaded with dots.

studies did not consider that adult women with classic CAH are less sexually active, less likely to be in a relationship, and less likely to actively pursue pregnancy (30,34,35). Pregnancy rates in treated women actively pursuing conception are as high as 91.3 percent in classic CAH with no difference between salt-wasting or simple virilizing forms (36). In NCCAH, pregnancy rates are mildly reduced compared to the normal population, ranging from 65 to 95 percent (37). These rates are biased towards the severe end of the NCCAH as many women are never diagnosed, nor seek medical attention.

The mechanisms of impaired fertility are multifactorial, predominantly as a result of adrenal androgen and progesterone excess. Adrenal androgens and their conversion to estrogens by aromatase may alter normal central hypothalamic-pituitary-gonadal (HPG) feedback. High circulating progesterone levels may impede ovulation and endometrial development and thicken cervical mucus, in the manner of contraceptives (30,34). The end result is chronic anovulation and endometrial dysfunction. Although the exact mechanism is unknown, women with primary adrenal insufficiency have reduced fertility and this likely plays a role in classic CAH (38). Aside from the hormonal contributors, woman with classic CAH may have impaired sexual/reproductive function related to their *in utero* androgen exposure. The effect on development of external genitalia or subsequent genital surgery can lead to difficult, painful, or even impede intercourse, reducing frequency and chance of pregnancy (30,34). Newer surgical techniques, revision of indications for intervention, and improvement in vaginal dilatation techniques have improved rates of sexual satisfaction to that of age-matched controls (39).

15.3.3 Management

The mainstay of management in classic CAH are glucocorticoid and mineralocorticoid replacement. These function to both replace deficient hormones and suppress ACTH-driven production of androgens (28). In adults, hydrocortisone 15–25 mg/d in 2–3 doses is recommended (28); alternatively, prednisolone can be used. As in other causes of AI, during pregnancy dexamethasone is contraindicated. Fludrocortisone is essential in classic CAH, to prevent salt-wasting crisis in more severe forms and treat subclinical deficiency in less severe. Maintaining adequate salt balance reduces vasopressin and ACTH secretion, allowing for lower doses of glucocorticoid (28). Fludrocortisone doses required in adulthood are similar to those in adrenal insufficiency. Treatment of NCCAH with glucocorticoids is recommended in adult women with patient-important hyperandrogenism or infertility (28).

Some women may require higher glucocorticoid doses to conceive despite adequate suppression of adrenal androgens. Prednisolone, 2–5 mg thrice daily suppresses circulating progesterone to <2 nmol/L during the follicular phase (36). In NCCAH, rates for spontaneous conception can be improved with low-dose glucocorticoid treatment. Additionally, this normalizes the higher rate of spontaneous miscarriage (37). As with polycystic ovarian syndrome, there is some evidence that metformin may suppress adrenal androgens in those with obesity and/or insulin resistance (40). Some women require ovulation induction with gonadotropins or clomiphene, or assisted reproductive technologies, as with non-affected women (30).

Preconception genetic counselling should be offered to all prospective parents/partners affected

by CAH (28). With the reported incidence rates, carrier status of 21-hydroxylase deficiency occurs in 1 in 50–60 (27,30). In couples with one affected parent and one carrier, the rate of 21-hydroxlase deficiency in a fetus is 50 percent, half of which will be female. Due to the strong genotype-phenotype correlation, noninvasive prenatal genotyping of maternally circulating fetal DNA can predict disease severity (29,41,42), however this is not widely available (28). The standard method of prenatal diagnosis is to obtain fetal or placental cells using amniocentesis or chorionic villous sampling, however both procedures carry a small risk of pregnancy loss (43). With *in vitro* fertilization, pre-implantation genetic testing can determine the presence of CAH and facilitate the transfer of unaffected embryos (44). Pre-natal treatment to prevent virilization in affected female fetuses with maternally administered dexamethasone is controversial with significant ethical concerns; therefore, it is considered experimental (28). There are long term metabolic and neurocognitive risks to children/adults exposed to excess glucocorticoids during gestation (45,46). Additionally, to be effective, treatment must begin early (prior to week 7) before the diagnosis can be confirmed (after 10 weeks), exposing the majority of fetuses unnecessarily (30).

Management of CAH through pregnancy can be challenging due to the previously mentioned changes in adrenal steroidogenesis interfering with usual monitoring. There do not appear to be higher rates of gestational diabetes, preeclampsia, or premature delivery; most pregnancies reported are uneventful (30). There is no consensus on glucocorticoid dosing during pregnancy and likely depends on the pre-conception dose. Guidelines recommend maintenance of pre-pregnancy doses and adjustment based on symptoms (28), those on dosing regimens similar to primary adrenal insufficiency will require at 20–40 percent increase in the third trimester. The fetus is protected from all but the most severe cases of hyperandrogenism due to placental aromatase, only two cases in the literature have been reported with evidence of virilization born to untreated/poorly treated mothers (34). Mineralocorticoid dosing may need adjustment as in other causes of primary AI.

In the setting of previous urogenital surgery, many women with classic CAH require delivery by cesarean section (C-section); however, spontaneous vaginal delivery is described in approximately one third of cases in the literature (30). Stress dosing of glucocorticoids during gestation and delivery should be approached as in other causes of AI described earlier. The rates of adrenal crisis are 4–6 per 100 patient years in CAH, but there are no pregnancy specific data (47).

15.3.4 Other Rare Types

Mutations occurring in other enzymes along the corticosteroid synthesis pathway cause alternate forms of CAH (48). Deficiency of 11β-hydroxylase impairs the final step in cortisol synthesis, leading to ACTH-driven androgen excess, and hypertension through buildup of the potent mineralocorticoid 11-deoxycorticosterone. Mutations in 17α-hydroxylase, cause impaired production of cortisol, adrenal androgens, and gonadal steroids with buildup of mineralocorticoids, of which corticosterone retains enough glucocorticoid activity to prevent adrenal crisis. These patients present with hypokalemic hypertension, undervirilization of 46XY newborns, primary amenorrhea in 46XX children, and absent pubertal development with hypergonadotropic hypogonadism. Steroid acute regulatory protein (StAR) facilitates transfer of cholesterol esters from the outer to inner mitochondrial membrane to allow formation of pregnenolone and is fundamental in steroid biosynthesis. Deficiency causes ACTH-driven toxic accumulation of intracellular cholesterol leading to worsening function and apoptosis. All steroid hormones are deficient, presenting with adrenal or salt-wasting crisis, female external genitalia in 46XY infants and enlarged adrenal glands filled with lipid (also known as lipoid CAH).

As with 21-hydroxylase deficiency, the mainstay of treatment in each of these conditions is glucocorticoids along with mineralocorticoid and sex steroid replacement if required (48).

A summary of all the reported pregnancies in rarer forms of CAH is presented in the review by Reisch (30).

15.4 Cushing's Syndrome

15.4.1 Diagnosis

Cushing's syndrome reduces fertility (49). Nonetheless, pregnancy may occur in women with active Cushing's syndrome and new onset Cushing's syndrome may be diagnosed during pregnancy. This requires clinical vigilance, since pregnancy is associated with clinical findings such as weight gain and new onset striae, as well as hypertension and disorders of glucose metabolism. Although recognized as features of Cushing's syndrome, these are more commonly due to other conditions, such as preeclampsia and gestational diabetes mellitus (Table 15.2). Clinical signs such as thinning of the skin, easy bruising, and proximal myopathy should be sought, as they are more specific for cortisol excess. Minimal trauma fracture is rare in pregnancy, and this is also an indication for exclusion of cortisol excess. The Endocrine Society Clinical Guidelines suggest

Table 15.2. Comparison of discriminatory clinical features of endocrine causes of hypertension in pregnancy

More suggestive of gestational hypertension	More suggestive of preeclampsia	More suggestive of PPGL	More suggestive of PA	More suggestive of Cushing's syndrome
• Onset >20 weeks' gestation without associated features of preeclampsia or other disorders	• Proteinuria • Peripheral and/or facial edema • Renal/liver impairment • Thrombocytopenia • HELLP syndrome (hemolysis, increased liver enzymes, low platelets)	• Presentation <20 weeks but as noted above, can present at any time and symptoms often increase peripartum • Paroxysmal hypertension • Orthostatic hypotension • Other symptoms such as flushing and sweating	• Hypokalemia • Pre-existing diagnosis	• Skin thinning • Easy bruising • Proximal myopathy • Minimal trauma fracture • Florid presentation with hypokalemia, muscle wasting and virilization is concerning for ACC

three possible screening tests for the diagnosis of Cushing's syndrome – the 1 mg dexamethasone suppression test (DST), 24 hour urinary free cortisol (24h UFC), and late night salivary cortisol (LNSC) (50). The interpretation of the 1 mg DST is problematic because of the normal increase in serum cortisol during pregnancy, and there are insufficient data to establish a definitive cutoff to distinguish Cushing's syndrome from normal (51). Additionally, dexamethasone suppression of cortisol is reduced during pregnancy, leading to potential false positive results. Trimester-specific data exist for serum cortisol, 24h UFC (8), and LNSC [52]. Therefore, when suggestive clinical features of glucocorticoid excess are combined with a 24h UFC >2.4× Upper Limit of Normal (ULN) (second trimester) or >3× ULN (third trimester), a diagnosis of Cushing's syndrome should be strongly considered. Serum free cortisol rises significantly during pregnancy, indicating that the increase in total serum cortisol is not solely accounted for by increased CBG production. LNSC is a measure of free cortisol and also progressively increases during pregnancy, to approximately three fold the nonpregnant state by the third trimester (52).

15.4.2 Etiology

All forms of Cushing's syndrome may present in pregnancy (pituitary, ectopic, and adrenal). Adrenal causes comprise 60 percent of cases, significantly more frequently than in the nonpregnant population where Cushing's disease (ACTH-secreting pituitary adenoma) predominates (49,51). Despite the primary adrenal pathology, ACTH may be incompletely suppressed in around 50 percent of cases (53), due to placental secretion of CRH, relative resistance of ACTH to elevated cortisol levels, and possible interference in some ACTH assays due to the marked pregnancy related increases in corticotrophin like intermediate peptide (CLIP) and proopiomelanocortin (POMC). This may be due to an adrenal adenoma or rarely an adrenal carcinoma. In addition, a condition of "pregnancy-induced" Cushing's syndrome exists (51,54). This may be associated with adrenal hyperplasia and is caused by the elevated human chorionic gonadotrophin (hCG) interacting with aberrant Luteinizing hormone (LH) receptors expressed on the adrenal cortex leading to subsequent hypercortisolism. This

condition is associated with the worst fetal outcomes (49), resolves on delivery and may recur during subsequent pregnancies (54).

Magnetic resonance imaging (MRI) without contrast may be undertaken from the late first trimester/early second trimester to assist in localizing the source of the Cushing's syndrome. If the woman has ACTH-dependent Cushing's syndrome, she is statistically seven times more likely to have Cushing's disease than ectopic ACTH production (49), and a pituitary MRI is indicated. Bilateral inferior petrosal sinus sampling is regarded as the gold standard for distinguishing pituitary from an ectopic source of ACTH excess, but is rarely undertaken during pregnancy. However, a peripheral CRH test (100 μg) may be safely performed during pregnancy. Administration of exogenous CRH to a patient with an ACTH-secreting pituitary adenoma results in a significant rise in plasma ACTH (55), but usually no rise is seen in cases of ectopic ACTH secretion. There are rare exceptions to this rule, when an ectopic neuroendocrine tumour expresses the CRH receptor. High dose (8mg) dexamethasone suppression testing is useful if it results in >50 percent cortisol suppression, as this would then be highly suggestive of a pituitary lesion (55). However, the converse is not true and failure to suppress cortisol with high dose dexamethasone does not definitively diagnose ectopic ACTH secretion.

15.4.3 Management

If the woman has ACTH-independent Cushing's syndrome and a clear unilateral adrenal mass on imaging, surgery should be undertaken during the second trimester to provide a definitive cure. For Cushing's disease, a 2018 review found only 13 reported cases of trans-sphenoidal surgery for Cushing's disease in the literature, undertaken between 10–23 weeks' gestation (56). Eight women entered remission, there were two intra-uterine deaths and two neonatal deaths (56). In the rare instance of a vision-threatening pituitary macroadenoma secreting ACTH, urgent trans-sphenoidal decompression may be required. Medical management results in lowering of the cortisol excess and allows for definitive localization studies to be performed postpartum. However, surgical treatment of Cushing's syndrome during pregnancy (combining adrenalectomy and pituitary surgery) has been associated with reduced fetal loss compared to medical management and no treatment in a systematic review (49).

Cabergoline, a dopamine-2 receptor agonist commonly prescribed in the treatment of prolactinoma, has been successfully used for Cushing's disease in pregnancy in doses of 2–3.5 mg per week (55). It is safe, generally well tolerated, and will not result in adrenal insufficiency but the likely prevention of lactation must be explained to the patient.

Metyrapone, an inhibitor of 11β-hydroxylase, the final step in cortisol synthesis, is the usual drug of choice for medical management of Cushing's syndrome in pregnancy (55), quickly and effectively reducing cortisol production (57). The usual starting dose is 500 mg two to three times per day. Monitoring is straightforward if using mass spectrometry assay methodology for serum and urinary free cortisol, but immunoassays usually have significant cross reactivity between cortisol and 11-deoxycortisol. Metyrapone also results in an increase in the active mineralocorticoid metabolite deoxycorticosterone. In pregnancy this may cause a clinical issue with hypertension/hypokalaemia (55,58) but this seems to be uncommon, perhaps due to the mineralocorticoid receptor antagonism by elevated progesterone.

Ketoconazole inhibits androgen production as well as cortisol. It is teratogenic in animal studies, raising concerns regarding its use in the presence of a male fetus (55). However, case reports in which ketoconazole has been used during pregnancy have not demonstrated such an effect (59,60). The aim of medical management should be to maintain the 24h UFC within the trimester-specific reference range – to less than 2.4 fold the nonpregnant range during the second trimester and 3 fold the nonpregnant range in the third trimester (8).

15.5 Primary Aldosteronism

Primary aldosteronism (PA), with its characteristic clinical features of hypertension, elevated aldosterone, and suppressed plasma renin, is the most common secondary cause of hypertension (61) with a reported prevalence of 3–13 percent amongst general populations with hypertension, increasing to 20 percent in those patients considered to have "treatment resistant" hypertension (61). Older clinical reports required the presence of hypokalemia to raise suspicion of PA, but it is now clear that, when systematic testing of hypertensive patients is performed, serum potassium is normal in the majority (60–80 percent) of PA cases (62).

15.5.1 Etiology

Excess aldosterone production arises from one or both adrenal glands and may be caused by germline variants or develop *de novo* (63). Familial hyperaldosteronism Type 1 (also known as glucocorticoid remediable hyperaldosteronism) is a rare autosomal dominant form of PA (<1 percent of PA cases) with marked phenotypic heterogeneity (64), generally effectively treated by glucocorticoids. This variant will not be further considered in the current discussion. Despite PA being a common recognized cause of hypertension outside pregnancy, case reports during pregnancy are sporadic, suggesting under diagnosis and/or publication bias (65).

15.5.2 Diagnosis

The physiologic changes of pregnancy make definitive diagnosis of PA during gestation difficult. As noted earlier, both aldosterone and renin levels rise substantially but not in direct proportion, so the aldosterone:renin ratio (the most commonly used screening test for PA) may give both false positive and false negative results (65). Hypokalemia in association with pregnancy related hypertension may raise clinical suspicion of PA (Table 15.2), but it has also been noted that, in women with a known pre-pregnancy diagnosis of PA, potassium levels may normalize due to the aldosterone antagonism by high progesterone levels (65). Malha et al. have reported that elevated aldosterone with plasma renin activity $< 4 \, \text{ng} / \text{mL} /$ hour is suggestive of PA in pregnancy, but these results are likely assay dependent (66). Ultrasound and MRI may be used to define unilateral versus bilateral disease. More definitive testing using saline infusions and fludrocortisone has rarely been performed during pregnancy and localization using adrenal vein sampling is contraindicated due to the level of radiation exposure (65).

15.5.3 Management

PA carries a high risk of pregnancy complications (10,65,67) and all treatment recommendations appear empirical. If a unilateral aldosterone secreting adenoma is diagnosed pre-pregnancy, then adrenalectomy prior to pregnancy is indicated (10). In nine reported cases of laparoscopic adrenalectomy during pregnancy, biochemical cure of PA was obtained, but complications including intrauterine growth restriction (2), pre-term delivery (1), and fetal death in utero (1) occurred frequently (65).

Medical therapy for PA is commonly used in patients with bilateral adrenal hyperplasia, but the evidence base for use of specific medications during pregnancy remains sparse. Some authors recommend cessation of mineralocorticoid antagonists at least one month preconception followed by anti-hypertensive treatment with medications with a recognized pregnancy safety profile (e.g., alpha methyldopa and labetalol) (68). Spironolactone is not generally recommended for use in pregnancy due to its known antiandrogenic properties and concern regarding the potential for feminization of a male fetus. However the data supporting this potential risk of spironolactone treatment are limited to one animal study (69) and a single human case report (65). Amiloride has been used in a small number of pregnancies without reported adverse effects (65) and eplerenone is also favored by some authors, due to its lack of androgen receptor blockade (70).

In women with suspected PA first noted during pregnancy, the diagnosis should generally be reevaluated at three months postpartum using medications which do not affect the diagnostic tests (e.g., verapamil, prazosin, or hydralazine) as needed to control hypertension.

Whilst further research is clearly required to define the optimal management of PA during pregnancy, a clinically reasonable overall approach would be to use standard, pregnancy appropriate, antihypertensive therapy as first line treatment, especially in the first trimester then consider escalation of therapy with mineralocorticoid antagonists during the second and third trimesters if control of hypertension and/or hypokalemia is inadequate. Progression to surgical adrenalectomy should be reserved for severe, treatment resistant hypertension related to unilateral adrenal lesions.

15.6 Pheochromocytoma and Paraganglioma

Pheochromocytoma or paraganglioma (PPGL) are suggested to occur in 7/100,000 pregnancies (71).

Historically, maternal and fetal mortality were extremely high (~50 percent). In a systematic review examining case reports from 1998 to 2013, the overall maternal mortality rate was 9.8 percent in pheochromocytoma and 3.6 percent in paragangliomas, with fetal mortality 16 percent and 12 percent respectively (72). In a large case series of 89 pregnant women between 1968 and 2018, the greatest risk for adverse outcomes was absence of diagnosis. The 7 percent intrauterine fetal death rate at a median of 21 weeks, one maternal death at 38 weeks, and two severe maternal cardiac complications immediately postpartum occurred in women undiagnosed during pregnancy (73).

The majority of cases diagnosed around pregnancy are detected antenatally (~73 percent) and ~90 percent report at least one symptom antenatally (15). Symptoms reported are similar to the nonpregnant state, including hypertension (either persistent or paroxysmal), headache, sweating, palpitations, chest pain, nausea, vomiting, and flushing. The presenting symptoms can be similar to preeclampsia and can increase around the time of delivery, possibly due to mechanical compression from the gravid uterus, contractions, or administration of anaesthesia. Presentation can also be due to a hypertensive crisis, pulmonary edema, or cardiomyopathy. Clinical differentiation from preeclampsia can be difficult (Table 15.2). Some features more common in preeclampsia include proteinuria and edema as well as features of the HELLP syndrome (hemolysis, elevated liver enzymes, low platelets). In contrast, pheochromocytoma and paraganglioma are less likely to present with proteinuria and oedema, but may suffer paroxysms of hypertension and orthostatic hypotension (74). Consideration of the potential for pheochromocytoma or paraganglioma needs to be given in the setting of such symptoms and testing for maternal plasma or urinary metanephrines undertaken.

15.6.1 Diagnosis

Catecholamine metabolism is not altered by pregnancy, and while in some patients with preeclampsia levels can be mildly increased, significant elevation is more suggestive of PPGL (75). Plasma free or urinary fractionated metanephrines and 3-methoxytyramine should be measured – these have a high negative predictive value (76). There can be assay interference from some drugs; for example, methyldopa and labetalol in electrochemical assays but not in liquid chromatography-mass spectrometry (LC-MS/MS) assays. Knowing the local method of analysis is important in interpreting the results. Other drugs can cause false positives through pharmacological effects. For example, tricyclic antidepressants elevate plasma normetadrenaline by reducing neuronal noradrenaline reuptake (76). These interferences are not altered by pregnancy. Blood tests should ideally be undertaken fasted and supine. Clonidine suppression tests are not routinely undertaken as part of the diagnostic work up in pregnancy due to risk of hypotension.

Outside pregnancy, computed tomography (CT), ^{123}I-metaiodobenzylguanidine (MIBG) scintigraphy, and ^{68}Ga-DOTATATE positron emission tomography (PET)/CT are important anatomical and functional imaging modalities but are not used in pregnancy. Noncontrast MRI can be used for imaging, though gadolinium is typically avoided in pregnancy due to theoretical concerns with limited data (75,77).

In most cases the primary tumour is adrenal (80 percent) in origin. A review of 89 cases in pregnancy between 1968 and 2018 reported that 42 percent had unilateral pheochromocytoma, 29 percent bilateral, 29 percent paraganglioma, 9 percent multifocal disease, and 8 percent metastatic (73).

15.6.2 Genetic Considerations

Up to 40 percent of all patients with PPGL have a germline mutation resulting in a genetic syndrome associated with these tumors (15). These mutated genes can be separated into two clusters: genes involved in the cellular response to hypoxia (cluster 1 – pseudohypoxic; *VHL, SDHx*), and those involved in intracellular kinase pathway signaling (cluster 2 – protein kinase; *RET, NF1, MAX*) (78). The individual genetic syndromes are associated with a range of associated pathologies, the clinical features of which should be sought at review. In pregnant women diagnosed with PPGL, genetic testing should be undertaken (15).

15.6.3 Management

Optimal management should involve a multidisciplinary team with medical, surgical, and obstetric expertise. Treatment should be with alpha-adrenergic receptor blockade, aiming to avoid significant hypotension which can compromise circulation to the uteroplacental unit. Phenoxybenzamine does cross the placenta and has been associated with neonatal complications such as respiratory depression and hypotension, so infants need close monitoring (74). Doxazosin has not been reported to have the same neonatal concerns around hypotension and respiratory depression (68). Surgery is the necessary definitive treatment, ideally during the second trimester. A case series of 12 women with adrenalectomy in pregnancy at a median of 20 weeks for a mixture of indications, including two with pheochromocytoma, reported that nine were undertaken via a lateral laparoscopic transabdominal route, and there was pre-term birth in seven cases (79).

15.6.4 Delivery

There is no definite consensus on delivery management. Delivery planning will depend significantly on obstetric history and the overall pregnancy situation at the time in which PPGL has been diagnosed. Decisions should be made in the multidisciplinary team setting with involvement of the patient and their support network. Successful vaginal deliveries have been reported in women who are appropriately blocked with alpha-adrenergic blocking agents and receive good pain relief (e.g., with epidural anesthesia). The case series of 89 women mentioned above reported that delivery was by cesarean section (C-section) in 44 percent, vaginal in 39 percent, with 6 percent elective termination and intrauterine fetal demise in 7 percent (73). In the C-section group there was one fetal death in a delivery at 22 weeks, with no complications in the vaginal deliveries. C-Section does not necessarily remove the risk of hypertensive crisis or delivery complications, as catecholamine excess can also be stimulated by abdominal surgery. A suggested management algorithm, updated from an earlier paper (80), has been included (Figure 15.4).

15.7 Adrenocortical Carcinoma

Adrenocortical carcinomas (ACC) are rare and aggressive tumors, with an estimated population incidence of 1–2 cases per million (81). There is a female predominance (55–60 percent), and although the peak age of incidence is 40–50 years,

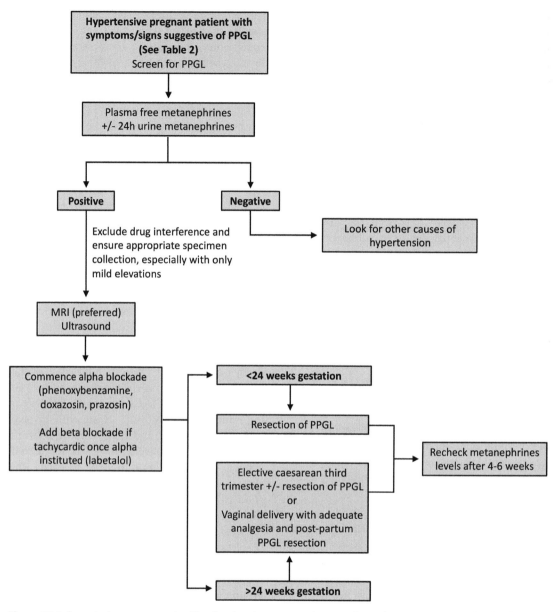

Figure 15.4 Suggested management algorithm for pheochromocytoma/paraganglioma during pregnancy. Updated with more recent evidence from original by Oliva and colleagues (80).

sporadic cases affect younger women and may thus complicate pregnancy (82). Overall prognosis is poor and varies according to tumor size. Localized primary tumors <5 cm diameter have a reported 10-year survival of 80 percent. Localized tumors >5 cm have a reported 60 percent 10-year survival, falling to 10 percent if distant metastatic spread is evident at diagnosis (83).

Limited *in vitro* data suggest that higher levels of estrogen and progesterone enhance tumor growth and may lead to a more aggressive clinical course during pregnancy (83). Small case series of ACC in pregnancy often describe larger tumors, with frequent features of florid Cushing's syndrome (~70 percent), often associated with pronounced hypokalemia (84), hypertension, diabetes, muscle wasting, and virilization (82).

15.7.1 Diagnosis

Diagnostic testing for cortisol excess should proceed as previously outlined. Ultrasound is generally recommended as the primary imaging modality, but MRI is almost invariably required to optimally define tumor size and signal characteristics and define local and metastatic spread (83).

15.7.2 Management

Medical therapy of Cushing's syndrome during pregnancy as previously outlined is generally recommended only as an urgent temporary measure designed to reduce marked cortisol hypersecretion in preparation for surgery. Mitotane is generally avoided in pregnancy due to its slow onset of action and teratogenic effects in animals (83).

Both laparoscopic and open surgical approaches to ACC resection have been attempted in second and early third trimesters. Immediate maternal complications appear rare, though early recurrence in the tumor bed in 4/6 cases in one series suggested incomplete primary excision (83). Pre-term birth is frequently reported (82,83).

Maternal mortality during or immediately following pregnancy appears rare in ACC patients. However, postpartum prognosis is very poor with 5-year survival of 13 percent reported (82), reflecting mortality four times higher than that of matched nonpregnant controls. However, in women with a previous diagnosis of ACC, a subsequent pregnancy does not appear to increase the risk of disease recurrence (85), although this may be largely due to self-selection and more favorable overall baseline clinical characteristics (83,85).

References

1. Rainey WE, Rehman KS, and Carr BR. Fetal and maternal adrenals in human pregnancy. *Obstet Gynecol Clin North Am.* 2004, 31(4):817–835, x.

2. Duthie L, and Reynolds RM. Changes in the maternal hypothalamic-pituitary-adrenal axis in pregnancy and postpartum: Influences on maternal and fetal outcomes. *Neuroendocrinology.* 2013, 98 (2):106–115.

3. Mastorakos G, and Ilias I. Maternal and fetal hypothalamic-pituitary-adrenal axes during pregnancy and postpartum. *Ann N Y Acad Sci.* 2003, 997:136–149.

4. Levin G, Elchalal U, and Rottenstreich A. The adrenal cortex: Physiology and diseases in human pregnancy. *Eur J Obstet Gynecol Reprod Biol.* 2019, 240:139–143.

5. Lindsay JR, and Nieman LK. The hypothalamic-pituitary-adrenal axis in pregnancy: challenges in disease detection and treatment. *Endocr Rev.* 2005, 26 (6):775–799.

6. Monticone S, Auchus RJ, and Rainey WE. Adrenal disorders in pregnancy. *Nat Rev Endocrinol.* 2012, 8 (11):668–678.

7. Soldin OP, Guo T, Weiderpass E, et al. Steroid hormone levels in pregnancy and 1 year postpartum using isotope dilution tandem mass spectrometry. *Fertil Steril.* 2005, 84(3):701–710.

8. Jung C, Ho JT, Torpy DJ, et al. A longitudinal study of plasma and urinary cortisol in pregnancy and postpartum. *J Clin Endocrinol Metab.* 2011, 96(5):1533–1540.

9. Challis JR, and Patrick JE. Changes in the diurnal rhythms of plasma cortisol in women during the third trimester of pregnancy. *Gynecol Obstet Invest.* 1983, 16 (1):27–32.

10. Landau E, and Amar L. Primary aldosteronism and pregnancy. *Ann Endocrinol.* 2016, 77(2):148–160.

11. Lumbers ER, and Pringle KG. Roles of the circulating renin-angiotensin-aldosterone system in human pregnancy. *Am J Physiol Regul Integr Comp Physiol.* 2014, 306(2): R91–101.

12. Levanovich PE, Diaczok A, and Rossi NF. Clinical and molecular perspectives of monogenic hypertension. *Curr Hypertens Rev.* 2020, 16(2):91–107.

13. Ehrhart-Bornstein M, Vukicevic V, Chung KF, et al. Chromaffin progenitor cells from the adrenal medulla. *Cell Mol Neurobiol.* 2010, 30 (8):1417–1423.

14. van Berkel A, Lenders JW, and Timmers HJ. Diagnosis of endocrine disease: Biochemical diagnosis of phaeochromocytoma and paraganglioma. *Eur J Endocrinol.* 2014, 170(3):R109–119.

15. Lenders JWM, Langton K, Langenhuijsen JF, et al. Pheochromocytoma and pregnancy. *Endocrinol Metab Clin North Am.* 2019, 48 (3):605–617.

16. Jaffe RB, Mesiano S, Smith R, et al. The regulation and role of fetal adrenal development in human pregnancy. *Endocr Res.* 1998, 24(3–4):919–926.

17. Else T, and Hammer GD. Genetic analysis of adrenal absence: Agenesis and aplasia. *Trends Endocrinol Metab.* 2005, 16(10):458–468.

18. Schneiderman M, Czuzoj-Shulman N, Spence AR, et al. Maternal and neonatal outcomes of pregnancies in

women with Addison's disease: A population-based cohort study on 7.7 million births. *BJOG*. 2017, 124 (11):1772–1779.

19. Bothou C, Anand G, Li D, et al. Current management and outcome of pregnancies in women with adrenal insufficiency: Experience from a multicenter survey. *J Clin Endocrinol Metab*. 2020, 105 (8):e2853–2863.

20. Suri D, Moran J, Hibbard JU, et al. Assessment of adrenal reserve in pregnancy: Defining the normal response to the adrenocorticotropin stimulation test. *J Clin Endocrinol Metab*. 2006, 91 (10):3866–3872.

21. Lebbe M, and Arlt W. What is the best diagnostic and therapeutic management strategy for an Addison patient during pregnancy? *Clin Endocrinol (Oxf)*. 2013, 78 (4):497–502.

22. Bornstein SR, Allolio B, Arlt W, et al. Diagnosis and treatment of primary adrenal insufficiency: An endocrine society clinical practice guideline. *J Clin Endocrinol Metab*. 2016, 101(2):364–389.

23. Anand G, and Beuschlein F. MANAGEMENT OF ENDOCRINE DISEASE: Fertility, pregnancy and lactation in women with adrenal insufficiency. *Eur J Endocrinol*. 2018, 178(2): R45–R53.

24. Murphy VE, Fittock RJ, Zarzycki PK, et al. Metabolism of synthetic steroids by the human placenta. *Placenta*. 2007, 28(1):39–46.

25. Prete A, Taylor AE, Bancos I, et al. Prevention of adrenal crisis: Cortisol responses to major stress compared to stress dose hydrocortisone delivery. *J Clin Endocrinol Metab*. 2020, 105(7):2262–2274.

26. Sacre K, Dehoux M, Chauveheid MP, et al.

Pituitary-adrenal function after prolonged glucocorticoid therapy for systemic inflammatory disorders: An observational study. *J Clin Endocrinol Metab*. 2013, 98(8):3199–3205.

27. Merke DP, and Auchus RJ. Congenital adrenal hyperplasia due to 21-hydroxylase deficiency. *N Engl J Med*. 2020, 383(13):1248–1261.

28. Speiser PW, Arlt W, Auchus RJ, et al. Congenital adrenal hyperplasia due to steroid 21-hydroxylase deficiency: An endocrine society* clinical practice guideline. *J Clin Endocrinol Metab*. 2018, 103 (11):4043–4088.

29. New MI, Abraham M, Gonzalez B, et al. Genotype-phenotype correlation in 1,507 families with congenital adrenal hyperplasia owing to 21-hydroxylase deficiency. *Proc Natl Acad Sci USA*. 2013, 110 (7):2611–2616.

30. Reisch N. Pregnancy in congenital adrenal hyperplasia. *Endocrinol Metab Clin North Am*. 2019, 48 (3):619–641.

31. Heather NL, Seneviratne SN, Webster D, et al. Newborn screening for congenital adrenal hyperplasia in New Zealand, 1994–2013. *J Clin Endocrinol Metab*. 2015, 100 (3):1002–1008.

32. Merke DP, and Bornstein SR. Congenital adrenal hyperplasia. *Lancet*. 2005, 365 (9477):2125–2136.

33. Mulaikal RM, Migeon CJ, and Rock JA. Fertility rates in female patients with congenital adrenal hyperplasia due to 21-hydroxylase deficiency. *N Engl J Med*. 1987, 316(4):178–182.

34. Lekarev O, Lin-Su K, and Vogiatzi MG. Infertility and reproductive function in patients with congenital adrenal hyperplasia: Pathophysiology, advances in management, and

recent outcomes. *Endocrinol Metab Clin North Am*. 2015, 44 (4):705–722.

35. Słowikowska-Hilczer J, Hirschberg AL, Claahsen-van der Grinten H, et al. Fertility outcome and information on fertility issues in individuals with different forms of disorders of sex development: Findings from the dsd-LIFE study. *Fertil Steril*. 2017, 108 (5):822–831.

36. Casteràs A, De Silva P, Rumsby G, et al. Reassessing fecundity in women with classical congenital adrenal hyperplasia (CAH): Normal pregnancy rate but reduced fertility rate. *Clin Endocrinol (Oxf)*. 2009, 70 (6):833–837.

37. Bidet M, Bellanné-Chantelot C, Galand-Portier M-B, et al. Fertility in women with nonclassical congenital adrenal hyperplasia due to 21-hydroxylase deficiency. *J Clin Endocrinol Metab*. 2010, 95 (3):1182–1190.

38. Erichsen MM, Husebye ES, Michelsen TM, et al. Sexuality and fertility in women with Addison's disease. *J Clin Endocrinol Metab*. 2010, 95 (9):4354–4360.

39. Nordenström A, Frisén L, Falhammar H, et al. Sexual function and surgical outcome in women with congenital adrenal hyperplasia due to CYP21A2 deficiency: Clinical perspective and the patients' perception. *J Clin Endocrinol Metab*. 2010, 95 (8):3633–3640.

40. Krysiak R, and Okopien B. The effect of metformin on androgen production in diabetic women with non-classic congenital adrenal hyperplasia. *Exp Clin Endocrinol Diabetes*. 2014, 122 (10):568–571.

41. Vermeulen C, Geeven G, de Wit E, et al. Sensitive monogenic noninvasive prenatal diagnosis by targeted

haplotyping. *Am J Hum Genet.* 2017, 101(3):326–339.

42. Simpson JL, and Bischoff F. Novel non-invasive prenatal diagnosis as related to congenital adrenal hyperplasia. *Adv Exp Med Biol.* 2011, 707:37–38.

43. McCann-Crosby B, Placencia FX, Adeyemi-Fowode O, et al. Challenges in prenatal treatment with dexamethasone. *Pediatr Endocrinol Rev.* 2018, 16(1):186–193.

44. Besser AG, Blakemore JK, Grifo JA, et al. Transfer of embryos with positive results following preimplantation genetic testing for monogenic disorders (PGT-M): Experience of two high-volume fertility clinics. *J Assist Reprod Genet.* 2019, 36 (9):1949–1955.

45. Wallensteen L, Zimmermann M, Thomsen Sandberg M, et al. Sex-dimorphic effects of prenatal treatment with dexamethasone. *J Clin Endocrinol Metab.* 2016, 101 (10):3838–3846.

46. Hirvikoski T, Nordenström A, Wedell A, et al. Prenatal dexamethasone treatment of children at risk for congenital adrenal hyperplasia: The Swedish experience and standpoint. *J Clin Endocrinol Metab.* 2012, 97(6):1881–1883.

47. Reisch N, Willige M, Kohn D, et al. Frequency and causes of adrenal crises over lifetime in patients with 21-hydroxylase deficiency. *Eur J Endocrinol.* 2012, 167(1):35–42.

48. Balsamo A, Baronio F, Ortolano R, et al. Congenital adrenal hyperplasias presenting in the newborn and young infant. *Front Pediatr.* 2020, 8:593315.

49. Caimari F, Valassi E, Garbayo P, et al. Cushing's syndrome and pregnancy outcomes: A systematic review of published cases. *Endocrine.* 2017, 55(2):555–563.

50. Nieman LK, Biller BM, Findling JW, et al. The diagnosis of Cushing's syndrome: An endocrine society clinical practice guideline. *J Clin Endocrinol Metab.* 2008, 93(5):1526–1540.

51. Brue T, Amodru V, and Castinetti F. MANAGEMENT OF ENDOCRINE DISEASE: Management of Cushing's syndrome during pregnancy: Solved and unsolved questions. *Eur J Endocrinol.* 2018, 178(6): R259–R266.

52. Lopes LM, Francisco RP, Galletta MA, et al. Determination of nighttime salivary cortisol during pregnancy: Comparison with values in non-pregnancy and Cushing's disease. *Pituitary.* 2016, 19(1):30–38.

53. Lindsay JR, and Nieman LK. Adrenal disorders in pregnancy. *Endocrinol Metab Clin North Am.* 2006, 35(1):1–20, v.

54. Achong N, D'Emden M, Fagermo N, et al. Pregnancy-induced Cushing's syndrome in recurrent pregnancies: Case report and literature review. *Aust N Z J Obstet Gynaecol.* 2012, 52(1):96–100.

55. Machado MC, Fragoso M, and Bronstein MD. Pregnancy in patients with Cushing's syndrome. *Endocrinol Metab Clin North Am.* 2018, 47 (2):441–449.

56. Jolly K, Darr A, Arlt W, et al. Surgery for Cushing's disease in pregnancy: Our experience and a literature review. *Ann R Coll Surg Engl.* 2019, 101(1): e26–e31.

57. Close CF, Mann MC, Watts JF, et al. ACTH-independent Cushing's syndrome in pregnancy with spontaneous resolution after delivery: Control of the hypercortisolism with metyrapone. *Clin Endocrinol (Oxf).* 1993, 39 (3):375–379.

58. Connell JM, Cordiner J, Davies DL, et al. Pregnancy complicated by Cushing's syndrome: Potential hazard of metyrapone therapy. *Case report. Br J Obstet Gynaecol.* 1985, 92(11):1192–1195.

59. Zieleniewski W, and Michalak R. A successful case of pregnancy in a woman with ACTH-independent Cushing's syndrome treated with ketoconazole and metyrapone. *Gynecol Endocrinol.* 2017, 33 (5):349–352.

60. Berwaerts J, Verhelst J, Mahler C, et al. Cushing's syndrome in pregnancy treated by ketoconazole: Case report and review of the literature. *Gynecol Endocrinol.* 1999, 13 (3):175–182.

61. Yang Y, Reincke M, and Williams TA. Prevalence, diagnosis and outcomes of treatment for primary aldosteronism. *Best Pract Res Clin Endocrinol Metab.* 2020, 34(2):101365.

62. Mulatero P, Stowasser M, Loh KC, et al. Increased diagnosis of primary aldosteronism, including surgically correctable forms, in centers from five continents. *J Clin Endocrinol Metab.* 2004, 89 (3):1045–1050.

63. Prada ETA, Burrello J, Reincke M, et al. Old and new concepts in the molecular pathogenesis of primary aldosteronism. *Hypertension.* 2017, 70 (5):875–881.

64. Sanga V, Lenzini L, Seccia TM, et al. Familial hyperaldosteronism type 1 and pregnancy: Successful treatment with low dose dexamethasone. *Blood Press.* 2021, 1–5.

65. Morton A. Primary aldosteronism and pregnancy. *Pregnancy Hypertens.* 2015, 5 (4):259–262.

66. Malha L, and August P. Secondary hypertension in pregnancy. *Curr Hypertens Rep.* 2015, 17(7):53.

67. Zelinka T, Petrák O, Rosa J, et al. Primary aldosteronism and pregnancy. *Kidney Blood Press Res.* 2020, 45(2):275–285.

68. Corsello SM, and Paragliola RM. Evaluation and management of endocrine hypertension during pregnancy. *Endocrinol Metab Clin North Am.* 2019, 48 (4):829–842.

69. Hecker A, Hasan SH, and Neumann F. Disturbances in sexual differentiation of rat foetuses following spironolactone treatment. *Acta Endocrinol (Copenh).* 1980, 95 (4):540–545.

70. Riester A, and Reincke M. Progress in primary aldosteronism: Mineralocorticoid receptor antagonists and management of primary aldosteronism in pregnancy. *Eur J Endocrinol.* 2015, 172(1):R23–30.

71. Harrington JL, Farley DR, van Heerden JA, et al. Adrenal tumors and pregnancy. *World J Surg.* 1999, 23(2):182–186.

72. Wing LA, Conaglen JV, Meyer-Rochow GY, et al. Paraganglioma in pregnancy: A case series and review of the literature. *J Clin Endocrinol Metab.* 2015, 100(8):3202–3209.

73. Bancos I, Atkinson E, Eng C, et al. Maternal and fetal outcomes in phaeochromocytoma and pregnancy: A multicentre retrospective cohort study and systematic review of literature. *Lancet Diabetes Endocrinol.* 2021, 9(1):13–21.

74. Manoharan M, Sinha P, and Sibtain S. Adrenal disorders in pregnancy, labour and postpartum – An overview. *J Obstet Gynaecol.* 2020, 40 (6):749–758.

75. Affinati AH, and Auchus RJ. Endocrine causes of hypertension in pregnancy. *Gland Surg.* 2020, 9(1):69–79.

76. Lenders JW, Duh QY, Eisenhofer G, et al. Pheochromocytoma and paraganglioma: An endocrine society clinical practice guideline. *J Clin Endocrinol Metab.* 2014, 99 (6):1915–1942.

77. Guidelines for Diagnostic Imaging During Pregnancy and Lactation. Committee Opinion No. 723. *Obstet Gynecol.* 2017, 130(2): e210–216.

78. Crona J, Taïeb D, and Pacak K. New perspectives on pheochromocytoma and paraganglioma: Toward a molecular classification. *Endocr Rev.* 2017, 38 (6):489–515.

79. Gaujoux S, Hain É, Marcellin L, et al. Adrenalectomy during pregnancy: A 15-year experience at a tertiary referral center. *Surgery.* 2020, 168(2):335–339.

80. Oliva R, Angelos P, Kaplan E, et al. Pheochromocytoma in pregnancy: A case series and review. *Hypertension.* 2010, 55 (3):600–606.

81. Fassnacht M, Kroiss M, and Allolio B. Update in adrenocortical carcinoma. *J Clin Endocrinol Metab.* 2013, 98(12):4551–4564.

82. Abiven-Lepage G, Coste J, Tissier F, et al. Adrenocortical carcinoma and pregnancy: Clinical and biological features and prognosis. *Eur J Endocrinol.* 2010, 163 (5):793–800.

83. Raffin-Sanson ML, Abiven G, Ritzel K, et al. Adrenocortical carcinoma and pregnancy. *Ann Endocrinol.* 2016, 77(2):139–147.

84. Zhang Y, Yuan Z, Qiu C, et al. The diagnosis and treatment of adrenocortical carcinoma in pregnancy: A case report. *BMC Pregnancy Childbirth.* 2020, 20(1):50.

85. de Corbière P, Ritzel K, Cazabat L, et al. Pregnancy in women previously treated for an adrenocortical carcinoma. *J Clin Endocrinol Metab.* 2015, 100 (12):4604–4611.

Chapter

16

Hormones and Multiple Pregnancy

Viola Seravalli, Noemi Strambi, and Mariarosaria Di Tommaso

16.1 Hormone Levels in Multiple Pregnancies

The levels of hormones in multiple pregnancies have been compared to singleton pregnancies in a limited number of studies (1–5). While in some cases increased concentrations seem to confer an advantage, as in the case of human chorionic gonadotropin (hCG), in other cases, higher levels of certain hormones have been linked to an increased risk of developing complications, such as gestational diabetes or cholestasis, in multiple pregnancies compared to singletons.

16.1.1 Human Chorionic Gonadotropin (hCG)

In multiple gestations, the levels of hCG are significantly higher compared to singleton pregnancies (6,7). In the first trimester, the levels of β-hCG measured in maternal blood are more than two-fold higher in twin pregnancies (3). The hCG in pregnancy has multiple functions: It contributes to the maintenance of the ovarian corpus luteum in early pregnancy, it regulates fetal and placental steroidogenesis, and it promotes maternal immune tolerance and trophoblast differentiation required for a successful pregnancy (8). The observation of higher circulating levels of hCG in women carrying a twin pregnancy is probably related to the number of feto-placental units and a larger placental mass, and it might explain the lower incidence of early pregnancy loss observed after assisted reproduction in twins compared to singleton pregnancies (9,10).

16.1.2 Steroid Hormones
16.1.2.1 Estrogens
Higher serum levels of estradiol (E2) and estriol (E3) have been detected in serum and urine in mothers carrying twins compared to singletons

(1–5,11) (Table 16.1). At 20 weeks of gestation, reported mean estrogen serum levels are roughly 1.5 times higher in twin gestations compared to singletons (2). A significant difference is also observed at 26 weeks, when E2 and E3 levels are 1.4 and 1.9 times higher in twin gestations, respectively (4), and at the time of delivery (2). When monozygotic twin pregnancies are compared to dizygotic pregnancies, no significant differences in estrogen concentration in maternal blood are found (2), suggesting that zygosity does not influence maternal hormonal levels in twin gestations.

The higher levels of estrogens in multiple pregnancies may play a role in the increased risk of some pregnancy complications. The prevalence of intrahepatic cholestasis of pregnancy (ICP) is four to five times greater in twin pregnancies compared to singletons (11,12), and this could be related to higher levels of estrogens, as evidence suggests that estrogens are involved in the pathogenesis of ICP in genetically predisposed women (13–15). In experimental animal models, administration of estrogen derivatives is able to induce ICP, which appears to be related to the impaired expression and/or function of specific transporter proteins (16). Multiple pregnancies are also believed to be associated with greater insulin resistance and a higher risk of developing gestational diabetes mellitus (17,18). Although higher age and greater weight gain in mothers carrying twins may contribute to this association, this effect has mainly been attributed to increased levels of hormones such as estrogens, progesterone, and human placental lactogen that may influence the frequency of gestational diabetes through their insulin antagonistic effects (18).

16.1.2.2 Progesterone
Concentrations in twin pregnancies are reported to be 1.5–1.8 times higher than in singletons at 20 and 26 weeks, respectively, and also at the time

183

Table 16.1. Studies comparing maternal serum levels of steroid hormones in twin and singleton pregnancies

Study	Hormones tested	Time of sampling	Number of subjects	Main findings (in twin pregnancies compared to singletons)
Kuijper et al. 2015 (2)	Estrogens (E1, E2, E3), Progesterone	18–22 weeks and at delivery	Singletons: 247 Twins: 203	Increased levels of E1, E2, E3, and P ($p < 0.05$)
Smith et al. 2009 (4)	Estrogens (E2, E3), Progesterone	26 weeks	Singletons: 456 Twins: 10	Increased levels of E2, E3, and P ($p < 0.05$)
Houghton et al. 2019 (1)	Estrogens (E2, E3), Testosterone	Third trimester and at delivery	Singletons: 62 Twins: 41	Increased levels of E2, E3 and T ($p < 0.05$) (differences not exceeding 20 percent) No significant difference in testosterone levels
Póvoa et al. 2018 (3)	Estrogens (E2)	8–9^{+6} weeks	Singletons: 50 Twins: 47	Increased levels of E2 ($p < 0.05$)
Thomas et al. 1998 (5)	Estrogens (E2) and Testosterone	6–20 weeks	Singletons: 115 Twins: 11	Increased levels of E2 and T ($p < 0.05$)

E1 = estrone, E2 = estradiol; E3 = estriol; P = progesterone; T = Testosterone

of delivery (Table 16.1) (2,4). As for estrogens, a larger placental volume, and therefore an increased steroid-producing capacity, probably accounts for the higher levels of progesterone in mothers carrying twins.

16.1.2.3 Testosterone

Data on testosterone levels in twin pregnancies are more limited and contradictory (Table 16.1). While maternal serum testosterone concentrations at 6–20 weeks were found to be higher in women carrying twins compared to women carrying a singleton gestation (5), a larger, more recent study failed to find a significant difference in testosterone concentrations in the third trimester and at delivery (1).

16.1.3 Corticotropin Releasing Hormone (CRH)

During pregnancy, the placenta synthetizes CRH and releases it into maternal circulation at increasing levels over the course of gestation, with a dramatic increase during the 5–6 weeks preceding the onset of labor (19). CRH has been linked to numerous functions. It is involved in the signaling systems that control uterine contractions and the timing of birth, as it stimulates prostaglandin synthesis in fetal membranes and placenta

(8). During pregnancy, CRH is also released in response to fetal stress and an increase in maternal CRH levels has been described in pregnancies complicated by pre-term labor, fetal growth restriction, preeclampsia, and fetal asphyxia.

Higher CRH levels have been found in mothers of twins compared to singletons in the third trimester, and also at term, although data are based on a limited number of subjects (4,19). In addition, the rapid rise in plasma CRH levels which occurs near term in singleton gestation seems to occur earlier in twin gestations, even when twin pregnancies complicated by pre-term labor are removed from the analysis (4,19). It seems likely that the early rise in maternal plasma CRH and the high levels seen in twin gestations may contribute to the increased incidence of pre-term labor observed in multiple gestations, in addition to mechanical factors such as the increased uterine volume and increased uterine wall tension.

16.1.4 Human Placental Lactogen (HPL)

The HPL is an insulin-antagonist produced by the syncytiotrophoblast, and it is thought to mediate the diabetogenic effect of pregnancy. It antagonizes insulin action, inducing glucose intolerance, lipolysis, and proteolysis in the maternal system, and favoring the transfer of glucose and amino acids to the fetus. It seems to exert its metabolic effects through stimulation of IGF-1. The levels of HPL have been demonstrated to be significantly higher in twins compared to singletons (20), and this, combined with the increase in estrogen levels, might contribute to the higher risk of developing gestational diabetes in multiple compared to singleton pregnancies (21).

16.1.4.1 Effect of Hormonal Profiles of Twin Pregnancies on the Offspring

Some studies have suggested a number of effects of prenatal hormone exposure on the offspring in twin pregnancies. In particular, it was suggested that a higher estrogen exposure in dizygotic twins could play a role in the development of hormone-related tumors such as breast, prostate, or testicular cancer (22,23). Kuijper et al. (2) collected maternal serum around mid-pregnancy and at the time of delivery, and umbilical cord blood at birth from a large cohort of twin pregnancies and singleton control subjects. Surprisingly, they found that both estrogens and progesterone were lower in the umbilical cord blood of twin neonates compared to singletons, challenging the general assumption that maternal serum hormone levels are a reflection of actual fetal hormone exposure and that twins are overexposed to estrogens and progesterone at time of birth (2).

Another issue related to hormonal levels in twins that is still controversial is the possible influence of a twin of a certain sex on the hormonal status of a co-twin of the other sex during pregnancy, deriving from the observation of reproductive and behavioral differences between same-sex and opposite-sex female twins. The hypothesis of an overexposure to androgens and consequent masculinization of the female fetus in opposite-sex twins (24) has not been confirmed in studies on cord blood sample from dizygotic twins, where girls of an opposite sex twin did not show higher serum androgen concentrations compared with same-sex twin girls (2,25). It is possible that the masculinizing effects reported in opposite-sex twin girls are caused by factors that are not reflected by the measurement of cord blood hormone levels at birth. The issue of the possible influence of a twin of a certain sex on the hormonal status of a co-twin of the other sex during gestation remains a matter of debate.

It is noteworthy that the cord blood concentration of certain hormones measured at birth is a surrogate marker of the actual fetal hormonal levels, which cannot be measured directly in the fetus during gestation without significant risks for the pregnancy. Although it might not precisely reflect fetal steroid exposure during pregnancy, the collection of cord blood at birth is currently the most practical method of approximating circulating fetal hormones in normal pregnancy, as long as proper assay is employed and confounding factors, such as the possible influence of obstetric and perinatal factors, are taken into account (26).

16.2 Pathophysiology of Pre-term Delivery in Multiple Pregnancies

16.2.1 Epidemiology and Pathophysiology of Pre-term Birth in Multiple Pregnancies

Multiple pregnancies have a higher risk of pre-term delivery (PTD), defined as delivery before 37 completed weeks of gestation. More than half of twin pregnancies deliver pre-term, accounting for up to 20 percent of all pre-term births in Europe and United States. These include both spontaneous and medically indicated PTD. The multifactorial pathophysiology of spontaneous PTD remains partly unknown, even in singletons, also because the ultimate mechanisms leading to the onset of labor are incompletely understood. Physiologically, when pregnancy reaches term, the increased volume and wall tension of the uterus, the augmented production of CRH by the placenta and the increased surfactant protein secreted by the mature fetal lung act as signals for the initiation of parturition, stimulating the release of cytokines. The activation of inflammatory signaling determines an increased expression of gap junctions, prostaglandin and oxytocin receptors in the myometrium, and changes in progesterone receptor expression, which determines a functional progesterone withdrawal. Multiple pathological mechanisms including intrauterine infection, stress, and uterine over-distension may induce premature activation of this process with consequent PTD.

Although the association between multiple pregnancy and pre-term birth has been largely

185

recognized, it is yet not fully understood what factors predispose an early delivery of multiple pregnancies and if the risk factors and pathological mechanisms that are associated with pre-term birth in singleton pregnancies also apply to multiple gestations.

16.2.2 Hormonal Profiles and Pre-term Delivery in Multiple Gestations

Higher circulating levels of CRH, likely derived from the larger placental mass, and higher CRH percentage daily change, have been described in twin pregnancies (4,27) and this, in conjunction with the higher uterine volume, may contribute to the substantial increase in PTD rate in twins (28). CRH effects on the onset of labor are mediated by the increase in estrogen release and the altered progesterone/estrogen ratio induced by CRH, and also by the effect that it has on myometrial contractility. CRH also has a pro-inflammatory action, it induces the release of chemokines and cytokines in the myometrium at term, and it modulates prostaglandin production by the placenta and fetal membranes (8).

In singletons pregnancies, high salivary estriol and lower saliva progesterone concentrations have been associated with spontaneous pre-term delivery (29,30). When analyzed in twin pregnancies, serial progesterone and estrogen levels in saliva and serum were not significantly different between women delivering at term and those delivering pre-term (31). Furthermore, no correlation between plasma steroid hormone concentrations and cervical length or gestational age at delivery has been found (32). These findings suggest that twin and singleton pregnancies present intrinsic differences in the hormone trajectories. It is possible that the higher median hormone concentrations in twins make the differences between pregnancies delivering pre-term and those delivering at term less evident than in singletons (31).

During pregnancy, uterine quiescence is maintained by progesterone, and functional progesterone receptors inactivation is involved in the initiation of human labor and parturition. For this reason, progesterone has been introduced to treat women at risk of PTD, and it has been shown to be effective in patients with singleton gestations and a history of PTD and in pregnancies with a detected short cervix in the second trimester (33,34). However, its efficacy has not been confirmed in twin pregnancies (35,36), and one study showed that 200 mg vaginal progesterone treatment does not increase the circulating progesterone concentration in twin pregnancies (35). As already discussed, progesterone concentrations in twin pregnancies have found to be higher than in singletons throughout gestation. However, ratios of P/E2, P/E3, and E3/E2 were surprisingly shown to be similar up to the early third trimester of pregnancy. A clinical consequence for progesterone supplementation in twin pregnancies is that to provide a similar P/E3 ratio to that seen in term singleton pregnancies, (where?) a higher dose may be required (4).

The greater degree of stretch to which the myometrium in a multiple pregnancy is exposed compared to singleton pregnancies, due to the over-distension created by accommodating an extra fetus, is often presented as one of the main factors leading to pre-term labor in twin pregnancies. However, supporting data for this hypothesis is lacking, and there appears to be very little research comparing myometrium from singleton and multiple pregnancy groups. In nonlaboring myometrium from singleton and multiple pregnancies, no difference in gap junction proteins and no effect of stretch on the expression of such proteins were observed (37).

Some authors have suggested that the predisposition of twin pregnancy to premature labor may be the result of a different expression of oxytocin receptors in the myometrium (38). The hypothesis that the uterus during a twin pregnancy might be more receptive to oxytocin at an earlier gestational age comes from the *in vitro* observation that frequency of contractions and responses to oxytocin are increased in myometrium from twin pregnancies (than compared to?) myometrium from singletons. The contractile activity was also found to correlate with the increasing levels of stretch (39). Further studies on larger samples and also on laboring myometrium would be needed to explore differences in the expression pattern of a number of proteins associated with contraction and its modulation in twins. More information could be acquired using newer advanced technologies to study gene expression, for a better understanding of the uterine physiology and application of this information to problems in pregnancy and labor (40).

16.3 Conclusions

The biological mechanism by which pre-term delivery occurs might be different in twin and singleton pregnancies. Further research should focus on singleton-twin differences in placental hormones profiles and in the mechanisms involved in twin pre-term delivery, which may require different preventive and therapeutic strategies compared to singleton pregnancies.

References

1. Houghton LC, Lauria M, Maas P, et al. Circulating maternal and umbilical cord steroid hormone and insulin-like growth factor concentrations in twin and singleton pregnancies. *J Dev Orig Health Dis.* 2019, 10 (2):232–236.

2. Kuijper EA, Twisk JW, Korsen T, et al. Mid-pregnancy, perinatal, and neonatal reproductive endocrinology: A prospective cohort study in twins and singleton control subjects. *Fertil Steril.* 2015, 104 (6):1527–15234.e1–9.

3. Póvoa A, Xavier P, Matias A, et al. First trimester β-hCG and estradiol levels in singleton and twin pregnancies after assisted reproduction. *J Perinat Med.* 2018, 46(8):853–856.

4. Smith R, Smith JI, Shen X, et al. Patterns of plasma corticotropin-releasing hormone, progesterone, estradiol, and estriol change and the onset of human labor. *J Clin Endocrinol Metab.* 2009, 94(6):2066–2074.

5. Thomas HV, Murphy MF, Key TJ, et al. Pregnancy and menstrual hormone levels in mothers of twins compared to mothers of singletons. *Ann Hum Biol.* 1998, 25(1):69–75.

6. Fridström M, Garoff L, Sjöblom P, et al. Human chorionic gonadotropin patterns in early pregnancy after assisted reproduction. *Acta Obstet Gynecol Scand.* 1995, 74(7):534–538.

7. Norman RJ, McLoughlin JW, Borthwick GM, et al. Inhibin and relaxin concentrations in early singleton, multiple, and failing pregnancy: Relationship to gonadotropin and steroid profiles. *Fertil Steril.* 1993, 59 (1):130–137.

8. Seravalli V, Di Tommaso M, Challis JR, et al. *Endocrinology of maternal-placental axis.* In: Petraglia F, C FB, (Eds.). *Female Reproductive Dysfunction.* 2020; 397–410. Springer, Cham.

9. Lambers MJ, Mager E, Goutbeek J, et al. Factors determining early pregnancy loss in singleton and multiple implantations. *Hum Reprod.* 2007, 22(1):275–279.

10. Matias A, La Sala GB, and Blickstein I. Early loss rates of entire pregnancies after assisted reproduction are lower in twin than in singleton pregnancies. *Fertil Steril.* 2007, 88 (5):1452–1454.

11. Gonzalez MC, Reyes H, Arrese M, et al. Intrahepatic cholestasis of pregnancy in twin pregnancies. *J Hepatol.* 1989, 9(1):84–90.

12. Gardiner FW, McCuaig R, Arthur C, et al. The prevalence and pregnancy outcomes of intrahepatic cholestasis of pregnancy: A retrospective clinical audit review. *Obstet Med.* 2019, 12(3):123–128.

13. Arrese M, and Reyes H. Intrahepatic cholestasis of pregnancy: A past and present riddle. *Ann Hepatol.* 2006, 5 (3):202–205.

14. Lammert F, Marschall HU, Glantz A, et al. Intrahepatic cholestasis of pregnancy: Molecular pathogenesis, diagnosis and management. *J Hepatol.* 2000, 33 (6):1012–1021.

15. Reyes H, and Simon FR. Intrahepatic cholestasis of pregnancy: An estrogen-related disease. *Semin Liver Dis.* 1993, 13(3):289–301.

16. Wagner M, and Trauner M. Transcriptional regulation of hepatobiliary transport systems in health and disease: Implications for a rationale approach to the treatment of intrahepatic cholestasis. *Ann Hepatol.* 2005, 4(2):77–99.

17. Alkaabi J, Almazrouei R, Zoubeidi T, et al. Burden, associated risk factors and adverse outcomes of gestational diabetes mellitus in twin pregnancies in Al Ain, UAE. *BMC Pregnancy Childbirth.* 2020, 20(1):612.

18. Schwartz DB, Daoud Y, Zazula P, et al. Gestational diabetes mellitus: Metabolic and blood glucose parameters in singleton versus twin pregnancies. *Am J Obstet Gynecol.* 1999, 181 (4):912–914.

19. Warren WB, Goland RS, Wardlaw SL, et al. Elevated maternal plasma corticotropin releasing hormone levels in twin gestation. *J Perinat Med.* 1990, 18(1):39–44.

20. Spellacy WN, Buhi WC, and Birk SA. Human placental lactogen levels in multiple pregnancies. *Obstet Gynecol.* 1978, 52(2):210–212.

21. Roach VJ, Lau TK, Wilson D, et al. The incidence of gestational diabetes in multiple pregnancy. *Aust N Z J Obstet Gynaecol.* 1998, 38(1):56–57.

22. Swerdlow AJ, De Stavola BL, Swanwick MA, et al. Risks of breast and testicular cancers in young adult twins in England

and Wales: Evidence on prenatal and genetic aetiology. *Lancet.* 1997, 350 (9093):1723–1728.

23. Trichopoulos D. Hypothesis: Does breast cancer originate in utero? *Lancet.* 1990, 335 (8695):939–940.

24. Tapp AL, Maybery MT, and Whitehouse AJ. Evaluating the twin testosterone transfer hypothesis: A review of the empirical evidence. *Horm Behav.* 2011, 60(5): 713–722.

25. Galiano V, Solazzo G, Rabinovici J, et al. Cord blood androgen levels of females from same sex and opposite sex twins – A pilot study. *Clin Endocrinol (Oxf).* 2021, 94 (1):85–89.

26. Hollier LP, Keelan JA, Hickey M, et al. Measurement of androgen and estrogen concentrations in cord blood: accuracy, biological interpretation, and applications to understanding human behavioral development. *Front Endocrinol (Lausanne).* 2014, 5:64.

27. TambyRaja RL, and Ratnam SS. Plasma steroid changes in twin pregnancies. *Prog Clin Biol Res.* 1981;69a:189–195.

28. Stock S, and Norman J. Preterm and term labour in multiple pregnancies. *Semin Fetal Neonatal Med.* 2010, 15 (6):336–341.

29. Heine RP, McGregor JA, Goodwin TM, et al. Serial salivary estriol to detect an increased risk of preterm birth.

Obstet Gynecol. 2000, 96 (4):490–497.

30. Lachelin GC, McGarrigle HH, Seed PT, et al. Low saliva progesterone concentrations are associated with spontaneous early preterm labour (before 34 weeks of gestation) in women at increased risk of preterm delivery. *BJOG.* 2009, 116 (11):1515–1519.

31. Lim H, Powell S, McNamara HC, et al. Placental hormone profiles as predictors of preterm birth in twin pregnancy: A prospective cohort study. *PLoS ONE.* 2017, 12(3):e0173732.

32. Johnsson VL, Pedersen NG, Worda K, et al. Plasma progesterone, estradiol, and unconjugated estriol concentrations in twin pregnancies: Relation with cervical length and preterm delivery. *Acta Obstet Gynecol Scand.* 2019, 98(1):86–94.

33. da Fonseca EB, Bittar RE, Carvalho MH, et al. Prophylactic administration of progesterone by vaginal suppository to reduce the incidence of spontaneous preterm birth in women at increased risk: A randomized placebo-controlled double-blind study. *Am J Obstet Gynecol.* 2003, 188(2):419–424.

34. Hassan SS, Romero R, Vidyadhari D, et al. Vaginal progesterone reduces the rate of preterm birth in women with a sonographic short cervix: A multicenter, randomized, double-blind,

placebo-controlled trial. *Ultrasound Obstet Gynecol.* 2011, 38(1):18–31.

35. Norman JE, Mackenzie F, Owen P, et al. Progesterone for the prevention of preterm birth in twin pregnancy (STOPPIT): A randomised, double-blind, placebo-controlled study and meta-analysis. *Lancet.* 2009, 373(9680):2034–2040.

36. Rouse DJ, Caritis SN, Peaceman AM, et al. A trial of 17 alpha-hydroxyprogesterone caproate to prevent prematurity in twins. *N Engl J Med.* 2007, 357(5):454–461.

37. Lyall F, Lye S, Teoh T, et al. Expression of Gsalpha, connexin-43, connexin-26, and EP1, 3, and 4 receptors in myometrium of prelabor singleton versus multiple gestations and the effects of mechanical stretch and steroids on Gsalpha. *J Soc Gynecol Investig.* 2002, 9(5):299–307.

38. Turton P, Neilson JP, Quenby S, et al. A short review of twin pregnancy and how oxytocin receptor expression may differ in multiple pregnancy. *Eur J Obstet Gynecol Reprod Biol.* 2009, 144 Suppl 1:S40–44.

39. Turton P, Arrowsmith S, Prescott J, et al. A comparison of the contractile properties of myometrium from singleton and twin pregnancies. *PLoS ONE.* 2013, 8(5):e63800.

40. Wray S. Insights from physiology into myometrial function and dysfunction. *Exp Physiol.* 2015, 100 (12):1468–1476.

Chapter

17

Hormones in Pregnancy and the Developmental Origins of Health and Disease

John R. G. Challis, Felice Petraglia, Deborah M. Sloboda,
Victor K. M. Han, and Judith G. Hall

17.1 Introduction

An adversely altered developmental trajectory is a major contributor to the global proliferation of noncommunicable diseases (NCD). The United Nations General Assembly has recognized that many noncommunicable diseases are inherently preventable. The COVID-19 pandemic has brought into focus the interactions between infection, the importance of maintaining a "One Health" approach to global population health, the environment including climate controls, and implications for manifestation of NCD's.

In this chapter we discuss the influences of pregnancy, the hormones and physiological adaptations of pregnancy, to Developmental Origins of Health and Disease (DOHaD). We will examine ways of predicting predisposition to noncommunicable conditions and begin to suggest how that knowledge might be applied to the diagnosis, avoidance, intervention, and prevention of noncommunicable disease in newborns, children, adolescents, and youth, as well as in adults across health disciplines. The discussion applies to Indigenous and immigrant populations as well as non-Indigenous sectors in a manner that addresses social inequities in health provision, altered clinical practice, and informed government policy.

17.2 Early Background

The role of pregnancy and of the placenta in fetal development and later life noncommunicable diseases gathered increased attention following the observations of David Barker and Clive Osmond in the late 1980's (1,2). These researchers showed an inverse relationship between weight at birth, measured within the normal birth weight range, in several cohorts of individuals in the 1920's, with their blood pressure and risk of death from cardiovascular disease in later life at age 60+. This inverse relationship persisted for relative risk of developing glucose intolerance or diabetes. Barker's observations were initially greeted with some skepticism but were substantiated in many other studies, most importantly in the US Nurses Cohort (3). In addition, Barker found that the birth weight/placental weight relationship predicted, on a population basis, systolic blood pressure in later life. Those individuals with higher birth weight and low placental weight had lower systolic blood pressures at age 50, whereas individuals with low birth weight and higher placental weight had substantially elevated blood pressure. It was as though the placenta underwent hypertrophy in an attempt to support the fetus and ensure its survival in an apparently compromised intra-uterine environment.

A major criticism of Barker's original observations was that while they demonstrated an association between birth weight and later life blood pressure, experimental evidence in support of the observations was lacking. Soon, however, Langley-Evans and colleagues (4) showed that pregnant rats fed a diet that was low (9 percent) in the protein casein, compared to 18 percent casein controls, delivered pups with lower birth weight and increased placental weight. These low-birth-weight pups (of mothers fed low protein diets) at 16 weeks' postnatal age had increased systolic blood pressure and were insulin resistant. These experimental findings recapitulated the epidemiological observations of Barker. They showed that birth weight was in effect, a surrogate measure for the intra-uterine environment that altered fetal growth and development, and not a "cause" of later life disease. Later Lillycrop et al. (5) showed that the low protein diet produced methylation changes in critical genes in the liver of pups from these underfed pregnancies, opening the door to an epigenetic basis for understanding developmental programming. In landmark papers, Meaney et al. (6) proposed an epigenetic basis for the effects of maternal undernutrition on fetal birth weights and the subsequent later life predisposition to metabolic and cardiovascular disease.

In addition to nutritional deprivation, experimental studies showed that maternal stress, mimicked in part by administering the synthetic glucocorticoid betamethasone to normally fed pregnant rats, produced intrauterine growth restriction and increased blood pressure in the offspring at 16 weeks of age (7). In other studies, inhibition of placental 11 beta hydroxysteroid dehydrogenase 11beta hydroxysteroid dehydrogenase2 (11beta HSD2) enzyme, resulted in intra uterine growth restriction (IUGR). Placental 11beta HSD2 metabolizes maternal corticosteroid and regulates the transplacental transfer of active corticosteroid from mother to fetus. In its absence or with reduced activity, more maternal corticosterone (in the rat) or cortisol (in human pregnancy) crosses the placenta from mother to fetus. In pregnant rats, there was no effect of placental 11beta HSD inhibition after maternal adrenalectomy, but the growth restriction again occurred with maternal glucocorticoid administration. Hence, maternal under-nutrition and maternal stress both impaired fetal growth, resulting in lower birth weight and later life predisposition towards hypertension. These may be separate actions, or the effects of nutrition may be exacerbated by maternal stress or mediated by stress responses, of mother and/or fetus (8,9).

To recapitulate, the DOHaD paradigm refers to an adaptation during development that predisposes an individual or population to later life chronic disorder or disease. Others quickly showed that there may be sex differences in these responses and profound inter-generational epigenetic effects, which in humans are most evident in vulnerable populations and amongst Indigenous groups. The vulnerability varies during the life course and contributes to health inequities.

17.3 Human Studies

Tessa Roseboom and colleagues in Amsterdam conducted an extensive series of studies in which they have been able to observe the impact of extreme malnutrition in a human population (10). During the Dutch Hunger winter of 1944–1945, more than 22,000 persons, including women at various stages of pregnancy, were subjected to extreme famine and cold. If hunger occurred in women during the first trimester of pregnancy, the offspring had an increased risk of developing hypertension as adults. In contrast, if hunger occurred in women later in pregnancy, their offspring were born low birth weight and, as adults, had increased adiposity and glucose intolerance.

Later it became clear from studies in Helsinki, that the effects of the intrauterine environment in pregnancy were interwoven with growth and metabolism in the early postnatal years (11). Hence, children with low body mass indices (BMI) at 2 years of age who developed higher BMI at 11 years were at far greater risk of developing coronary heart disease as adults than children with higher BMI at 2 years who maintained similar BMI ratios at 11 years. Returning to the neonatal (up to 28 days after birth) and early infancy period, these and other findings challenge the practice of promoting rapid weight gain in underweight babies – "catch-up growth" – placing them on an inappropriate developmental trajectory, with associated risk of their becoming glucose intolerant at a later stage of life (12).

Collectively, these observations support the thesis advanced by Gluckman and Hanson of "Match – Mismatch" (13,14). Gluckman and Hanson posited that the fetus in utero adjusts to its environment in a manner that is predictive of the anticipated environment ex utero. This is clearly of evolutionary significance. If, for example, diet is compromised in pregnancy, the fetus adjusts its metabolism and physiology accordingly, and if diet continues to be restricted after birth, that individual has a lower risk of developing hypertension and diabetogenic response than the individual undernourished during pregnancy and exposed to excess nutrition or high fat diet postnatally.

17.4 The Role of the Placenta

The placenta has a central role in mediating these responses through nutrient transfer and selective barrier mechanisms (15). As discussed throughout this volume, the placenta regulates transfer of nutrients, gases, and hormones between mother and fetus. Placental size and morphology are regulated by cell number, barrier thickness, surface, and volume density that determine the impact of blood flow changes and vascular resistance. Placental transporters such as GLUT-1-3 and the System A transporter determine glucose and amino acid fluxes and, as discussed, enzymes such as 11 beta HSD regulate glucocorticoid transfer between mother and fetus (15,16). In turn, the placenta produces hormones including sex steroids and placental lactogen that alter maternal metabolism and the availability of maternal nutrients to the feto-maternal unit. Recent studies have shown clearly that the placenta adapts to the pregnancy environment with altered morphology, developmental markers, and transport proteins, in response to undernutrition for example, or to exposure of pregnant animals to a high fat diet (17).

One example of such an adaptation is the Placental System A amino acid transporter, located in the syncytiotrophoblast, that transports small unbranched neutral amino acids between mother and fetus (18). It is composed of at least three isoforms SNAT1, SNAT2, SNAT4, encoded by different genes. Placental System A is critically associated with fetal growth. In the human, its activity is reduced in the placenta of pregnancies with growth restricted fetuses, and in animals, inhibition of System A activity across gestation results in reductions in fetal weight. Furthermore, pregnant mice treated with dexamethasone at 13.5 and 14.5 days of pregnancy (term is ~20 days) have reduced System A transporter activity during the remainder of gestation (19). This suppressive action was similar for placentae of both male and female fetuses. Of interest, however, was the finding that although there is a progressive increase in System A activity in normal pregnancy, which is associated with increased expression of SNAT genes, the decrease in activity after dexamethasone was not associated with changes in gene expression. It was postulated that the action of the glucocorticoid might be exerted at the level of translation or incorporation of the transporter protein into the trophoblast membrane.

17.5 Stress and Glucocorticoids

In essentially every animal species that has been studied, there is an increase in biologically active glucocorticoid in the fetal circulation in late pregnancy, and evidence is accumulating that this rise is associated with pre-partum activation of the fetal HPA axis (20,21). Fetal glucocorticoids modulate a developmental switch, moving away from cellular proliferation towards cellular differentiation, thus promoting maturation of key organ systems, including the lungs, brain, and kidney, that are necessary for extra-uterine survival. However, the HPA axis itself is a target of programming. Administration of small amount of synthetic glucocorticoid to sheep during the first one third of pregnancy produced prolonged changes in fetal HPA axis activity and adrenal responses (22). Altered function of the fetal HPA axis may lead to impaired growth and altered neurologic, metabolic, and cardiovascular activity, effects that are observed in subsequent generations with transmission through either maternal or paternal lineages (23). For example, Reynolds and colleagues (24), in a series of pioneering studies, showed in adult men and women that high fasting cortisol levels and increased adrenal responsiveness to ACTH stimulation was associated with low birth weight, decades earlier. These effects on the HPA axis result from actions on the fetal epigenome and may include changes in DNA methylation, histone acetylation, and microRNAs, to alter gene expression (24,25).

Almost 20 years ago, Bloomfield et al. (26) showed that after pregnant sheep were mildly undernourished from before conception and for the first 30 days of pregnancy, there was a high incidence of pre-term birth. Those lambs born early had a precocious increase in fetal hypothalamic-pituitary adrenal (HPA) function, expressed as rises in fetal plasma adrenocorticotropic hormone (ACTH) and cortisol concentrations and increased pro-opiomelanocortin (POMC) gene expression, surprisingly in the fetal pituitary *pars intermedia* rather than the *pars distalis* (27). In the placentae, expression of 11beta HSD2 (converting active cortisol to inactive cortisone) was reduced after periconceptional undernutrition, resulting in significantly higher cortisol concentrations in the fetal circulation compared to control animals (28). This cortisol must have come from the mother, after transplacental transfer, because the fetal adrenal is known to be relatively inactive at this stage of gestation. In pregnancies with a singleton fetus, periconceptional undernutrition resulted in reduced methylation of the promoter region of the hypothalamic glucocorticoid receptor (GR) and corresponding increase in hypothalamic GR mRNA expression in the fetuses at term (29). Concurrently there was a decrease in hypothalamic DNA methyltransferase activity. These changes were programmed such that at 4 years after birth, GR mRNA expression was still elevated in hypothalamus of adult male and female sheep born from mothers that had been undernourished at the beginning of pregnancy (30). Importantly, this change was associated with a decrease in expression of POMC, an anorectic precursor protein, in these mature animals. Thus, maternal periconceptional nutritional status at the beginning of pregnancy appears to program permanent changes in gene expression in term fetuses and adult animals at four years of age. This is associated with a decrease in cortisol metabolizing activity in the placenta, a response replicated in preliminary studies of placental 11betaHSD2 protein levels in women who dieted to lose weight before conception (31).

The above studies indicate an important role of fetal glucocorticoids in programming and of regulating fetal glucocorticoid concentrations by different mechanisms during pregnancy. Fetal adrenocortical activity can be increased in response to hypoxia, for example at high altitude, with decreased umbilical or uterine blood flow, as well as placental insufficiency and in human clinical conditions such as preeclampsia (20). Maternal nutritional status contributes to "fetal nutrition," but this relationship is complicated by alterations in uterine and umbilical blood flows as well as in the expression of placental transporters. Maternal undernutrition as well as other maternal stressors will elevate maternal glucocorticoid concentrations, which may affect fetal glucocorticoid levels directly and/or fetal adrenal maturation (32). Maternal undernutrition also decreases placental 11beta HSD2 activity and alters availability of bioactive glucocorticoid in the placenta (for example in affecting placental CRH gene expression), as well as in the fetus (33,34). These responses are replicated in cases of maternal infection, with hypoxemia, preeclampsia, by maternal ingestion of Liquorice (which inhibits 11beta HSD2 activity), and with elevation of different lipoxygenase metabolites.

Hence, regulation of the placental 11beta HSD2 enzyme that normally serves as a metabolic protector to maintain cortisol values in the fetus at lower levels than the mother, is a critical gatekeeper of fetal development and developmental trajectories (35). The actions of placental 11beta HSD2 can be bypassed by the administration to the mother of synthetic glucocorticoids that are not metabolised by this enzyme. Alexander et al. (36) showed the effects of small changes in fetal glucocorticoid on neurological responses and potentially neurobehavioral development in children. They showed that term born children of mothers treated with betamethasone – a synthetic glucocorticoid in late pregnancy – had increased stress responses, measured as plasma cortisol in a Trier Social Stress Test (TSST) at 6–11 years of age. The effect was more pronounced in girls than in boys. While a single-course antenatal corticosteroid therapy provides substantial benefit to infants delivered preterm, subtle long term effects remain a concern. There is limited information on the impact of exposure to synthetic glucocorticoids of the human fetus at the current dosages used at times in multiple doses at different stages of pregnancy, especially with respect to long term development of the HPA axis, and the neurobehavioral outcomes (37).

Collectively, these observations illustrate that glucocorticoids administered to women in mid- to late-pregnancy may have long term effects in the offspring (15). The reason for sex differences in later responses are unclear but worthy of examination; they emphasize the importance of detailed observations in children of mothers pregnant at different stages of pregnancy during a pandemic such as COVID-19 (38). They emphasize the potential long term effects of toxic stress in both the prenatal and neonatal environment (39,40). Prenatal stress is likely compounded by postnatal physical or mental stress. They are consistent with altered stress responses of children born to mothers who were pregnant during major life-course events including ice storms, earthquakes, forest fires, war/refugee, and other environmental and psychological stresses (41). In a study of the parental rearing behavior of former Swiss indentured child laborers, their offspring reported more physical abuse, higher psychopathology, and higher childhood trauma (42); similar results of children with an almost two-fold increase in developmental vulnerabilities were found in high-risk Aboriginal families compared to healthy families (43). Studies from the Kobor laboratory in Vancouver, and the GUSTO cohort in Singapore (44,45) have shown differential methylation among adolescents whose parents reported high levels of stress during their children's early lives, and the patterning of such epigenetic marks varied by the children's gender. Hence, these responses suggest cross-generational effects, but further longitudinal studies are required.

Importantly, developmental programming can also occur ex utero in the early postnatal environment. In rats, natural variations in maternal grooming activity alters the newborn stress responses through long term changes in gene expression (46). Maternal licking and grooming increases glucocorticoid receptor expression in the hippocampus of pups. The mechanisms include increased histone acetylation mediated by nerve growth factor-inducible protein and can be reversed by postnatal cross fostering and pharmacological manipulations.

In pregnancy, alterations in the developing brain epigenome can result from maternal or fetal stress and from exposure to maternal synthetic glucocorticoids. In an elegant series of studies from the Matthews laboratory in Toronto (47,48), late pregnant guinea pigs were treated with glucocorticoids given in a manner that mimics the human experience of steroid treatment of women presenting in pre-term labor. Differential gene expression was observed in the prefrontal cortex in successive generations (F1, F2, F3) of offspring. A total of 1148 genes were differentially expressed in the F1 generation – 432 in F2 and 438 in F3. There were 22 genes that were differentially regulated in all three generations, with either increased or decreased expression from F1 to F3. Various other reports have shown long lasting altered DNA methylation signatures in brain tissues after stress or glucocorticoid treatment of parental generations, confirming similar changes in methylation responses and neuroendocrine development in successive generations and supporting intergenerational transmission as a critical aspect of neurobehavioral programming, mood, brain disorders, and anxiety responses.

17.6 Reproductive Function

The impact of early life events on later life reproductive health is of signal importance to individuals and to societal progression. Ibanez et al. (49) showed that girls of low birth weight progressively gained more body fat and abdominal fat mass than girls with birth weights appropriate for gestational age. Girls born LGA had decreased levels of SHBG and adiponectin in childhood, FSH hypersecretion in adolescence, and early pubertal onset and early menarche. Slododa and colleagues (50,51) showed that low birth weight and high BMI at eight years of age independently predicted early age at menarche. Girls that were smaller at birth with higher BMI at eight years had earlier menarche whereas, in girls that were larger at birth with lower BMI at eight years, menarche was delayed.

In experimental studies from the Sloboda laboratory (52), offspring of rats that were undernourished during pregnancy entered puberty, but had almost twice the number of irregular reproductive cycles as young adults and showed distinct characteristics of early reproductive ageing compared to controls, including an early loss of ovarian antral follicles. But in western society, overnutrition as well as undernutrition may impact development. In similar studies, offspring of mothers fed a high fat diet had early puberty and disrupted reproductive cyclicity with only 19 percent of offspring showing regular cycles compared to 72 percent controlled offspring (53). Again, these observations are indicators of early ovarian aging. It may be that these impairments in reproductive function are set in place during fetal life. Tsoulis et al. (54) showed that offspring of mothers fed a high fat diet had a reduced number of fetal oocytes and that the number of fetal oocytes was negatively correlated with maternal fat mass. Furthermore, the numbers of pre-pubertal atretic follicles were higher in offspring of mothers fed a high fat diet compared to their control counterparts. Collectively these observations are consistent with an important influence of maternal diet on reproductive performance of female offspring. Further studies are required to determine whether there are critical times in gestation for this activity and whether epigenetic changes in critical pituitary genes are involved.

Low birth weight and pre-term labor are also associated with the development of endometriosis in adult life in an Italian population (55). In the same study, the use of formula feeding was associated with development of endometriosis during reproductive life, with dysmenorrhea and infertility. In agreement, these results have been confirmed in a Chinese population, also showing a positive correlation with neonatal vaginal bleeding and paternal smoking (56). The association between low birth weight and the high risk of developing endometriosis was also shown in a French population (57). Further influences of intrauterine development on the later occurrence of polycystic ovary syndrome (PCOS) have also been described and reflect hormonal and metabolic affects (58).

17.7 Microbiome

Our understanding of what happens to the mother's microbiome during pregnancy is still relatively unclear and unchartered (59,60). The role that the microbiome plays in maternal adaptation to pregnancy is a new area of research; key host-microbe relationships may potentially govern glucose and insulin resistance in pregnancy. But little data exist as yet that outline the mechanisms of action. Some research suggests that maternal microbiome changes rapidly at the beginning of pregnancy, but this is not a consistent finding. What is consistent, is the profound influence of the maternal diet on the pregnant mother's microbiome (61). The microbiome influences and is further influenced by maternal obesity, a critical indicator of obesity in early childhood. An emerging area of interest, especially since it is a potential route of intervention, is how the maternal microbiota affects fetoplacental development, and how that might be altered at different stages of gestation, in a manner that benefits life-long newborn developmental processes (61). Amongst healthy infants, formula-fed infants, compared with breastfed infants, had increased richness of microbiota species, with overrepresentation of *Clostridium difficile*. Infants born by elective cesarean delivery show much lower bacterial diversity, but the long term outcomes are still unclear. The impact of antibiotic treatment during pregnancy and in the postnatal lactation period on the maternal and neonatal gut microbiota and its subsequent effects on childhood development require examination. Concern has been expressed recently about the impact of the COVID-19 pandemic on the microbiota of infected and uninfected individuals, the relationship to fetal development

in women pregnant during the pandemic and the longer term consequences of stress, of altered schooling and family interaction, of pre-existing conditions on adolescence, and exacerbation of societal inequities during and as a consequence of this period of time (62).

17.8 Concluding Comments

This brief chapter has focused primarily on two aspects of developmental programming: malnutrition, manifest as either too little or too much dietary intake; and stress, directly or indirectly impacting the developing fetus, and replicated in part through exogenous glucocorticoid administration. Developmental programming can clearly proceed along many other axes, and in many cases, through interconnected or interdependent pathways. A recent study examined the major risk and resiliency factors in early life that are associated with adult-onset disease pathways that could be used to predict health and disease trajectories (63). These included early life nutrition, maternal/paternal health, maternal/paternal psychological exposure, toxicants, and social determinants. It stressed the importance of studying resiliency factors and their interaction with risk factors to inform interventions to prevent or to mitigate adverse health outcomes. The majority of studies in the current literature are on populations from developed countries where interventions such as antenatal steroids to improve neonatal morbidity and mortality may have different impact and outcomes than in populations from low- and middle-income countries (LMIC). There is a substantial shortage of studies from LMIC, and with identified Indigenous and disadvantaged populations, suggesting that the effects of early life exposures on life-course health outcomes in these populations needs much further research. A recent series of reviews in Lancet (64,65) has summarized the importance of the periconceptional time window, the potential for intervention and the evidence for promoting early childhood development. As evidenced from the present article, interventions will require better understanding of the timing during the life course of a primary adverse event and of a later effector and will need to address these multiple causal pathways that alter a child's ability to achieve a full developmental potential.

References

1. Barker DJP, Winter PD, Osmond C, et al. Weight in infancy and death from ischaemic heart disease. *Lancet.* 1989, 8663:577–580.

2. Barker DJP, Bull AR, Osmond C, et al. Fetal and placental size and the risk of hypertension in adult life. *Br Med J.* 1990, 301:259–262.

3. Rich-Edwards JW, Stampfer MJ, Manson JE, et al. Birthweight and risk of cardiovascular disease in a cohort of women followed up since 1976. *Br Med J.* 1997, 315:396–400.

4. Langley-Evans SC, Gardner D, and Jackson AA. Maternal protein restriction influences the programming of the rat hypothalamic-pituitary adrenal axis. *J Nutrition.* 1996, 126:1578–1585.

5. Lillycrop KA, Phillips ES, Jackson AA, et al. Dietary protein restriction of pregnant rats induces, and folic acid supplementation prevents epigenetic modification of hepatic gene expression in the offspring. *J. Nutrition.* 2005, 135:1382–1386.

6. Meaney MJ, S Zyf M, and Seckl JR. Epigenetic mechanisms of perinatal programming of hypothalamic-pituitary adrenal function and health. *Trends Mol Med.* 2007, 2007:269–277.

7. Langley-Evans SC. Hypertension induced by foetal exposure to a maternal low-protein diet, in the rat, is prevented by pharmacological blockade of maternal glucocorticoid synthesis. *J. Hypertension.* 1997, 15:537–544.

8. Reynolds RM, Labad J, Buss C, et al. Transmitting biological effects of stress in utero: Implications for mother and offspring. *Psychoneuroendocrinology.* 2013, 38:1843–1849.

9. Meaney MJ. Maternal care, gene expression and the transmission of individual differences in stress reactivity across generations. *Ann Rev Neurosci.* 2001, 24:1161–1192.

10. Roseboom TJ, van der Meulen JH, Osmond C, et al. Coronary heart disease after prenatal exposure to the Dutch famine, 1944–45. *Heart.* 2000, 84:595–598.

11. Eriksson JG. Early growth, and coronary heart disease and type 2 diabetes: Experiences from the Helsinki birth cohort. *Int J Obesity.* 2006, 30:S18–S22.

12. Ozanne SE, and Hales NC. Peer fetal growth followed by rapid catch-up growth leads to premature death. *Mech Ageing Dev.* 2005, 126:852–854.

13. Gluckman PD, Hanson MA, Beedle AS, et al. Predictive adaptive responses in perspective. *Trends Endocrinol Metab.* 2008, 19:109–110.

14. Gluckman PD, Hanson MA, and Low FM. Evolutionary and developmental mismatches are consequences of adaptive developmental plasticity in humans and have implications for later disease risk. *Phil Trans Royal Society B.* 2019. https://doi.org/10.1098/rstb.2018.0109.

15. Braun T, Challis JR, Newnham JP, et al. Early life glucocorticoid exposure: The hypothalamic-pituitary-adrenal axis, placental function and long-term disease risk. *Endocr Rev.* 2013, 34:885–916.

16. Seckl JR, Benediktsson R, Linsay RS, et al. Placental 11b-hydroxysteroid dehydrogenase and the programming of hypertension. *J Steroid Biochem Mol Biol.* 1995, 55:447–450.

17. Connor KL, Kibschull M, Matysiak-Zablocki E, et al. Maternal malnutrition impacts placental morphology and transporter expression: An origin for poor offspring growth. *J Nutr Biochem.* 2020, 78:108329.

18. Regnault TR, Friedman JE, Wilkening RB, et al. Fetoplacental transport and utilization of amino acids in IUGR – A review. *Placenta.* 2005. Suppl A; S52–S62.

19. Audette MC, Challis JRG, Jones RL, et al. Antenatal dexamethasone treatment in mid-gestation reduces system A transporter activity in the late gestation murine placenta. *Endocrinology.* 2011. 152:3561–3570.

20. Challis JRG, Matthews SG, Gibb W, et al. Endocrine and paracrine regulation of birth at term and preterm. *Endocr Rev.* 2000. 21:514–550.

21. Challis JRG, and Brooks AN. Maturation and activation of hypothalamic-pituitary-adrenal function in fetal sheep. *Endocr Rev.* 1989, 10:182–204.

22. Braun T, Li S, Sloboda DM, et al. Effects of maternal dexamethasone treatment in early pregnancy on pituitary-adrenal axis in fetal sheep. *Endocrinology.* 2009 150:5466–5477.

23. Painter RC, Roseboom TJ, and de Rooij SR. Long-term effects of prenatal stress and glucocorticoid exposure. *Birth Defects Res Embryo Today.* 2021, 96:315–324.

24. Reynolds RM. Glucocorticoid excess and the developmental origins of disease; two decades of testing the hypothesis. *Psychoneuroendocrinology.* 2013, 38:1–11.

25. Waterland RA, and Jirtle RL. Early nutrition, epigenetic changes at transposons and imprinted genes, and enhanced susceptibility to adult chronic diseases. *Nutrition.* 2004, 20:63–68.

26. Bloomfield F, Oliver M, Hawkins P, et al. A periconceptional nutritional origin for non-infectious

preterm birth. *Science.* 2003, 300:606.

27. Bloomfield FH, Oliver MH, Hawkins P, et al. Periconceptional undernutrition in sheep accelerates maturation of the fetal hypothalamic-pituitary-adrenal axis in late gestation. *Endocrinology.* 2004, 145:4278–4285.

28. Connor KL, Challis JRG, vanZijl P, et al. Do alterations in placental 11beta-hydroxysteroid dehydrogenase (11betaHSD) activities explain differences in fetal hypothalamic-pituitary-adrenal (HPA) function following periconceptional undernutrition or twinning in sheep. *Reprod Sci.* 200916:1201–1212.

29. Begum G, Stevens A, Connor K, et al. Epigenetic changes in fetal hypothalamic energy regulating pathways are associated with maternal undernutrition and twinning. *FASEB J.* 2012, 26:1694–1703.

30. Begum G, Davies A, Stevens A, et al. Maternal undernutrition programs tissue-specific epigenetic changes in the glucocorticoid receptor in adult offspring. *Endocrinology.* 2013, 154:4560–4569.

31. Johnstone JF, Godfrey KM, Zelsman M, et al. *The relationship between placental 11β HSD-2 and maternal body composition, age and dieting status.* 2005 Society for Gynecologic Investigation Annual Meeting, Los Angeles, 2005.

32. Braun T, Li S, Sloboda DM, et al. Effects of maternal dexamethasone treatment in early pregnancy on pituitary-adrenal axis in fetal sheep. *Endocrinology.* 2009, 150:5466–5477

33. Constantinof A, Moisiadis VG, and Matthews SG. Programming of stress pathways: A transgenerational perspective. *J Steroid Biochem Mol Biol.* 2016, 160; 175–180.

34. Petraglia F, Imperatore A, and Challis JRG, Neuroendocrine mechanisms in pregnancy and parturition. *Endocr Rev.* 2010, 31:783–816.

35. Sun K, Yang K, and Challis JRG. Differential expression of 11betahydroxysteroid dehydrogenase types 1 and 2 in human placenta and foetal membranes. *J. Clin Endocr Metab.* 1997, 82:300–305.

36. Alexander N, Rosenlocher F, and Stadler T. Impact of antenatal synthetic glucocorticoid exposure on endocrine stress reactivity in term-born children. *J Clin Endocr Metab.* 2012, 97:3538–3544.

37. Asztalos EV, Murphy KE, and Matthews SG. A growing dilemma: Antenatal corticosteroids and long-term consequences. *Am J Perinatol.* 2020, https://doi.org/10.1055/s-0040-1718573.

38. Roseboom TJ, Ozanne SE, Godfrey KM, et al. Unheard, unseen and unprotected: DOHaD Council's call for action to protect the younger generation from the long-term effects of COVID-19. *J. Develop Orig Health Dis.* 2021, https://doi.org/10.1017/S2040174420000847.

39. Shenk CE, O'Donnell KJ, Pokhvisneva I, et al. Epigenetic age acceleration and risk for posttraumatic stress disorder following exposure to substantiated child maltreatment. *J Clin Child Adolesc Psychol.* 2021, 1–11.

40. Franke HA. Toxic stress: Effects, prevention and treatment. *Children.* 2014, 1:390–402.

41. Anda RF, Felitti VJ, Bremner JD, et al. The enduring effects of abuse and related adverse experiences in childhood: A convergence of evidence from neurobiology and epidemiology. *Eur Arch Psychiat Clin Neurosci.* 2006, 256:174–186.

42. Kuffer AL, Thoma MV, and Maercker A. Transgenerational aspects of former Swiss child laborers: Do second generations suffer from their parents' adverse early-life experiences. *Eur J. Psychotraumatol.* 2016, 7: https://doi.org/10.3402/ejptv7.30804.

43. Strobel NA, Richardson A, Shepherd CCJ, et al. Modelling factors for Aboriginal and Torres Strait Islander child neurodevelopment outcomes: A latent class analysis. *Paediatr Perinat Epidemiol.* 2019, 00:1–12. https://doi.org/10.1111/ppe.12616.

44. Boyce WT, and Kobor MS. Development and the epigenome: The 'synapse' of gene – Environment interplay. *Develop Sci.* 2015, 18:1–23.

45. Chen L, Pan H, Tuan TA, et al. GUSTO Study Group. Brain-derived Neurotrophic Factor (BDNF) val66met polymorphism influences the association of the methylome with maternal anxiety and neonatal brain volumes. *Develop Psychopathol.* 2015, 271:137–150.

46. Meaney MJ. Maternal care, gene expression, and the transmission of individual differences in stress reactivity across generations. *Ann Rev Neurosci.* 2001, 24:1161–1192.

47. Moisiadis VG, and Matthews SG. Glucocorticoids and fetal programming part1: Outcomes. *Nat Rev Endocrinol.* 2014, 10:391–402.

48. Moisiadis VG, and Matthews SG. Glucocorticoids and fetal programming part 2: Mechanisms. *Nat Rev Endocrinol.* 2014, 10:403–411.

49. Ibanez L, Potau N, Ferrer A, et al. Reduced ovulation rate in adolescent girls born small for gestational age. *J Clin Endocrinol Metab*. 2002, 87:3391–3393.

50. Sloboda DM, Hickey M, and Hart R. Reproduction in females: The role of early life environment. *Hum Reprod Update*. 2011, 17:210–227.

51. Sloboda DM, Hart R, Doherty DA, et al. Age at menarche: Influences of prenatal and postnatal growth. *J Clin Endocrinol Metab*. 2007, 92:46–50.

52. . Sloboda DM, Howie GJ, Gluckman PD, et al. Pre-and postnatal nutritional histories influence reproductive maturation and ovarian function in the rat. *PLoS ONE*. 2009, 4:e6744.

53. Jazwiec P, and Sloboda DM. Nutritional adversity, sex and reproduction: Thirty years on from Barker and what have we learned? *J Endocrinol*. 2019, 242:T51–T68.

54. Tsoulis M, Chang, P Moore CJ, et al. Maternal high fat diet induced loss of fetal oocytes is associated with compromised follicle growth in adult offspring. *Biol Reprod*. 2016, 94:94.

55. Vannuccini S, Lazzeri L, Orlandini C, et al. Potential influence of in utero and early neonatal exposures on the later development of endometriosis. *Fertil Steril*. 2016105:997–1002.

56. Liu S, Cui H, Zhang Q, et al. Influence of early-life factors on the development of endometriosis. *Eur J Contracept Reprod Health Care*. 2019, 24:216–221.

57. Borghese B, Sibiude J, Santulli P, et al. Low birth weight is strongly associated with the risk of deep infiltrating endometriosis: Results of a 743 case-control study. *PLoS ONE*. 2015, 10:e0117387.

58. Dumesic DA, Goodarzi MO, Chazenbalk GD, et al. Intrauterine environment and polycystic ovary syndrome. *Semin Reprod Med*. 2014, 32:159–165.

59. Flint HJ, Scott KP, Louis P, et al. The role of gut microbiota in nutrition and health. *Nat Rev Gastroenterol Hepatol*. 2012, 9:577–589.

60. Gohir W, Ratcliffe EM, and Sloboda DM. Of the bugs that shape us: Maternal obesity, the gut microbiome and longterm disease risk. *Pediatr Res*. 2014, 77:196–204.

61. Gohir W, Whelan FJ, Surette MG, et al. 2015. Pregnancy-related changes in the maternal gut microbiota are dependent upon the mother's periconceptional diet. *Gut Microbiobes*. 6:310–320.

62. Finlay BB, Amato KR, Azad M, et al. The hygiene hypothesis, the COVID pandemic, and consequences for the human microbiome. *Proc Natl Acad Sci*. 2021, 118:e2010217118.

63. Abdul-Hussein A, Kareem A, Tewari S, et al. Early life risk and resiliency factors and their influences on developmental outcomes and disease pathways: A rapid evidence review of systematic reviews and meta-analyses. *J Develop Orig Health Dis*. 2021 (in press).

64. Britto PR, Lye SJ, Proulx K, et al. Nurturing care: Promoting early childhood development. *Lancet*. 2017, 389:91–102.

65. Daelmans B, Darmstadt GL, Lombardi J, et al. Early childhood development, the foundation of sustainable development. *Lancet*. 2017, 389:9–11.

Index